2025

ADVANCES IN
MOLECULAR PATHOLOGY

EDITOR-IN-CHIEF
Ahmad Abou Tayoun, PhD, FACMG

SECTION EDITORS
Erin Graf, PhD, D(ABMM)
Yuan Ji, MS, PhD, MBA
Jeremiah Karrs, DO
Marilyn M. Li, MD
Ann M. Moyer, MD, PhD
Stefan Rentas, PhD, FACMG

ELSEVIER

Publishing Director, Medical Reference: Dolores Meloni
Editor: Taylor Hayes
Developmental Editor: Malvika Shah

© 2025 Elsevier Inc. All rights are reserved, including those for text and data mining, AI training, and similar technologies.

This periodical and the individual contributions contained in it are protected under copyright by Elsevier and the following terms and conditions apply to their use:

Photocopying
Single photocopies of single articles may be made for personal use as allowed by national copyright laws. Permission of the Publisher and payment of a fee is required for all other photocopying, including multiple or systematic copying, copying for advertising or promotional purposes, resale, and all forms of document delivery. Special rates are available for educational institutions that wish to make photocopies for non-profit educational classroom use.
For information on how to seek permission visit www.elsevier.com/permissions or call: (+44) 1865 843830 (UK)/(+1) 215 239 3867 (USA).

Derivative Works
Subscribers may reproduce tables of contents or prepare lists of articles including abstracts for internal circulation within their institutions. Permission of the Publisher is required for resale or distribution outside the institution. Permission of the Publisher is required for all other derivative works, including compilations and translations (please consult www.elsevier.com/permissions).

Electronic Storage or Usage
Permission of the Publisher is required to store or use electronically any material contained in this periodical, including any article or part of an article (please consult www.elsevier.com/permissions). Except as outlined above, no part of this publication may be reproduced, stored in a retrieval system or transmitted in any form or by any means, electronic, mechanical, photocopying, recording or otherwise, without prior written permission of the Publisher.

Notice
Journals published by Elsevier comply with applicable product safety requirements. For any product safety concerns or queries, please contact our authorized representative, Elsevier B.V., at productsafety@elsevier.com.

Practitioners and researchers must always rely on their own experience and knowledge in evaluating and using any information, methods, compounds or experiments contained herein. Health care practitioners must exercise their professional judgement and make all treatment-related decisions based solely on the specific conditions of each patient. Because of rapid advances in the medical sciences, independent verification of diagnoses and drug dosages should always be made. The content is provided "as-is" and Elsevier makes no representations or warranties, whether express or implied, as to the accuracy, completeness, or adequacy of any content. To the fullest extent permitted by law, Elsevier assumes no responsibility for any damages, adverse events, or liability arising from use of information contained herein including for any injury and/or damage to persons or property, whether as a matter of product liability, negligence or otherwise.

Inclusion of any advertising material in this publication does not constitute a guarantee or endorsement of the quality or value of such product or service or of any of the representations or claims made by the advertiser.

Publisher's note: Elsevier takes a neutral position with respect to territorial disputes or jurisdictional claims in its published content, including in maps and institutional affiliations.

For accessibility purposes, images in this journal are accompanied by alt text descriptions provided by Elsevier.

Reprints: For copies of 100 or more of articles in this publication, please contact the Commercial Reprints Department, Elsevier Inc., 360 Park Avenue South, New York, NY 10010-1710. Tel: 212-633-3874; Fax: 212-633-3820; E-mail: reprints@elsevier.com.

Publishing Office:
Elsevier, Inc.
1600 John F. Kennedy Boulevard,
Suite 1600
Philadelphia, PA 19103
United States

International Standard Serial Number: 2589-4080
International Standard Book Number: 13: 978-0-443-42929-3

ADVANCES IN MOLECULAR PATHOLOGY

EDITOR-IN-CHIEF

AHMAD ABOU TAYOUN, PhD, FACMG
Associate Professor of Genetics, Dubai Health,
Director, Dubai Health Genomic Medicine Center,
Dubai, UAE

SECTION EDITORS

ERIN GRAF, PhD, D(ABMM) – Infectious Disease
Director of Microbiology, Laboratory Medicine and Pathology, Associate Professor, Laboratory Medicine and Pathology, Mayo Clinic Arizona, Phoenix, AZ, USA

YUAN JI, MS, PhD, MBA - Hot Topics
Professor, Department of Pathology, University of Utah School of Medicine, Medical Director of Genetics and Genomics, ARUP Laboratories, Salt Lake City, UT, USA

JEREMIAH KARRS, DO - Hematopathology
Assistant Director, Clinical Genomics and Advanced Technologies, Assistant Professor, Department of Pathology, Dartmouth-Hitchcock, Lebanon, NH, USA

MARILYN M. LI, MD - Solid Tumors
Professor, Department of Pathology and Laboratory Medicine, The Children's Hospital of Philadelphia, University of Pennsylvania, Philadelphia, PA, USA

ANN M. MOYER, MD, PhD – Pharmacogenomics
Professor of Laboratory Medicine and Pathology, Division of Laboratory Genetics and Genomics, Mayo Clinic, Rochester, MN, USA

STEFAN RENTAS, PhD, FACMG - Genetics
Assistant Director, Division of Molecular Pathology, Genetics and Genomics, Assistant Professor of Pathology, Duke University School of Medicine, Durham, NC, USA

CONTRIBUTORS

AUTHORS

PATRICK BENOIT, MD, FRCPC
Fellow, Department of Laboratory Medicine, University of California, San Francisco, San Francisco, California, USA

BENJAMIN A. BLEIBERG, MD
Fellow, Division of Hematology-Oncology, Department of Internal Medicine, Hospital of the University of Pennsylvania, Philadelphia, Pennsylvania, USA

BENJAMIN T. BRADLEY, MD, PhD
Assistant Professor, Department of Pathology, University of Utah, Medical Director, ARUP Laboratories, Salt Lake City, Utah, USA

ANDREW BRYAN, MD, PhD
Associate Professor, Department of Laboratory Medicine and Pathology, Mayo Clinic, Phoenix, Arizona, USA

KAJIA CAO, PhD
Assistant Clinical Professor, Department of Pathology and Laboratory Medicine, University of California, Los Angeles, California, USA

DREW T. DICKINSON, PharmD, MPH
Assistant Professor, Department of Pharmacy, Mayo Clinic, Phoenix, Arizona, USA

LIAM L. DONNELLY, MD
Assistant Professor of Pathology and Laboratory Medicine, Dartmouth Hitchcock Medical Center, Geisel School of Medicine, Lebanon, New Hampshire, USA

CYNTHIA L. GONG, PharmD, PhD
Senior Research Associate, Curta Inc., Seattle, Washington, USA

TRISTAN R. GRAMS, PhD
Fellow, Department of Pathology, University of Utah, ARUP Laboratories, Salt Lake City, Utah, USA

KATHLEEN GWILLIAM, PhD
Laboratory of Genetics and Genomics Fellow, Department of Pathology, Virginia Commonwealth University, Richmond, Virginia, USA

EVANN E. HILT, M(ASCP) CM, PhD, D(ABMM)
Assistant Professor, Department of Laboratory Medicine and Pathology, University of Minnesota, Assistant Medical Director, Infectious Diseases Diagnostic Laboratory, M Health Fairview, Minneapolis, Minnesota, USA

CATHERINE A. HOGAN, MD, MSc, FRCPC
Clinical Assistant Professor, Department of Pathology and Laboratory Medicine, University of British Columbia, Medical Microbiologist, Public Health Laboratory, BC Centre for Disease Control, Vancouver, British Columbia, Canada

DAN ILGES, PharmD
Assistant Professor, Department of Pharmacy, Mayo Clinic, Phoenix, Arizona, USA

YUAN JI, MS, PhD, MBA
Professor, Department of Pathology, University of Utah School of Medicine, Medical Director of Genetics and Genomics, ARUP Laboratories, Salt Lake City, Utah, USA

VAIDEHI JOBANPUTRA, MS, PhD, FACMG
Chief Diagnostic Officer, Molecular Diagnostics, New York Genome Center, Professor, Department of Pathology and Cell Biology, Director Precision Genomics Laboratory, Columbia University Irving Medical Center, New York, New York, USA

JEREMIAH KARRS, DO
Assistant Director, Clinical Genomics and Advanced Technologies, Assistant Professor, Department of Pathology, Dartmouth-Hitchcock, New Hampshire, USA

PRABHJOT KAUR, MD
Associate Professor, Department of Pathology, Dartmouth Hitchcock Medical Center, Geisel School of Medicine, Lebanon, New Hampshire, USA

MARILYN M. LI, MD
Professor, Department of Pathology and Laboratory Medicine, The Children's Hospital of Philadelphia, University of Pennsylvania, Philadelphia, Pennsylvania, USA

FUMIN LIN, PhD
Assistant Clinical Professor, Department of Pathology and Laboratory Medicine, University of California, Los Angeles, California, USA

SIMRAN D.S. MAGGO, PhD
Assistant Professor, Department of Pharmacy, Bernard J. Dunn School of Pharmacy, Shenandoah University, Winchester, Virginia, USA

MELINA E. MARMARELIS, MD
Assistant Professor, Division of Hematology-Oncology, Department of Internal Medicine, Hospital of the University of Pennsylvania, Philadelphia, Pennsylvania, USA

KENDALL E. MARTIN, PhD
Laboratory of Genetics and Genomics Fellow, Department of Pathology, Virginia Commonwealth University, Richmond, Virginia, USA

JENNY Q. NGUYEN, PharmD
Clinical Pharmacogenomics Specialist Pharmacist, Personalized Care Program, Children's Hospital Los Angeles, Los Angeles, California, USA

SALVATORE F. PRIORE, MD, PhD
Assistant Professor, Division of Precision and Computational Diagnostics, Department of Pathology and Laboratory Medicine, Hospital of the University of Pennsylvania, Philadelphia, Pennsylvania, USA

ELENA A. REPNIKOVA, PhD, FACMG
Associate Professor of Pathology, University of Missouri Kansas City Medical School, Assistant Director of Cytogenetics and Molecular Genetics, Children's Mercy, Kansas City, Missouri, USA

ANNAPURNA SAKSENA, MBBS, MD
Assistant Professor, Division of Hematopathology, Department of Pathology and Laboratory Medicine, Hospital of the University of Pennsylvania, Philadelphia, Pennsylvania, USA

T. NIROSHI SENARATNE, PhD
Assistant Clinical Professor, Department of Pathology and Laboratory Medicine, University of California, Los Angeles, California,
USA

SHERIN SHAABAN, MD, PhD, FACMG
Associate Professor, Department of Pathology, University of Utah School of Medicine, Medical Director, ARUP Laboratories, Salt Lake City, Utah, USA

PARTH S. SHAH, MD
Assistant Professor of Medicine, Dartmouth Hitchcock Medical Center, Geisel School of Medicine, Lebanon, New Hampshire, USA

LINGHUI DAVID SU, BSc
Research Scientist, Public Health Laboratory, BC Centre for Disease Control, Vancouver, British Columbia, Canada

MADINA SUKHANOVA, PhD, FACMG
Associate Professor of Pathology, Co-Medical Director of Cytogenetics, Assistant Technical Director of Molecular Diagnostics, Feinberg School of Medicine, Northwestern University, Chicago, Illinois, USA

AMANDA THOMAS-WILSON, MS, PhD, FACMG
Director, Molecular Diagnostics/CLIA Lab, New York Genome Center, New York, New York, USA

SCOTT A. TURNER, PhD, FACMG
Associate Professor, Department of Pathology, Virginia Commonwealth University, Richmond, Virginia, USA

LAUREN M. WAINMAN, PhD
Supervisor, Department of Pathology and Laboratory Medicine, Dartmouth Hitchcock Medical Center, Geisel School of Medicine, Lebanon, New Hampshire, USA

JULIA WANG, MD, PhD
Hematopathology Fellow, Hospital of the University of Pennsylvania, Philadelphia, Pennsylvania, USA

DEREK WONG, PhD
Assistant Professor, Division of Genomic Diagnostics, Department of Pathology and Laboratory Medicine, The Children's Hospital of Philadelphia, University of Pennsylvania Perelman School of Medicine, Philadelphia, Pennsylvania, USA

FANG ZHAO, MD, PhD
Assistant Professor, Department of Pathology and Laboratory Medicine, University of Cincinnati, College of Medicine, Cincinnati, Ohio, USA

CONTENTS

VOLUME 8 • 2025

Editorial Board, *iii*

Contributors, *v*

Preface: Advances in Molecular Pathology: Precision Diagnostics Across the Spectrum, *xvii*
By Ahmad Abou Tayoun

SECTION: GENETICS

Advances in Inherited Bone Marrow Failure Syndromes: Clinical Manifestations, Genetics, and Diagnostic Approaches, *1*
By Fumin Lin, Kajia Cao, T. Niroshi Senaratne, and Marilyn M. Li

Inherited bone marrow failure syndromes (IBMFS) are a group of phenotypically and genetically heterogeneous diseases requiring precise and timely diagnosis. This review summarizes the history, clinical features, and genetic mechanisms of both classic and newly identified IBMFS entities. Clonal hematopoiesis, a somatic event in patients with IBMFS, is increasingly recognized for its dual role in either facilitating adaptive genetic rescue or promoting maladaptive malignant transformation. While targeted panels and exome sequencing remain the most popular sequencing modalities, each has distinct advantages and limitations and should be incorporated into a comprehensive diagnostic strategy for IBMFS.

Introduction, *1*
History of inherited bone marrow failure syndromes discovery, *2*
Clinical and genomic characteristics of inherited bone marrow failure syndromes, *3*
Fanconi anemia, 3
Telomere biology disorders/dyskeratosis congenita, 7
Diamond Blackfan anemia, 7
Shwachman Diamond syndrome, 7
Severe congenital neutropenia, 8
GATA2 deficiency syndrome, 8
SAMD9/SAMD9L syndrome, 8
Congenital amegakaryocytic thrombocytopenia, 8
Thrombocytopenia absent radii syndrome, 8
RUNX1 familial platelet disorder with associated myeloid malignancies, 8
ERCC6L2-related disease, 8
AMeD syndrome, 9
Somatic conversion and clonal hematopoiesis, *9*
Diagnostic tools, *9*
Functional screening, 9
Genetic testing, 10
Recommendation of diagnostic algorithm, *12*
Summary, *12*
Disclosure, *12*

Advances in Prenatal Genomic Sequencing, *15*
By Amanda Thomas-Wilson and Vaidehi Jobanputra

Genome sequencing (GS) is redefining prenatal genetic diagnostics by offering a comprehensive, single-test approach to detect a wide array of genetic variation. Compared with conventional methods like karyotyping, chromosomal microarray, and exome sequencing, GS demonstrates higher diagnostic yield in cases with and without fetal anomalies detected by ultrasound scan. This article reviews current evidence, challenges, and future directions, emphasizing GS as a transformative tool for precision prenatal care.

Introduction, *15*
History of prenatal testing, *16*
Background and Evolution Toward Genome Sequencing as a First-Tier Test, 17

Current Evidence of Diagnostic and Incremental Yield of Prenatal Genome Sequencing, 20
Challenges of prenatal genome sequencing, *21*
Technical Challenges of Short-Read Genome Sequencing, 21
Interpretation and Reporting Challenges, 21
Maternal Cell Contamination, Mosaicism, and Mitochondrial Heteroplasmy, 21
Counseling and Consent Complexity, 22
Future directions, *22*
Long-Read Sequencing, 22
Transcriptome Sequencing (RNA Sequencing), 22
Noninvasive Genome Sequencing via Cell-Free DNA, 22
Discussion, *22*
Summary, *23*
Clinics care points, *23*
Disclosure, *23*

SECTION: HEMATOPATHOLOGY

Role of Long-read Sequencing in Comprehensive Genomic Profiling of Hematolymphoid Malignancies, *27*
By Lauren M. Wainman, Liam L. Donnelly, Prabhjot Kaur, Parth S. Shah, and Jeremiah Karrs

Long-read sequencing (LRS) technologies have emerged as powerful tools in genomic analysis. This review explores the applications of LRS in hematolymphoid neoplasms (myeloid and lymphoid neoplasms), where genomic complexity and structural alterations play significant roles in pathogenesis, diagnosis, and treatment selection. We discuss the technical principles of various LRS platforms, complex structural variants, and haplotype phasing in hematologic malignancies. Current clinical applications are reviewed with examples demonstrating how LRS has resolved diagnostically challenging cases in leukemias and lymphomas and extended biologic insight. Furthermore, we address implementation challenges, including bioinformatic analysis, validation requirements, and cost considerations for clinical laboratories.

Introduction, *27*
Fundamentals of long-read sequencing technologies, *28*
Technical principles and platforms, 28
Comparative advantages and limitations of long-read sequencing versus short-read sequencing, 28
Implementation and wet laboratory considerations, 30
Bioinformatic pipelines and packages for variant detection, 30
Applications of long-read sequencing in hematolymphoid neoplasms, *31*
Detection of structural variants and gene fusions, 31
Analysis of repetitive regions and difficult-to-sequence genes, 32
Haplotype phasing and compound heterozygosity, 33
Full-length transcript analysis, 34
Epigenetic marker analysis, 34
Summary, *35*
Clinics care points, *35*
Declaration of artificial intelligence and artificial intelligence-assisted technologies in the writing process, *36*

DNA Methylation-Based Profiling in Mature B-cell Neoplasms, *41*
By Julia Wang and Annapurna Saksena

This article reviews the role of DNA methylation profiling in B-cell tumors, particularly focusing on its impact in mature B-cell lymphomas. DNA methylation patterns are critical for regulating gene expression and maintaining cell identity, and disruptions in this system contribute to neoplastic transformation. The article highlights how DNA methylation signatures can be used to classify tumor subtypes and predict clinical outcomes, emphasizing their potential for guiding personalized treatment approaches in hematologic cancers. Understanding these modifications paves the way for targeted therapies based on specific epigenetic profiles.

Introduction, *41*

Chronic Lymphocytic Leukemia/Small Lymphocytic Lymphoma, 43
Mantle Cell Lymphoma, 43
Waldenström s Macroglobulinemia, 44
Follicular Lymphoma, 44
Diffuse Large B-cell Lymphoma, 45
Burkitt Lymphoma, 45
Multiple Myeloma, 46
Potential of DNA methylation-based profiling as a mitotic clock, *46*
DNA methylation-based classification of mature B-cell neoplasms, *47*
Potential advantages of DNA methylation-based classification, *48*
Potential clinical applications of DNA methylation-based profiling in mature B-cell neoplasms, *48*
Summary and future directions, *49*
Clinics care points, *49*
Disclosures, *49*

SECTION: SOLID TUMORS

Emerging Biomarkers in Non–small Cell Lung Cancer: *ERBB2* and *MET* Amplifications, *53*

By Benjamin A. Bleiberg, Melina E. Marmarelis, and Salvatore F. Priore

Gene amplification is a common molecular mechanism in cancer that results in overexpression of oncogenic proteins. Gene amplification can be a primary oncogenic driver, secondarily acquired after treatment, or both. This article will review gene amplifications that occur in non–small cell lung cancer with a focus on *ERBB2* and *MET* amplifications and discuss various techniques to identify them and their advantages and limitations. Gene amplifications have clinical implications for patient management and are an active area of interest for clinical trials and novel therapy development.

Introduction, *53*
Techniques for Assessing Gene Copy Number Gains, 54
Advantages and Limitations of Testing Methods, 55
Gene Amplification in Non small Cell Lung Cancer, 57
Clinics care points, *65*
Disclosure, *66*

Perspectives on Homologous Recombination Repair Deficiency (HRD): Updates on Testing to Treatments, *69*

By Kathleen Gwilliam, Kendall E. Martin, and Scott A. Turner

Homologous recombination (HR) is required for high-fidelity repair of DNA double-stranded breaks. When the homologous recombination repair (HRR) pathway is deficient an accumulation of DNA damage can lead to genomic instability and facilitate tumorigenesis. Homologous recombination deficiency (HRD) occurs when pathogenic variants or epigenetic alterations impact the function of genes in the HRR pathway (*BRCA1*, *BRCA2*, and so forth). HRD status can be assayed by identifying variants in the HRR pathway or by measuring the amount of genomic scarring caused by the loss of this repair mechanism. HRD status has implications for the treatment of breast, ovarian, prostate, and pancreatic cancers. Treatment by FDA-approved therapies, including platinum-based chemotherapy and PARP inhibitors, results in cell death through mechanisms such as synthetic lethality and has shown improved response in HRD-positive tumors. While HRD limitations remain, including testing inconsistencies, lack of standardization, and limited establishment of clinical cutoffs, the clinical utility of this biomarker is promising, with several clinical trials for existing and novel therapeutics underway.

Introduction, *69*
Homologous recombination repair pathway, *70*
Homologous recombination deficiency, *70*
Testing to identify homologous recombination deficiency, *71*
Identification of Genomic Scarring, 71
Testing for Germline and/or Somatic Variants in Homologous Recombination Deficiency, 72
Testing of Homologous Recombination Repair Gene Promoter Methylation, 72

Testing for RAD51 Foci Formation, 72
Alternative Methods in Development, 73
Therapeutics for homologous recombination deficiency-positive cancers, *74*
Homologous Recombination Deficiency Targeted Therapeutics and Synthetic Lethality, 74
Platinum-Based Therapies, 74
Poly (ADP-Ribose) Polymerase Inhibitors, 74
Polymerase Theta Inhibitors, 74
BRCA1 and/or BRCA2 Variant Reversion After Treatment, 75
Treatment guidelines for homologous recombination repair deficiency-positive cancers, *76*
Breast Cancer, 76
Ovarian Cancer, 76
Prostate Cancer, 77
Pancreatic Cancer, 77
Challenges and summary, *77*
Clinics care points, *78*
Disclosure, *78*

A Review of Molecular Techniques and Biomarkers for the Diagnosis of Tumors of the Central Nervous System, *83*
By Derek Wong

Tumors of the central nervous system (CNS) are a heterogenous group of neoplasms that each have a unique genomic landscape that can be associated with distinct clinical outcomes. Therefore, accurate diagnosis and molecular profiling of these tumors is crucial for guiding clinical management and providing information on patient prognosis. In this article, we review current and future molecular techniques useful for CNS tumor diagnostics and summarize key molecular features, biomarkers, and algorithms used by the World Health Organization classification of CNS tumors to establish an integrated histologic diagnosis.

Introduction, *83*
Current techniques, *84*
Immunohistochemistry and fluorescence in situ hybridization, 84
Polymerase chain reaction and Sanger sequencing, 84
Methylation analysis, 84
Array-based technologies, 85
Next-generation sequencing, 86
RNA fusion, 86
Emerging techniques, *88*
Methylation profiling, 88
RNA sequencing, 88
Cell-free tumor DNA profiling, 88
Third-generation sequencing, 88
Tumor entities, *88*
Adult diffuse glioma, 88
Meningioma, 89
Pediatric low-grade glioma, 89
Pediatric high-grade glioma, 91
Ependymoma, 91
Medulloblastoma, 92
Other tumors, 92
Summary, *92*
Clinics care points, *92*
Disclosure, *93*

SECTION: PHARMACOGENOMICS

Economic Analysis of Pharmacogenomics: Challenges and Progress, *97*
By Simran D.S. Maggo, Jenny Q. Nguyen, and Cynthia L. Gong

Pharmacogenomic (PGx) testing identifies genetic variations affecting drug metabolism, enhancing medication efficacy and safety by reducing adverse events and improving clinical outcomes. Despite clinical benefits, widespread adoption remains hindered by economic barriers and health care system challenges, including high upfront costs, inconsistent reimbursement policies, and implementation difficulties. This targeted review (2014–2024) evaluates economic studies of PGx testing across multiple therapeutic areas, including psychiatry, cardiology, oncology, and hypersensitivity reactions. Addressing implementation barriers through provider education, multidisciplinary collaboration, clear clinical guidelines, and efficient patient communication is critical for integrating PGx into routine practice.

Introduction, *97*
Methods, *98*

Search Strategy, 98
Abstract and Title Screening, 98
Data Extraction, 98
Data Analysis, 98
Review of literature, *98*
Pharmacogenomic Testing, 99
Economic Approach, 106
Discussion, *107*
Methodological Considerations, 107
Limitations and Variability in Pharmacogenomic Test Specifications, 107
Clinical and Policy Considerations, 108
Summary, *109*
Clinics care points, *109*
Disclosures, *109*

SECTION: INFECTIOUS DISEASE

A Beginner's Guide to Assay Development for Emerging Pathogens, *113*

By Tristan R. Grams and Benjamin T. Bradley

This article provides clinical laboratories with a comprehensive guide for developing diagnostic assays in response to emerging infectious pathogens. It systematically addresses essential considerations throughout assay development, including preanalytical factors such as pathogen biology, patient populations, specimen selection, and regulatory timing; analytical decisions involving target identification, testing platform selection, and internal control strategies; and postanalytical elements like clear reporting practices, data sharing, collaboration with public health agencies, and managing testing surges. Incorporating real-life experiences from previous outbreaks, the guide highlights practical examples of successful strategies as well as common pitfalls encountered, offering critical insights for future assay design.

Introduction, *113*
Preanalytical considerations, 114
Analytical considerations, 118
Postanalytical considerations, 121
Summary, *126*
Clinics care points, *127*
Disclosure, *127*

Current State of Metagenomics for Infectious Diseases Diagnosis: Limitations and Future Directions, *131*

By LingHui David Su, Patrick Benoit, Evann E. Hilt, and Catherine A. Hogan

With advancements in sequencing technology and recognition of limitations of conventional microbiology testing, metagenomic next-generation sequencing (mNGS) has expanded from research laboratories to clinical settings. The hypothesis-free nature of this technology offers unique diagnostic potential, particularly for the investigation of challenging syndromes where infection is high on the differential diagnosis. However, the broader implementation and clinical use of mNGS remain limited. In this article, we review the testing availability and performance of mNGS across various sample types in North America including for immunocompromised and pediatric populations. We discuss current challenges and provide insights into future avenues for research and clinical applications.

Introduction, *131*
The current state of testing and its clinical impact, *132*
Blood/Plasma, *132*
Bronchoalveolar Lavage, *133*
Cerebrospinal Fluid, *133*
Other Sample Types, *134*
The utility of metagenomic next-generation sequencing across patient populations and clinical syndromes, *135*
Immunocompromised Hosts, 135
Pediatrics, 136
Other infections and/or clinical syndromes, *136*
Parasitic Infections, 136
Blood Culture-Negative Endocarditis, 136
Use as a Complementary Rule-Out Test, 136
Integration with Stewardship, 137
Current challenges and future avenues, *137*
Laboratory challenges, *138*
Future avenues, *138*
Summary, *139*
Clinics care points, *139*
Disclosure, *139*

Molecular Detection of Antimicrobial Resistance Markers, Clinical Application, and Limitations, *145*

By Drew T. Dickinson, Dan Ilges, and Andrew Bryan

In this review, we describe common molecular resistance determinants that are included in Food and Drug Administration-approved syndromic panels and targeted assays. We propose a framework for the implementation of rapid molecular diagnostic testing and provide guidance on suggested actions based upon the detection or absence of specific resistance markers. The data supporting the use of these panels to inform patient care are reviewed, with a particular focus on the need for coupling robust laboratory reporting and antimicrobial stewardship. We include a call for multidisciplinary collaboration for proper implementation of rapid molecular resistance assays and interpretation of results.

Introduction, *145*
Framework for clinical application of rapid molecular diagnostics, *145*
Specific resistance determinants, *148*
mecA/C, 148
vanA/B, 148
CTX-M, 148
Carbapenemases (KPC, IMP, VIM, NDM, and OXA), 149
When No Specific Resistance Determinants Are Detected, 149
Blood culture test systems, *150*
Lower respiratory tract test systems, *155*
Bone and joint-related specimens, *158*
Swabs and direct isolate testing, *158*
Summary and future directions, *158*
Clinics care points, *159*
Disclosure, *159*

SECTION: HOT TOPICS

Health Disparities and Precision Medicine, *163*

By Sherin Shaaban and Yuan Ji

In the last few decades, precision medicine has taken strides toward personalizing patient care and offered hope about its potential to transform medicine and health care and to improve population health. The lack of inclusion of ethnic minorities and socially disadvantaged population subgroups in precision medicine research and implementation could potentially further exacerbate the already existing health disparities. Innovative and practical approaches for better understanding of health disparities causes and mechanisms are needed to develop strategies to eliminate them within the context of precision medicine efforts.

Introduction, *163*
Health disparities related to race, ethnicity, and genetic ancestry, *164*
Health disparities related to sex and gender, *166*
Health disparities related to age, *167*
Health disparities and artificial intelligence, *168*
Health disparities related to socioeconomic status, *168*
Health disparities related to geographic location, *169*
Summary, *169*
Funding, *170*
Disclosure, *170*

The Near Future of Cancer Cytogenetics: Whole Genome Sequencing, Long-Read Sequencing, or Optical Genome Mapping?, *175*

By Madina Sukhanova and Elena A. Repnikova

The field of genetic diagnostics has experienced significant advancements since its inception, evolving from traditional chromosome analysis in cultured preparations to the complex whole-genome technologies available today. Given the substantial progress in diagnostic technologies, a pertinent question arises regarding the potential for these molecular methodologies to serve as stand-alone tests in cancer diagnostics and whether it is time to move away from conventional cytogenetics. This review seeks to evaluate and compare the clinical utility of whole genome DNA-based methods and to assess the ongoing relevance of traditional chromosome analysis in contemporary diagnostics.

Introduction, *175*
Conventional Cytogenetic Methods, 176
Implementation of Whole-Genome Methods in Current Clinical Practice, 177
Landscape of the Modern Whole-Genome Methods, 177
Summary, *184*
Clinics care points, *185*
Disclosure, *185*

Economics of Molecular Pathology, *189*
By Fang Zhao and Yuan Ji

The economics of molecular pathology plays a crucial role in shaping health care decisions and patient outcomes. This review examines the key players in the financial landscape, including health care providers, payers, and patients. It explores the economic value and health benefits of molecular testing, highlighting its role in precision medicine. The article also covers coding complexities, financial considerations for test implementation, and the challenges of securing reimbursement. Finally, it addresses challenges and strategies for sustainability, concluding with future directions focused on artificial intelligence powered tools to improve efficiency and value-based reimbursement models shaping the economics of molecular pathology.

Introduction, *189*
Discussion, *189*
Key players within the economic landscape of molecular pathology, 189
Economic value and health benefits of molecular testing, 190
Coding for molecular pathology, 191
Economic considerations for molecular test implementation, 192
Essential tools for economic evaluation of molecular testing, 193
Challenges and strategies in the health economics of molecular testing, 194
Future directions, *195*
Summary, *195*
Clinics care points, *195*
Declaration of AI and AI-assisted technologies in the writing process, *195*
Disclosure, *196*

Advances in Molecular Pathology 8 (2025) xvii–xviii
ADVANCES IN MOLECULAR PATHOLOGY

Preface

Advances in Molecular Pathology: Precision Diagnostics Across the Spectrum

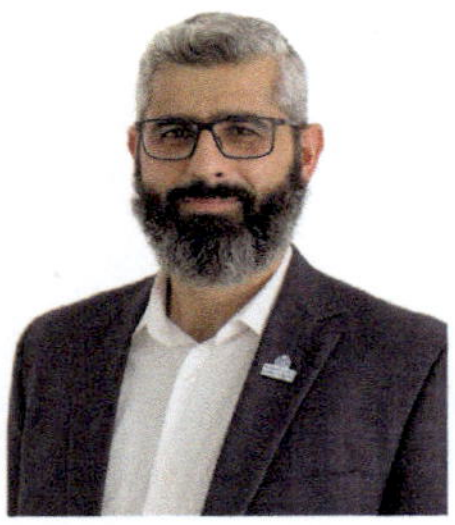

Ahmad Abou Tayoun, PhD, FACMG,
Editor-in-Chief

The field of molecular pathology has undergone a remarkable transformation over the past decade, driven by rapid technological advances and deeper integration of genomics into clinical care. As diagnostic precision becomes an essential pillar of modern medicine, molecular pathology stands at the crossroads of innovation and implementation, guiding diagnosis, prognosis, and treatment decisions across diverse clinical domains.

Advances in Molecular Pathology brings together leading experts across key subspecialties to highlight current progress, evolving challenges, and future directions in this dynamic field. The issue is organized into thematic sections, each reflecting major arenas of clinical relevance. The *Genetics* section opens with insights into inherited bone marrow failure syndromes and the expanding role of prenatal genomic sequencing, both of which exemplify the shift toward early, comprehensive diagnostics. In the *Hematopathology* section, the adoption of long-read sequencing and methylation profiling is reshaping our understanding of hematolymphoid malignancies, offering refined classification and prognostic stratification.

The *Solid Tumors* section captures the expanding biomarker landscape, from *ERBB2* and *MET* amplifications in non–small cell lung cancer to homologous recombination repair deficiency and molecular markers in CNS tumors. These advances are not only redefining diagnosis but also aligning with targeted therapies. The *Pharmacogenomics* section introduces an important economic perspective, essential for the sustainable integration of personalized medicine.

The *Infectious Disease* section addresses the growing role of molecular tools in pathogen detection, metagenomics, and antimicrobial resistance, highlighting lessons learned from recent global health challenges.

https://doi.org/10.1016/j.yamp.2025.07.005
2589-4080/25/ © 2025 Published by Elsevier Inc.

Finally, the *Hot Topics* section explores timely and critical themes, including the impact of health disparities on precision medicine, emerging cytogenomic technologies, and the broader economics that underpin molecular pathology practice.

As chief editor, I am honored to present this comprehensive issue that reflects the scientific rigor, translational focus, and collaborative spirit of our contributors. We hope this volume serves as a valuable resource for pathologists, researchers, and clinicians navigating the evolving landscape of molecular diagnostics.

DISCLOSURES

None.

Ahmad Abou Tayoun, PhD, FACMG
Dubai Health Genomic Medicine Center
Department of Genetics
Dubai Health, Dubai, UAE

E-mail address: Ahmad.Tayoun@dubaihealth.ae

SECTION: GENETICS

Advances in Molecular Pathology 8 (2025) 1–14
ADVANCES IN MOLECULAR PATHOLOGY

Advances in Inherited Bone Marrow Failure Syndromes

Clinical Manifestations, Genetics, and Diagnostic Approaches

Fumin Lin, PhD[a,*], Kajia Cao, PhD[a], T. Niroshi Senaratne, PhD[a], Marilyn M. Li, MD[b,c,d]

[a]Department of Pathology and Laboratory Medicine, University of California, A6-210, CHS Building, 10833 Le Conte Avenue, Los Angeles, CA 90095, USA; [b]Department of Pathology and Laboratory Medicine, The Children's Hospital of Philadelphia, Philadelphia, PA, USA; [c]Department of Pediatrics, The Children's Hospital of Philadelphia, Philadelphia, PA, USA; [d]Perelman School of Medicine, University of Pennsylvania, 716-I ARC Building, 3615 Civic Center Boulevard, Philadelphia, PA 19104, USA

KEYWORDS

- Inherited bone marrow failure syndromes • Clinical presentation • Somatic conversion • Functional screening
- Genetic testing • Next-generation sequencing

KEY POINTS

- Inherited bone marrow failure syndromes (IBMFS) are phenotypically and genetically heterogeneous.
- Next-generation sequencing (NGS) is widely used for IBMFS diagnosis, revealing new candidate genes for known entities and uncovering new syndromes with highly variable manifestations.
- Clonal hematopoiesis is a common phenomenon in IBMFS patients, which can lead to either adaptive somatic genetic rescue or maladaptive changes contributing to malignancies.
- Targeted gene panels and exome sequencing, the most utilized NGS methods, each have their own advantages and limitations.
- A comprehensive workflow, instead of a single test, is recommended for the accurate and efficient diagnosis of IBMFS.

INTRODUCTION

Bone marrow failure syndromes (BMFS) are characterized by quantitative or qualitative defects in hematopoiesis, producing an insufficient amount of functional blood cells of one or several lineages [1]. Approximately 10% to 15% of all cases and 30% of pediatric cases of BMFS are associated with causal constitutional (germline) genetic alterations, collectively known as inherited BMFS (IBMFS) [2]. Aplastic anemia can be caused by inherited disorders such as IBMFS but can also be acquired most commonly by autoimmune disorders. Unlike acquired BMFS, IBMFS are typically associated with a high risk for early onset hematologic malignancies such as myelodysplastic syndrome (MDS) and/or acute myeloid leukemia (AML), and for certain solid tumors [3]. Therefore, early diagnosis of IBMFS is essential for the treatment of BMFS as well as the prevention or early detection of related cancers. Identification of causal gene variants is also important in selecting suitable donors and choosing an appropriate conditioning regimen for hematopoietic stem cell transplantation (HSCT), which is currently the only curative therapy for most IBMFS [4], as well as for genetic counseling and testing of at-risk family members.

Classic IBMFS such as Fanconi anemia (FA) and dyskeratosis congenita (DC) were initially recognized

*Corresponding author. 2212E UCLA West Medical Building, 1010 Veteran Avenue, Los Angeles, CA 90024. *E-mail address:* FuminLin@mednet.ucla.edu

https://doi.org/10.1016/j.yamp.2025.05.001 www.advancesinmolecularpathology.com
2589-4080/25/ © 2025 Elsevier Inc. All rights are reserved, including those for text and data mining, AI training, and similar technologies.

ABBREVIATIONS	
AML	acute myeloid leukemia
BMFS	bone marrow failure syndromes
CAMT	congenital amegakaryocytic thrombocytopenia
CH	clonal hematopoiesis
cnLOH	copy-neutral loss of heterozygosity
CNVs	copy number variants
DBA	Diamond–Blackfan anemia
DC	dyskeratosis congenital
eADA	erythrocyte adenosine deaminase
ES	exome sequencing
FA	Fanconi anemia
G-CSF	granulocyte colony stimulating factor
GD	GATA2 deficiency syndrome
GOF	gain-of-function
GS	genome sequencing
HNSCC	head and neck squamous cell cancer
HSC	hematopoietic stem cell
HSCT	hematopoietic stem cell transplantation
IBMFS	inherited bone marrow failure syndromes
LOF	loss-of-function
MDS	myelodysplastic syndrome
NGS	next-generation sequencing
PIDs	primary immunodeficiency diseases
PVs	pathogenic variants
RIC	reduced-intensity conditioning
RUNX1-FPDMM	RUNX1 familial platelet disorder with associated myeloid malignancies
SCN	severe congenital neutropenia
SDS	Shwachman–Diamond syndrome
SGR	somatic genetic rescue
SNV	single nucleotide variant
TAR	thrombocytopenia absent radii
TBD	telomere biology disorders
VAF	variant allele frequency
VAF	variant allele frequency
VUS	variants of uncertain significance

based on specific cytopenia patterns that typically manifest in childhood along with syndromic congenital anomalies. However, it was soon realized that IBMFS are phenotypically heterogeneous and may display incomplete penetrance and/or variable expressivity [5]. In addition, different IBFMS can exhibit similar hematological manifestations. Therefore, the phenotype and family history of IBMFS may be atypical and remain unrecognized until severe hematologic manifestations occur [6]. The genetic causes of IBMFS are also heterogeneous. Recent research has greatly advanced our understanding of molecular mechanisms underlying different IBMFS and the affected signaling pathways, leading to the development of corresponding functional/biological assays [1,7]. The emergence of next-generation sequencing (NGS) techniques and modern computational tools allows for the simultaneous interrogation of numerous genes across larger patient cohorts, leading to a surge in the identification of causal genes for IBMFS. Consequently, molecular findings have become a gold standard in IBMFS diagnosis. Both targeted gene panels and exome sequencing (ES) have been utilized, with each having their own advantages and limitations.

While the phenomenon of clonal hematopoiesis (CH) has been well-documented in healthy individuals, CH in patients with IBMFS has recently garnered more attention. Somatic clonal changes may compensate for the functional deficiencies caused by germline pathogenic variants (PVs) [8]. However, these changes can also activate oncogenic pathways, leading to an increased risk for hematologic malignancies. Somatic conversion as well as clonal expansion can alter the variant allele frequency (VAF) of germline PVs, so NGS assays for IBMFS require increased sensitivity/reportable range compared to tests for other germline diseases.

In this review, we provide an overview of the history of IBMFS discovery, describe both classic and newly identified entities of IBFMS, highlight the different phenotypes and genetic mechanisms underlying IBFMS and the complexity of molecular diagnosis, and recommend a diagnostic workflow.

HISTORY OF INHERITED BONE MARROW FAILURE SYNDROMES DISCOVERY

As shown in Fig. 1, the history of IBMFS is a fascinating journey spanning several decades of medical discovery, biological research, and advances in the understanding of genetics. Initially, classic IBMFS subtypes were identified by their unique hematologic deficiencies and related congenital abnormalities. With the development of cellular and molecular studies, defective cellular functions or changes in enzyme activity were discovered for certain IBMFS such as spontaneous chromosomal breakage in FA and elevated erythrocyte adenosine deaminase (eADA) activity in Diamond–Blackfan anemia (DBA). Furthermore, major advances in genetic research and DNA sequencing techniques led to the identification of specific genes responsible for various IBMFS. In particular, the advent of NGS techniques has greatly accelerated

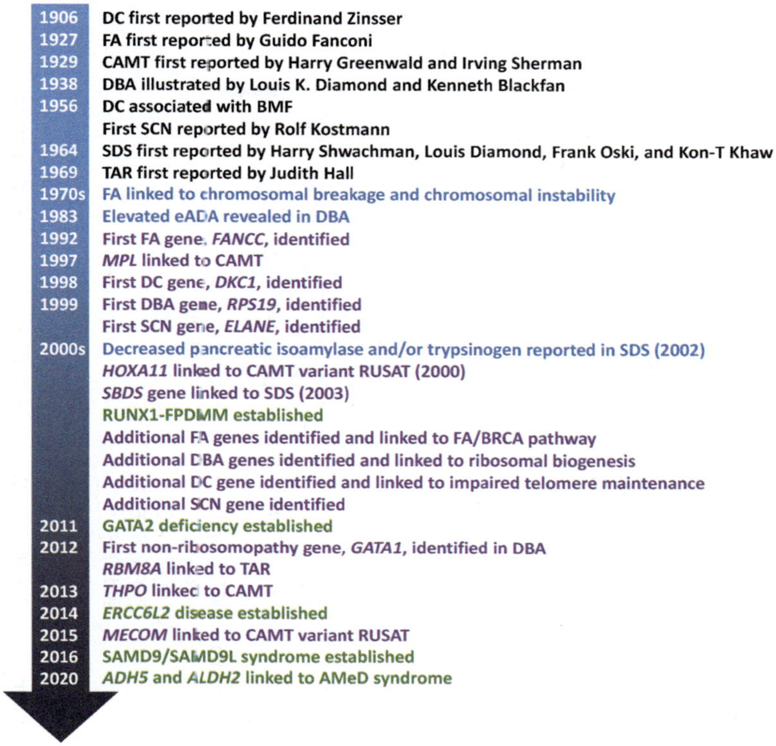

FIG. 1 Milestones in the discovery of IBMFS. Black: Phenotypes of specific entities recognized; Blue: defective cellular function or altered enzyme activity identified; Purple: disease genes identified in patients of corresponding entities; Green: entities established by PVs in the shared gene.

the process of new gene discovery, which in turn advances understanding of disease mechanisms. In addition, new entities are being established based on shared underlying genetic mechanisms despite a broad spectrum of associated phenotypes, such as GATA binding protein 2 (GATA2) deficiency syndrome (GD) and ERCC excision repair 6 like 2 (ERCC6L2) disease [9–11].

CLINICAL AND GENOMIC CHARACTERISTICS OF INHERITED BONE MARROW FAILURE SYNDROMES

Fanconi anemia

Patients with FA typically show congenital anomalies and childhood-onset pancytopenia, thrombocytopenia, or anemia with macrocytosis [12]. The bone marrow is usually hypocellular with prominent erythroid or multilineage dysplasia. Frequent congenital anomalies include short stature, radial ray anomalies (typically involving thumbs), hypo/hyperpigmentation, renal and gastrointestinal abnormalities, and others described in Table 1. Common malignancies associated with FA include MDS, AML, and head and neck squamous cell cancer (HNSCC), with younger onset compared to the general population [12]. However, substantial phenotypic heterogeneity has been reported; up to 40% of patients with FA may not present with congenital anomalies or BMF [13].

FA is caused by PVs in at least 23 genes involved in the FA/BRCA pathway, which is responsible for recognizing interstrand DNA crosslinks and repairing double-stranded DNA damage by homologous recombination [14]. Defective DNA repair triggers apoptosis via the *TP53* pathway, resulting in hematopoietic stem cell (HSC) depletion [15]. Most FA genes are associated with autosomal recessive inheritance, but X-linked recessive FA complementation group B (*FANCB*) and autosomal dominant inheritance RAD51 recombinase (*RAD51*) have been reported. The most common cause of FA is FA complementation group A (*FANCA*) PVs [16]. Different genetic causes also contribute to phenotypic heterogeneity. For

TABLE 1
Clinical, laboratory, and genetic features of inherited bone marrow failure syndromes

Syndrome	Hematological Characteristics	Other Features	Malignancies	Genes (Bold: Most Frequent)	Somatic Alterations	Treatment[a]
FA	Hypocellular marrow Pancytopenia, or cytopenia (macrocytic anemia, thrombocytopenia, leukopenia, and neutropenia)	Short stature, radial ray anomalies, hypo/hyperpigmentation, renal and gastrointestinal abnormalities, microcephaly, ophthalmic anomalies, hearing loss, developmental delay, cardiac anomalies, and clinodactyly Toxicities from chemotherapy or radiation due to DNA repair pathway defect	MDS, AML Solid tumors: SCC of head and neck, esophagus, and vulva; and brain, renal, and liver tumors	AR: *BRCA1, BRCA2, BRIP1, ERCC4, FAAP100,* ***FANCA, FANCC,*** *FANCD2, FANCE, FANCF,* ***FANCG,*** *FANCI, FANCL, FANCM, PALB2, RAD51C, MAD2L2, RFWD3, SLX4, UBE2T, XRCC2* XLR: *FANCB* AD: *RAD51*	+1q, back mutation, second-site variant High risk: +3q, −7/-7q, PVs of *RUNX1* and RAS pathway	Androgen therapy HSCT (RIC)
TBD/DC	Hypocellular marrow Microcytosis, thrombocytopenia, and later progressive pancytopenia	Nail dystrophy, mucosal leukoplakia, reticular skin pigmentation, pulmonary fibrosis, liver cirrhosis, early gray hair Decreased telomere length	MDS, AML Solid tumors: SCC of head and neck, skin; anogenital adenocarcinoma	XLR: *DKC1* AD: *NAF1, RPA1, TERC, TINF2, ZCCHC8* AR: *CTC1, NHP2, NOP10, POT1, STN1*, and *WRAP53* AD or AR: *ACD, PARN, RTEL1*, and *TERT*	+1q, back mutation, second-site variant, *TERT* promoter, cnLOH High risk: 7/7q, *TP53* PV	Androgen therapy HSCT (RIC)
DBA	Normocellular marrow, hypocellular with age and erythroblastopenia Macrocytic anemia with no other significant cytopenia	Growth restriction, developmental delay, anomalies of craniofacial skeleton, eyes, heart, visceral organs, and upper limb and hand (thumb) Elevated eADA	MDS, AML Solid tumor: osteosarcoma	AD: *RPL5, RPL9, RPL11, RPL15, RPL18, RPL26, RPL27, RPL31, RPL35, RPL35A, RPS7, RPS10, RPS15A, RPS17, RPS19, RPS24, RPS26, RPS27, RPS28, RPS29* XLR: *GATA1, TSR2*	Back mutation High risk: *TP53* PV	Corticosteroid treatment Red blood cell transfusion HSCT

SDS	Hypocellular marrow, myeloid dysplasia Neutropenia, macrocytosis	Recurrent infection, pancreatic dysfunction, growth restriction, skeletal abnormalities (dysplasia and osteoporosis), cardiac anomalies, and eczema Low pancreatic isoamylase and trypsinogen	MDS, AML	AR: *SBDS, DNAJC21, EFL1* AD: *SRP54*	−20q, i(7)(q10), *EIF6* LOF High risk: biallelic *TP53* PVs	G-CSF treatment HSCT
SCN	Promyelocyte maturation arrest in marrow Neutropenia	Recurrent infection	MDS, AML	AD: *ELANE, GFI1, SRP54, CLPB,* and *SEC61A1* AR: *HAX1, G6PC3, VPS45, CSF3R, JAGN1, SRP68* XLR: *WAS*	Back mutation, *CSF3R* PV High risk: *RUNX1* PV	G-CSF treatment HSCT
GD	Hypocellular marrow, megakaryocytic atypia, fibrosis Neutropenia, monocytopenia, and lymphopenia	Lymphedema, immunodeficiency, mycobacterial/ fungal/viral infections, pulmonary dysfunction, HPV-related disease	MDS, AML, and CMML	AD: *GATA2*	+8, +21q, der(1;7)(q10;p10), back mutation High risk: 7, PVs of *ASXL1, SETBP1*, and *STAG2*	HSCT
SAMD9/SAMD9L syndrome	Hypocellular marrow Ranging from thrombocytopenia to pancytopenia	MIRAGE (*SAMD9*): severe systemic infection, restriction of growth, adrenal hypoplasia, genital anomalies, and enteropathy Ataxia-pancytopenia syndrome (*SAMD9L*): cerebellar atrophy, dysmetria, ataxia, and nystagmus	MDS, AML	AD: *SAMD9* and *SAMD9L*	cnLOH of 7, second-site variant (LOF) High risk: 7/7q (could be transient), PVs of *SETBP1, ASXL1*, and *RUNX1*	HSCT

(*continued on next page*)

TABLE 1
(continued)

Syndrome	Hematological Characteristics	Other Features	Malignancies	Genes (Bold: Most Frequent)	Somatic Alterations	Treatment[a]
CAMT	Normocellular marrow with reduction/ absence of megakaryocytes Thrombocytopenia	Not common Radioulnar synostosis (*MECOM* or *HOXA11*)	N/A (MDS, AML rarely reported with *MECOM*)	AR: *MPL, THPO* AD: *MECOM, HOXA11*	N/A	HSCT (Thrombopoietin-receptor agonists instead of HSCT for *THPO*-mutated CAMT)
TAR	Decreased megakaryocytes in marrow Transient thrombocytopenia	Bilateral thumb-preserved radius aplasia, anomalies of skeleton, heart, and genitourinary system	N/A	AR: *RBM8A*	N/A	Mainly supportive, platelet counts improve spontaneously
RUNX1-FPDMM	Hypocellular or normocellular marrow for age, atypical megakaryocytes, and eosinophilia Thrombocytopenia (normal platelet size)	Prolonged bleeding and/or easy bruising, eczema, and psoriasis	MDS, AML, T-ALL or B-ALL, and lymphoma	AD: *RUNX1*	-7q, −11q High risk: second *RUNX1* PV, PVs of *SETBP1*, *ASXL1*, *FLT3*, *GATA2*, *SRSF2*, and *WT1*	Platelet transfusion HSCT
ERCC6L2-related disease	Hypocellular marrow with or without dysplasia Thrombocytopenia, anemia, and neutropenia	Not uniform (microcephaly, developmental delay?)	MDS, AML	AR: *ERCC6L2*	High risk: 7, *TP53* PV	HSCT
AMeD syndrome	Pancytopenia or thrombocytopenia/ anemia	Short stature, intellectual disability, microcephaly, abnormal skin pigmentation	MDS, AML	Digenic: *ADH5*/ *ALDH2*	+1q, −7, +8	HSCT

Abbreviations: HSCT, hematopoietic stem cell transplantation; RIC, reduced-intensity conditioning.
[a] Therapies for hematological issues.

example, FA patients with biallelic PVs in BRCA2 DNA repair associated (*BRCA2*) or partner and localizer of BRCA2 (*PALB2*) have early onset malignancies and embryonal tumors such as Wilms tumor and medulloblastoma that are typically not seen in FA caused by PVs in other genes [12,17]. Due to defective DNA repair, patients with FA are especially sensitive to genotoxic agents such as cyclophosphamide or busulfan in chemotherapy and ionizing radiation.

Telomere biology disorders/dyskeratosis congenita

DC, one of the prototypical telomere biology disorders (TBD), is characterized by a triad of nail dystrophy, mucosal leukoplakia, and reticular skin pigmentation. Affected individuals often have hypocellular bone marrow with thrombocytopenia and later progressive pancytopenia, and may show pulmonary fibrosis and other physical anomalies outlined in Table 1. People with DC have an increased risk for MDS, AML, and HNSCC. TBD including DC have a very broad phenotypic spectrum, ranging from almost asymptomatic to early onset BMF with significant neurodevelopmental delay [18].

Defects in telomere maintenance are the main cause underlying TBD [19]. Telomeres are critical structures that protect chromosome ends and therefore genomic integrity. When telomeres become extremely short, chromosome ends will be incorrectly recognized as DNA damage, triggering cell cycle arrest, or apoptosis of HSCs [20]. At least 16 genes functioning in telomere maintenance have been associated with TBD, showing autosomal dominant, autosomal recessive, and X-linked recessive inheritance. However, approximately 20% of patients with TBD remain genetically undefined [18]. Due to progressive telomere shortening, the genetic phenomenon of anticipation (earlier onset of more severe disease in successive generations) has been reported in families with DC [21]. Morbidity and mortality, including pulmonary and hepatic toxicity, are common in patients with TBD after transplantation, but reduced-intensity preparation for transplant improves outcomes [22].

Diamond–Blackfan anemia

DBA is characterized by profound normochromic and macrocytic anemia with normal leukocytes and platelets, usually presenting within the first year of life. However, the phenotypic spectrum ranges widely from mild or no anemia to fetal anemia and hydrops fetalis. The bone marrow is typically normocellular with pure red blood cell aplasia or hypoplasia and erythroblastopenia. Congenital anomalies such as short stature, growth deficiency, and craniofacial, upper limb (especially thumb), and heart malformations can be found in up to 50% of patients [23]. Patients with DBA are predisposed to MDS and AML, and certain solid tumors including osteosarcoma and gastrointestinal malignancies.

DBA was the first described ribosomopathy disease. Pathogenic single nucleotide variants (SNVs) and deletions of 20 ribosomal genes are associated with DBA, with *RPS19* being the most frequently mutated. The defective ribosomal proteins result in impaired ribosomal biogenesis, which in turn activates the *TP53* signaling pathway, cell cycle arrest, and apoptosis [24]. DBA is often inherited in an autosomal dominant manner, while *GATA1*-related and *TSR2*-related DBA are X-linked recessive. *GATA1*, the first nonribosomal protein gene associated with DBA, encodes an essential transcription factor for erythropoiesis and is usually insufficiently translated when ribosomal proteins are deficient [25]. However, the genetic cause is yet to be defined in approximately 20% of DBA patients [23].

Shwachman–Diamond syndrome

Shwachman–Diamond syndrome (SDS) is one of the most common IBMFS. Intermittent or persistent neutropenia is the most common hematologic feature, and it can be accompanied by anemia and thrombocytopenia [26]. The bone marrow typically shows variable degrees of hypocellularity with dysgranulopoietic features [26,27]. Childhood-onset exocrine pancreatic dysfunction is a characteristic finding, and other common features include growth failure, skeletal abnormalities, and recurrent infections due to neutropenia. However, fewer than 50% of patients show the classic combination of BMF and pancreatic insufficiency [27]. SDS also renders susceptibility to MDS and AML.

As an autosomal recessive disease, SDS is primarily caused by biallelic PVs of the *SBDS* gene. Biallelic PVs in *DNAJC21* and *EFL1* as well as heterozygous PVs of *SRP54* have also been reported. SBDS, interacting with elongation factor like GTPase 1 (EFL1), facilitates the release of eukaryotic translation initiation factor 6 (EIF6) that inhibits ribosomal maturation and the subsequent combination of ribosomal subunits into a functional ribosome. DnaJ Heat Shock Protein Family (Hsp40) Member C21 (DNAJC21) is involved in ribosome stabilization, while SRP54 is involved in protein trafficking [28]. As all these genes are related to ribosomal biogenesis or protein synthesis, SDS is also considered a ribosomopathy.

Severe congenital neutropenia

Severe congenital neutropenia (SCN) is characterized by profound chronic neutropenia and recurrent infections. Patients with SCN show characteristic myeloid maturation arrest in the bone marrow and are predisposed to MDS and AML, especially when treated with high-dose granulocyte colony stimulating factor (G-CSF) therapy [29]. SCN is one type of primary immunodeficiency diseases (PIDs) specifically impacting neutrophils, while other PIDs can affect different parts of the immune system, including antibody production, B/T cells, phagocytes, and complement proteins. Certain non-SCN PIDs may predispose to malignancies with lymphoma being the most common [30,31].

Heterozygous PVs in the elastase, neutrophil expressed (*ELANE*) gene occur in around 50% of patients with SCN [32]. Interestingly, some *ELANE* variants lead to cyclic neutropenia, conferring better response to G-CSF and lower risk of MDS and AML [33]. Less frequently, SCN can result from PVs in HCLS1 associated protein X-1 (*HAX1*), WASP actin nucleation promoting factor (*WAS*), growth factor independent 1 transcriptional repressor (*GFI1*), jagunal homolog 1 (*JAGN1*), glucose-6-phosphatase catalytic subunit 3 (*G6PC3*), colony stimulating factor 3 receptor (*CSF3R*), or other genes in Table 1.

GATA2 deficiency syndrome

GD is an autosomal dominant IBMFS with highly variable features including infections, cytopenias, pulmonary alveolar proteinosis, lymphedema, and increased risk of MDS and AML [34]. Patients usually show hypocellular bone marrow with fibrosis, megakaryocytic atypia, peripheral neutropenia, and monocytopenia [9].

GATA2 encodes a zinc finger transcription factor that is essential for HSC survival and self-renewal. Loss-of-function (LOF) variants or deletions of this gene result in insufficient GATA2 protein, leading to GD [10].

SAMD9/SAMD9L syndrome

Different from other IBMFS, sterile alpha motif domain containing 9 (SAMD9)/sterile alpha motif domain containing 9 like (SAMD9L) syndrome is caused by germline gain-of-function (GOF) variants in these 2 genes that negatively regulate cell proliferation. The phenotypic spectrum is broad and commonly includes cytopenia, immunodeficiency, infections, and susceptibility to MDS and AML. Growth impairment, infections, adrenal insufficiency, genital phenotypes, and enteropathy are commonly associated with pathogenic *SAMD9* variants, while pathogenic *SAMD9L* variants often involve progressive neurologic deficits. Both *SAMD9* and *SAMD9L* PVs are typically associated with hypocellular bone marrow and mild-to-severe cytopenias (including thrombocytopenia, macrocytic anemia, neutropenia, and lymphopenia) [35].

Congenital amegakaryocytic thrombocytopenia

Congenital amegakaryocytic thrombocytopenia (CAMT) is a severe form of thrombocytopenia characterized by markedly decreased or absent megakaryocytes in the bone marrow. Progression to MDS or AML has not been clearly described [36].

Most CAMT cases occur due to biallelic PVs resulting in loss of function of the *MPL* gene. *MPL* encodes the thrombopoietin receptor, which plays a crucial role in platelet production. Biallelic variants in thrombopoietin (*THPO*), encoding thrombopoietin, have also been reported. PVs of *HOXA11* or MDS1 and EVI1 complex locus (*MECOM*) cause radioulnar synostosis with amegakaryocytic thrombocytopenia, an autosomal dominant form of CAMT with the additional feature of radioulnar synostosis [36].

Thrombocytopenia absent radii syndrome

Thrombocytopenia absent radii (TAR) syndrome is characterized by bilateral thumb-preserved radius aplasia and generally transient thrombocytopenia. There is no clear evidence to link TAR with secondary malignancies. Anomalies of the skeletal, heart, and genitourinary system can also occur.

TAR is typically caused by a null allele (most often a deletion in 1q21.1) *in trans* with a hypomorphic allele in *RBM8A*, which is important for mRNA processing [37].

RUNX1 familial platelet disorder with associated myeloid malignancies

RUNX1 familial platelet disorder with associated myeloid malignancies (RUNX1-FPDMM) is caused by heterozygous LOF variants in *RUNX1* and is characterized by abnormal bruising or bleeding because of qualitative platelet defects and eczema. RUNX1-FPDMM is associated with increased risk of MDS, AML, acute lymphoblastic leukemias, and lymphomas [38].

ERCC6L2-related disease

ERCC6L2-related disease is a rare autosomal recessive form of IBMFS linked with LOF variants of the *ERCC6L2* gene, which functions in DNA damage repair including nucleotide excision repair and nonhomologous end joining. Common clinical features include hypocellular bone marrow with variable degrees of thrombocytopenia. Nearly one-third of patients initially present with MDS or AML [11].

AMeD syndrome

AMeD syndrome is a new form of IBMFS recently established from 10 cases of 8 unrelated families. It is characterized by growth restriction, short stature, developmental delay, intellectual disability, and early onset of bone marrow failure with pancytopenia, anemia, thrombocytopenia, and/or leukopenia. Patients with aplastic anemia, mental retardation, and dwarfism (AMeD) syndrome develop MDS during infancy or childhood. This syndrome shows unique digenic inheritance, caused by biallelic LOF variants in *ADH5* coupled with a heterozygous or homozygous LOF variant in *ALDH2* [39].

SOMATIC CONVERSION AND CLONAL HEMATOPOIESIS

While IBMFS are Mendelian diseases resulting from germline PVs, somatic alterations have been frequently reported. Generally, germline variants in IBMFS genes decrease the fitness of HSCs and impair differentiation and self-renewal. Because of the high turnover of hematopoiesis, somatic variants that restore HSC fitness will persist, a phenomenon known as somatic conversion [40]. A greater proportion of corresponding blood cells will be derived from those HSCs that gain a survival and/or proliferation advantage, leading to CH. Distinct from CH of indeterminate potential, which can be seen in the general population with increasing frequency by age and which usually involves epigenetic regulators such as DNA methyltransferase 3 alpha (*DNMT3A*), tet methylcytosine dioxygenase 2 (*TET2*), and ASXL transcriptional regulator 1 (*ASXL1*), CH in patients with IBMFS happens much earlier and more frequently and involves a different spectrum of genes [8,41,42]. Although CH provides fitness advantages for HSCs, it also presents varying risks for leukemic transformation depending on the underlying condition and the characteristics of the alteration [42]. With research advances and expanded application of NGS for IBMFS diagnosis, more accurate risk stratification has been applied to distinct CH variants [8]. Adaptive CH, also known as somatic genetic rescue (SGR), restores HSC fitness defects without activating leukemogenic pathways. Maladaptive CH typically compensates for HSC fitness defects by inhibiting tumor suppressor genes/pathways, leading to a higher risk for malignant transformation. However, some CH variants are of unknown clinical significance [8].

SGR can reverse mutated disease-causing genes back to the normal ("wild-type") genotype either through back mutation (SNV or indel at the same site of the germline PVs) or through copy-neutral loss of heterozygosity (cnLOH, replacing disease-causing allele with wild-type allele). These types of SGR have been reported in FA, TBD, DBA, RUNX1-FPDMM, SAMD9/SAMD9L syndrome, SCN, and GD, typically not increasing the risk of malignant transformation [43–49]. Somatic variants can also happen at a second site of affected genes to counteract the effect of germline variants, such as somatic truncating or missense LOF variants in *cis* to GOF germline variants in SAMD9/SAMD9L syndrome [48]. Somatic second-site variants are also reported in FA and TBD and are usually not associated with an increased risk for malignancies [50,51]. Chromosomal alterations can also attenuate the deleterious effects of germline PVs. Monosomy 7/7q can remove the GOF SAMD9/SAMD9L germline variants but also greatly increase the risk of developing leukemia [52]. In contrast, isochromosome 7q is a common somatic compensation mechanism in cases of SDS harboring a pathogenic *SBDS* splice variant, which rescues the deficiency but does not increase the risk of malignant transformation by duplicating the splice variant (which produces low-level normal SBDS protein) [53]. Somatic changes of different genes in the same signaling pathway as the constitutionally mutated gene are also reported, such as somatic activating *TERT* promoter variants in TBD and LOF of *EIF6* gene in SDS, both of which are considered adaptive CH [54–56]. HSCs can also acquire a proliferation advantage through inhibiting tumor-suppressor pathways or enhancing growth-promoting signals at a cost of increased risk of malignant transformation. Somatic PVs in *TP53* are recurrently observed in SDS and ERCC6L2 disease, with a higher allele frequency linked to the development of myeloid malignancies [11,55]. Although somatic mosaicism poses challenges to both phenotype-based and genotype-based diagnoses of IBFMS, it is crucial to recognize this phenomenon and ensure effective identification of these alterations.

DIAGNOSTIC TOOLS

Functional screening

Chromosomal breakage analysis

Due to defective DNA crosslink repair, patients with FA can be screened for increased chromosomal breakage and characteristic radial configurations in peripheral blood lymphocytes when exposed to DNA crosslinking agents such as mitomycin C or diepoxybutane. SGR may cause false-negative or equivocal results when testing blood or bone marrow cells, necessitating examination of skin fibroblasts. MDS, AML or recent chemotherapy may also complicate test results and interpretation [57].

Telomere length evaluation

Given the significantly shortened telomeres in patients with TBD, evaluation of telomere length in peripheral blood lymphocytes by flow fluorescence in situ hybridization should be considered. However, short telomeres have also been reported in FA, impacting assay specificity [58].

Erythrocyte adenosine deaminase activity analysis

Elevated eADA activity is observed in over 80% of patients with DBA; however, recent transfusion may affect testing results [59].

Serum trypsinogen and pancreatic isoamylase testing

Patients with SDS can be screened by deficiency of serum trypsinogen (before the age of 3 years) and decreased pancreatic isoamylase (after the age of 3 years), owing to characteristic childhood-onset exocrine pancreatic insufficiency [60,61].

It is important to note that functional screening assays are not available for all IBMFS entities and existing screening assays may not be entity-specific. Screening tests are often not amenable to multiplexing, leading to a potentially long and costly diagnostic journey; furthermore, these assays cannot reveal the underlying genetic cause, which is important for genetic counseling, donor selection for HSC transplant, downstream cascade testing, and family planning. Additionally, some assays, such as chromosomal breakage analysis and telomere length evaluation, are offered by fewer clinical laboratories; however, they are still useful tools to evaluate the pathogenicity of variants of uncertain significance (VUS) that are identified in genetic testing.

Genetic testing

As the genetic etiology has been revealed in the majority of IBMFS entities except for approximately 20% of patients with TBD and DBA [62], molecular analysis interrogating relevant genes has become the preferred approach for the diagnosis of IBMFS.

Historically, conventional sequencing techniques such as Sanger sequencing dominated the genetic diagnosis of IBMFS, investigating the gene(s) of interest based on clinical suspicion. While Sanger sequencing is highly accurate, the increasing number of causal genes and the significant phenotypic overlap between IBMFS entities make it less efficient as a diagnostic tool. Currently, Sanger sequencing is often used for NGS result confirmation and follow-up cascade testing for at-risk family members.

NGS enables sequencing of a massive amount of DNA fragments simultaneously, allowing analysis of many genes and samples in parallel. As a result, it has become the primary tool for IBMFS diagnosis. NGS techniques include targeted gene sequencing panels and ES, each with its own advantages and limitations. Panels focus on well-curated IBMFS-associated genes while ES provides a broad view of coding regions of all genes. Compared to ES, panels are more cost-effective, deliver faster results, and offer higher sequencing depth, making them a better option for detecting low-level mosaic variants and, therefore, an ideal testing modality for IBMFS. Higher sequencing depth also increases sensitivity for the identification of copy number variants (CNVs), as discussed later. Studies have shown that nearly half (37%–59%) of clinically diagnosed IBFMS cases have a genetic cause identified through panels [7,63–65], and even when used as a screening tool to rule out an IBMFS, panels show a diagnostic yield of 7.8% [66]. Meanwhile, ES is reported to identify causal variants in 47% to 48% of patients, slightly improving the diagnostic yield due to the analysis of a greater number of genes [65,67], and is commonly used in research to identify new candidate genes. ES can also be valuable in ruling out IBMFS by identifying causal variants in genes associated with other overlapping hematologic phenotypes, such as hereditary pyropoikilocytosis, glucose-6-phosphate dehydrogenase (G6PD) deficiency, pyruvate kinase deficiency, or other hereditary predispositions to myeloid malignancies. However, these genes can also be included in targeted panels to rule out common differential diagnoses [66]. A significant number of variants responsible for IBMFS are located in intronic regions, promoters, or enhancers, such as the *GATA2* c.1017 + 572C>T variant. Panels can identify these variants by adding probes to cover noncoding regions of interest. Modifying the target regions of ES is more challenging in comparison.

CNVs as causal genetic alterations or clinically significant CH markers in IBMFS are often underestimated, owing to challenges related to sequencing technology and bioinformatics. Detecting CNVs, particularly mosaic CNVs, is challenging with ES due to lower read depth. By integrating a single nucleotide polymorphism "back-bone" and employing advanced CNV calling algorithms and visualization tools, panels with deeper sequencing coverage outperform ES in identifying pathogenic CNVs [66]. Genome sequencing (GS), which sequences the entire genome, may be considered as an alternative due to the ability to identify noncoding variants and increased sensitivity for structural variants, and is being adopted in clinical settings. It is worth noting that small intragenic (exon-level) deletions/duplications identified by sequencing should be confirmed by orthogonal methods such as multiplex ligation-dependent probe amplification and droplet digital polymerase chain reaction.

When used for the study of germline changes, both ES and GS are typically designed to detect variants in the heterozygous or homozygous state (~50% or ~100% VAF) and, therefore, have limited sensitivity in detecting mosaic germline variants in peripheral blood due to SGR. In addition, low sequencing depth as well as the limitations of short-read sequencing makes it challenging for ES/GS to identify large indels and true PVs in GC-rich regions or genomic regions with high sequence homology to their pseudogenes, especially variants caused by gene conversion. For example, it has been reported that the *SBDS* c.183_184delinsCT variant is often missed by ES due to preferential alignment of sequencing reads to the pseudogene *SBDSP1* [68]. In addition, panels, with their high sensitivity for low-level mosaic somatic alterations, are better suited for monitoring patients with IBMFS over time for signs of malignant transformation.

As massively parallel sequencing methods, both ES/GS and panels generate a significant number of VUS. To establish the pathogenicity of a VUS, additional studies are needed, including but not limited to functional assays in cellular or animal models, other omics studies (such as transcriptomics and methylomics),

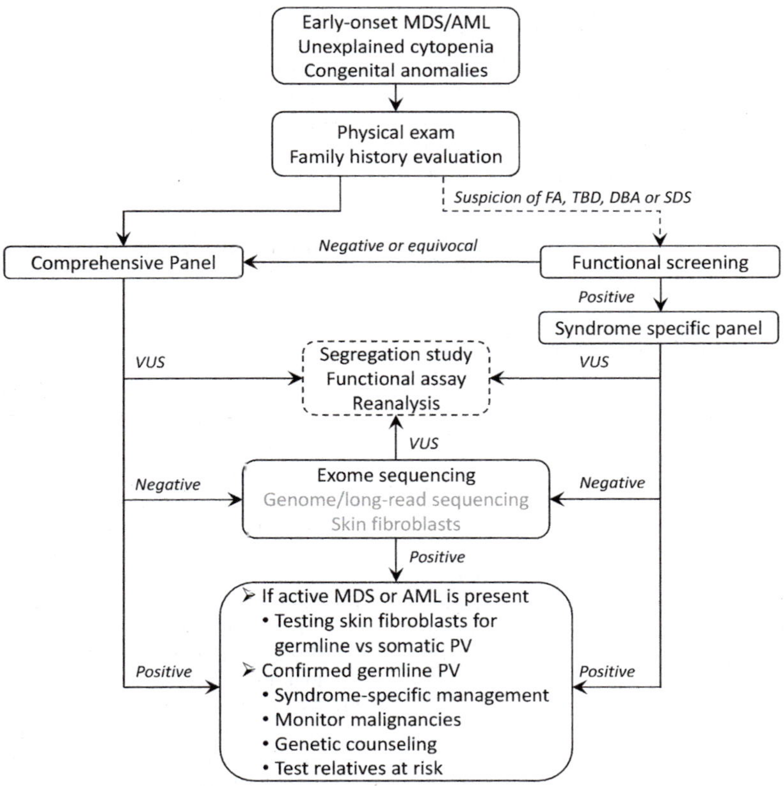

FIG. 2 Recommendation of a comprehensive approach for IBMFS diagnosis. Depending on confirmation or denial of the pathogenicity of VUS, procedures for diagnosed IBMFS or periodic reanalysis should be performed, respectively.

segregation analysis of affected and unaffected family members, genotype–phenotype correlation of large patient cohorts and controls, and periodic data reanalysis.

Recently novel approaches beyond DNA/RNA sequencing have been attempted for IBMFS diagnosis. One study has incorporated proteomic analysis in rapid IBMFS screening and showed identifiable proteomic clustering patterns for different IBMFS entities [69]. Computationally, a machine-learning algorithm was developed to help differentiate inherited and acquired BMF using 25 clinical and laboratory variables typically recorded at the initial clinical encounter [70].

RECOMMENDATION OF DIAGNOSTIC ALGORITHM

An evaluation for IBMFS should be initiated for patients with early onset MDS or AML, unexplained cytopenias, or associated congenital anomalies. The evaluation includes collecting family history, physical examination, blood and bone marrow studies, and functional and genetic testing. If FA, TBD, DBA, or SDS is suspected, a corresponding functional screen may be considered. Positive screening results can establish the diagnosis, and prompt syndrome-specific management, genetic counseling, and monitoring for related malignancies. Syndrome-specific NGS panels should still be recommended to identify a genetic etiology and confirm the diagnosis, as well as to allow testing of at-risk family members. If the clinical indication does not suggest a specific IBMFS entity, a more comprehensive IBMFS panel should be utilized. These panels should offer deep sequencing coverage enabling accurate CNV annotation and mosaic variant identification. If panels yield negative results, further testing with ES is indicated. Upon confirmation of a causal variant linked to IBMFS, the diagnosis is established, and appropriate clinical evaluations should follow. If PVs responsible for non-IBMFS hematologic disorders are revealed and align with clinical indications based on expert opinion, it is appropriate to discontinue the IBMFS workup. For VUS, familial segregation analysis and/or functional studies are recommended to assess pathogenicity. If both panels and ES return negative results, GS and/or long-read sequencing may be considered to identify structural variants, or testing a different tissue such as skin fibroblasts to identify potential somatic mosaicism (Fig. 2). Testing of an alternative tissue source will also be helpful in patients with an active hematologic malignancy, where distinguishing true germline variants from somatic changes will be challenging when testing blood. For example, a young patient with anemia and thrombocytopenia and later diagnosed with AML, has genetic testing on blood showing a *RUNX1* PV with a VAF at 41% and apparently nonmosaic trisomy 21, implying a Down syndrome-associated leukemia with somatic *RUNX1* PV. However, follow-up skin fibroblast testing shows this *RUNX1* PV was germline while trisomy 21 was somatic, consistent with a clinical diagnosis of RUNX1-FPDMM.

SUMMARY

Despite the heterogeneous nature of IBMFS, advances in molecular research and growing clinical awareness have greatly enhanced our understanding of these disorders, including atypical clinical presentations, rare candidate genes, and the phenomenon of somatic conversion. An accurate and timely diagnosis of IBMFS is essential for effective clinical management and better patient outcomes. As such, when IBMFS is suspected, a comprehensive workup should be conducted. This should include a thorough physical examination, complete blood count, bone marrow evaluation, family history assessment, relevant screening tests, and most importantly, genetic evaluation to ensure a precise diagnosis and guide appropriate management.

DISCLOSURE

All authors have no disclosures to declare in relation to this article.

REFERENCES

[1] West AH, Churpek JE. Old and new tools in the clinical diagnosis of inherited bone marrow failure syndromes. Hematology Am Soc Hematol Educ Program 2017; 2017:79–87.

[2] Moore CA, Krishnan K. Bone marrow failure. StatPearls. Treasure Island (FL) ineligible companies. Disclosure: Koyamangalath Krishnan declares no relevant financial relationships with ineligible companies. 2025.

[3] Alter BP, Giri N, Savage SA, et al. Cancer in the National Cancer Institute inherited bone marrow failure syndrome cohort after fifteen years of follow-up. Haematologica (Roma) 2018;103:30–9.

[4] Groarke EM, Young NS, Calvo KR. Distinguishing constitutional from acquired bone marrow failure in the hematology clinic. Best Pract Res Clin Haematol 2021;34:101275.

[5] Sorrow JM Jr, Hitch JM. Dyskeratosis congenita. First report of its occurrence in a female and a review of the literature. Arch Dermatol 1963;88:340–7.

[6] Keel SB, Scott A, Sanchez-Bonilla M, et al. Genetic features of myelodysplastic syndrome and aplastic anemia in pediatric and young adult patients. Haematologica (Roma) 2016;101:1343–50.
[7] Muramatsu H, Okuno Y, Yoshida K, et al. Clinical utility of next-generation sequencing for inherited bone marrow failure syndromes. Genet Med 2017;19: 796–802.
[8] Lundgren S, Keranen M, Wartiovaara-Kautto U, et al. Somatic compensation of inherited bone marrow failure. Semin Hematol 2022;59:167–73.
[9] Calvo KR, Hickstein DD. The spectrum of GATA2 deficiency syndrome. Blood 2023;141:1524–32.
[10] Crispino JD, Horwitz MS. GATA factor mutations in hematologic disease. Blood 2017;129:2103–10.
[11] Hakkarainen M, Kaaja I, Douglas SPM, et al. The clinical picture of ERCC6L2 disease: from bone marrow failure to acute leukemia. Blood 2023;141:2853–66.
[12] Mehta PA, Ebens C. Fanconi anemia. In: Adam MP, Feldman J, Mirzaa GM, et al, editors. GeneReviews ((R)). Seattle (WA)1993.
[13] Wilson DB, Link DC, Mason PJ, et al. Inherited bone marrow failure syndromes in adolescents and young adults. Ann Med 2014;46:353–63.
[14] D'Andrea AD, Grompe M. The Fanconi anaemia/BRCA pathway. Nat Rev Cancer 2003;3:23–34.
[15] Ceccaldi R, Sarangi P, D'Andrea AD. The Fanconi anaemia pathway: new players and new functions. Nat Rev Mol Cell Biol 2016;17:337–49.
[16] Savage SA, Walsh MF. Myelodysplastic syndrome, acute myeloid leukemia, and cancer surveillance in fanconi anemia. Hematol Oncol Clin N Am 2018;32:657–68.
[17] McReynolds LJ, Biswas K, Giri N, et al. Genotype-cancer association in patients with Fanconi anemia due to pathogenic variants in FANCD1 (BRCA2) or FANCN (PALB2). Cancer Genet 2021;258-259:101–9.
[18] Savage SA, Niewisch MR. Dyskeratosis congenita and related telomere biology disorders. In: Adam MP, Feldman J, Mirzaa GM, et al, editors. GeneReviews((R)). Seattle (WA) 1993.
[19] Grill S, Nandakumar J. Molecular mechanisms of telomere biology disorders. J Biol Chem 2021;296:100064.
[20] Townsley DM, Dumitriu B, Young NS. Bone marrow failure and the telomeropathies. Blood 2014;124: 2775–83.
[21] Vulliamy T, Marrone A, Szydlo R, et al. Disease anticipation is associated with progressive telomere shortening in families with dyskeratosis congenita due to mutations in TERC. Nat Genet 2004;36:447–9.
[22] Bhoopalan SV, Wlodarski M, Reiss U, et al. Reduced-intensity conditioning-based hematopoietic cell transplantation for dyskeratosis congenita: single-center experience and literature review. Pediatr Blood Cancer 2021;68:e29177.
[23] Sieff C. Diamond-blackfan anemia. In: Adam MP, Feldman J, Mirzaa GM, et al, editors. GeneReviews((R)). Seattle (WA)1993.
[24] Engidaye G, Melku M, Enawgaw B. Diamond Blackfan anemia: genetics, pathogenesis, diagnosis and treatment. EJIFCC 2019;30:67–81.
[25] Ludwig LS, Gazda HT, Eng JC, et al. Altered translation of GATA1 in Diamond-Blackfan anemia. Nat Med 2014;20:748–53.
[26] Nelson A, Myers K. Shwachman-diamond syndrome. In: Adam MP, Feldman J, Mirzaa GM, et al, editors. GeneReviews((R)). Seattle (WA)1993.
[27] Myers KC, Bolyard AA, Otto B, et al. Variable clinical presentation of Shwachman-Diamond syndrome: update from the North American Shwachman-Diamond syndrome registry. J Pediatr 2014;164:866–70.
[28] Bezzerri V, Cipolli M. Shwachman-diamond syndrome: molecular mechanisms and current perspectives. Mol Diagn Ther 2019;23:281–90.
[29] Klein C. Genetic defects in severe congenital neutropenia: emerging insights into life and death of human neutrophil granulocytes. Annu Rev Immunol 2011;29:399–413.
[30] Pai SY, Lurain K, Yarchoan R. How immunodeficiency can lead to malignancy. Hematology Am Soc Hematol Educ Program 2021;2021:287–95.
[31] Spoor J, Farajifard H, Rezaei N. Congenital neutropenia and primary immunodeficiency diseases. Crit Rev Oncol Hematol 2019;133:149–62.
[32] Boxer LA, Newburger PE. A molecular classification of congenital neutropenia syndromes. Pediatr Blood Cancer 2007;49:609–14.
[33] Makaryan V, Zeidler C, Bolyard AA, et al. The diversity of mutations and clinical outcomes for ELANE-associated neutropenia. Curr Opin Hematol 2015;22:3–11.
[34] Hsu AP, McReynolds LJ, Holland SM. GATA2 deficiency. Curr Opin Allergy Clin Immunol 2015;15:104–9.
[35] Sahoo SS, Erlacher M, Wlodarski MW. Genetic and clinical spectrum of SAMD9 and SAMD9L syndromes: from variant interpretation to patient management. Blood 2025;145:475–85.
[36] Tirthani E, Said MS, De Jesus O. Amegakaryocytic Thrombocytopenia. StatPearls. Treasure Island (FL) ineligible companies. Disclosure: Mina Said declares no relevant financial relationships with ineligible companies. Disclosure: Orlando De Jesus declares no relevant financial relationships with ineligible companies.2025.
[37] Petit F, Boussion S. Thrombocytopenia absent radius syndrome. In: Adam MP, Feldman J, Mirzaa GM, et al, editors. GeneReviews((R)). Seattle (WA)1993.
[38] Deuitch N, Broadbridge E, Cunningham L, et al. RUNX1 familial platelet disorder with associated myeloid malignancies. In: Adam MP, Feldman J, Mirzaa GM, et al, editors. GeneReviews((R)). Seattle (WA)1993.
[39] Oka Y, Hamada M, Nakazawa Y, et al. Digenic mutations in ALDH2 and ADH5 impair formaldehyde clearance and cause a multisystem disorder, AMeD syndrome. Sci Adv 2020;6.
[40] Revy P, Kannengiesser C, Fischer A. Somatic genetic rescue in Mendelian haematopoietic diseases. Nat Rev Genet 2019;20:582–98.

[41] Jaiswal S, Ebert BL. Clonal hematopoiesis in human aging and disease. Science 2019;366.
[42] Tsai FD, Lindsley RC. Clonal hematopoiesis in the inherited bone marrow failure syndromes. Blood 2020; 136:1615–22.
[43] Catto LFB, Borges G, Pinto AL, et al. Somatic genetic rescue in hematopoietic cells in GATA2 deficiency. Blood 2020;136:1002–5.
[44] Glembotsky AC, Marin Oyarzun CP, De Luca G, et al. First description of revertant mosaicism in familial platelet disorder with predisposition to acute myelogenous leukemia: correlation with the clinical phenotype. Haematologica (Roma) 2020;105:e535.
[45] Gross M, Hanenberg H, Lobitz S, et al. Reverse mosaicism in Fanconi anemia: natural gene therapy via molecular self-correction. Cytogenet Genome Res 2002;98: 126–35.
[46] Jongmans MC, Verwiel ET, Heijdra Y, et al. Revertant somatic mosaicism by mitotic recombination in dyskeratosis congenita. Am J Hum Genet 2012;90:426–33.
[47] Liu Q, Zhang L, Shu Z, et al. Two paternal mosaicism of mutation in ELANE causing severe congenital neutropenia exhibit normal neutrophil morphology and ROS production. Clin Immunol 2019;203:53–8.
[48] Sahoo SS, Pastor VB, Goodings C, et al, European Working Group of MDS in Children EWOG-MDS. Clinical evolution, genetic landscape and trajectories of clonal hematopoiesis in SAMD9/SAMD9L syndromes. Nat Med 2021;27:1806–17.
[49] Venugopal P, Moore S, Lawrence DM, et al. Self-reverting mutations partially correct the blood phenotype in a Diamond Blackfan anemia patient. Haematologica (Roma) 2017;102:e506–9.
[50] Sharma R, Sahoo SS, Honda M, et al. Gain-of-function mutations in RPA1 cause a syndrome with short telomeres and somatic genetic rescue. Blood 2022;139: 1039–51.
[51] Waisfisz Q, Morgan NV, Savino M, et al. Spontaneous functional correction of homozygous fanconi anaemia alleles reveals novel mechanistic basis for reverse mosaicism. Nat Genet 1999;22:379–83.
[52] Wong JC, Bryant V, Lamprecht T, et al. Germline SAMD9 and SAMD9L mutations are associated with extensive genetic evolution and diverse hematologic outcomes. JCI Insight 2018;3.
[53] Minelli A, Maserati E, Nicolis E, et al. The isochromosome i(7)(q10) carrying c.258+2t>c mutation of the SBDS gene does not promote development of myeloid malignancies in patients with Shwachman syndrome. Leukemia 2009;23:708–11.
[54] Gutierrez-Rodrigues F, Donaires FS, Pinto A, et al. Pathogenic TERT promoter variants in telomere diseases. Genet Med 2019;21:1594–602.
[55] Kennedy AL, Myers KC, Bowman J, et al. Distinct genetic pathways define pre-malignant versus compensatory clonal hematopoiesis in Shwachman-Diamond syndrome. Nat Commun 2021;12:1334.
[56] Maryoung L, Yue Y, Young A, et al. Somatic mutations in telomerase promoter counterbalance germline loss-of-function mutations. J Clin Investig 2017;127:982–6.
[57] Peffault de Latour R, Soulier J. How I treat MDS and AML in Fanconi anemia. Blood 2016;127:2971–9.
[58] Alter BP, Giri N, Savage SA, et al. Telomere length in inherited bone marrow failure syndromes. Haematologica (Roma) 2015;100:49–54.
[59] Fargo JH, Kratz CP, Giri N, et al. Erythrocyte adenosine deaminase: diagnostic value for Diamond-Blackfan anaemia. Br J Haematol 2013;160:547–54.
[60] Ip WF, Dupuis A, Ellis L, et al. Serum pancreatic enzymes define the pancreatic phenotype in patients with Shwachman-Diamond syndrome. J Pediatr 2002; 141:259–65.
[61] Rothbaum R, Perrault J, Vlachos A, et al. Shwachman-Diamond syndrome: report from an international conference. J Pediatr 2002;141:266–70.
[62] Dokal I, Tummala H, Vulliamy T. Inherited bone marrow failure in the pediatric patient. Blood 2022; 140:556–70.
[63] Galvez E, Vallespin E, Arias-Salgado EG, et al. Next-generation sequencing in bone marrow failure syndromes and isolated cytopenias: experience of the Spanish network on bone marrow failure syndromes. Hemasphere 2021;5:e539.
[64] Ghemlas I, Li H, Zlateska B, et al. Improving diagnostic precision, care and syndrome definitions using comprehensive next-generation sequencing for the inherited bone marrow failure syndromes. J Med Genet 2015; 52:575–84.
[65] Lee JM, Kim HS, Yoo J, et al. Genomic insights into inherited bone marrow failure syndromes in a Korean population. Br J Haematol 2024;205:1581–9.
[66] Lin F, Cao K, Chang F, et al. Uncovering the genetic etiology of inherited bone marrow failure syndromes using a custom-designed next-generation sequencing panel. J Mol Diagn 2024;26:191–201.
[67] Bluteau O, Sebert M, Leblanc T, et al. A landscape of germ line mutations in a cohort of inherited bone marrow failure patients. Blood 2018;131:717–32.
[68] Yamada M, Uehara T, Suzuki H, et al. Shortfall of exome analysis for diagnosis of Shwachman-Diamond syndrome: mismapping due to the pseudogene SBDSP1. Am J Med Genet 2020;182:1631–6.
[69] Wakamatsu M, Muramatsu H, Sato H, et al. Integrated proteogenomic analysis for inherited bone marrow failure syndrome. Leukemia 2024;38:1256–65.
[70] Gutierrez-Rodrigues F, Munger E, Ma X, et al. Differential diagnosis of bone marrow failure syndromes guided by machine learning. Blood 2023;141:2100–13.

Advances in Molecular Pathology 8 (2025) 15–26
ADVANCES IN MOLECULAR PATHOLOGY

Advances in Prenatal Genomic Sequencing

Amanda Thomas-Wilson, MS, PhD[a], Vaidehi Jobanputra, MS, PhD[a,b,*]
[a]Molecular Diagnostics/CLIA Lab, New York Genome Center, 101 6th Avenue, New York, NY 100013, USA; [b]Department of Pathology and Cell Biology, Columbia University Irving Medical Center, 630W 168 Street, New York, NY 10032, USA

KEYWORDS
• Prenatal genome sequencing • Fetal anomaly • Fetal diagnostic testing

KEY POINTS

- Significant advancements in prenatal screening and diagnostics have developed in the past decades.
- The availability of guidance for prenatal and neonatal interventions, therapies, and management is also rapidly evolving for many congenital disorders.
- Prenatal genome sequencing (GS) is a comprehensive test that is capable of detecting most variants previously requiring sequential testing and multiple methodologies.
- Preliminary data and comparative studies suggest GS could become a first-tier test for prenatal screening and diagnosis of genetic disorders.
- Prenatal GS has the potential to revolutionize personalized care during pregnancy and enable specific management and therapies for fetuses affected with genetic disorders.

INTRODUCTION

Advances in obstetrics and maternal fetal medicine have expanded prenatal imaging and screening capabilities, while development of next-generation sequencing (NGS) has increased the accuracy and scope of prenatal genetic testing. Prenatal genome sequencing (GS) is the most comprehensive test available for diagnosis of genetic etiologies in pregnancies with fetal structural anomalies. More recently, its use has expanded to include prenatal diagnosis in nonanomalous pregnancies. GS refers to the comprehensive analysis of the entire DNA sequence of an individual's genome, allowing for the detection of a wide range of variant types in a single test.

GS can detect variants ranging from a single nucleotide change to full chromosome aneuploidies, small and large insertion-deletion variants, copy number changes, repeat expansions, and mitochondrial DNA variants [1–4]. In recent years, GS has gained traction as a first-tier test for suspected genetic disorders in undiagnosed disease, offering higher diagnostic yields compared with other testing modalities [1–4]. GS can be used as an all-in-one diagnostic test on direct and cultured chorionic villus samples (CVS), direct and cultured amniotic fluid samples, and products of conception (POC) in pregnancies affected by fetal structural anomalies. Although prenatal GS is still relatively new, comparative studies in many prenatal and postnatal cohorts demonstrate that GS reliably detects all variants previously requiring multiple sequential methodologies [1–4], and has been used to end long diagnostic odysseys with identification of variants missed by other tests because of methodological limitations [5–7].

*Corresponding author. Department of Pathology & Cell Biology, Columbia University Irving Medical Center, 630W 168 Street, New York, NY 10032. *E-mail address:* vj2004@cumc.columbia.edu

https://doi.org/10.1016/j.yamp.2025.07.001
www.advancesinmolecularpathology.com
2589-4080/25/ © 2025 Elsevier Inc. All rights are reserved, including those for text and data mining, AI training, and similar technologies.

ABBREVIATIONS

array CGH	array comparative genomic hybridization
ASD	autism spectrum disorder
cfDNA	cell-free DNA
CMA	chromosomal microarray
CNV	copy number variant
CVS	chorionic villus samples
ES	exome sequencing
FISH	fluorescent in situ hybridization
GS	genome sequencing
MCC	maternal cell contamination
MLPA	multiplex ligation-dependent probe amplification
mtDNA	mitochondrial DNA
NGS	next-generation sequencing
NIPS	noninvasive prenatal screening
NIPT	noninvasive prenatal testing
POC	products of conception
qPCR	quantitative polymerase chain reaction
SNV	single nucleotide variant
SOC	standard of care
VUS	variant of uncertain significance

The past decade has also seen significant advancements in fetal therapies, interventions, and guidance for pregnancy and delivery management in fetuses with a variety of genetic disorders, leading to the proposal of a treatable fetal findings list containing genes for which prenatal and neonatal treatments are available [8]. Rapid sequencing in critically ill infants has shown that a genetic diagnosis can significantly reduce morbidity, mortality, and overall cost of treatment in ill neonates, infants, and pediatric patients [9,10], and by extension a genetic diagnosis in the prenatal period would be expected to have similar overall outcomes. Given this, identification of disease-causing variants in prenatal diagnostics has become increasingly important in anomalous and nonanomalous pregnancies for prenatal management as well as neonatal treatments and therapies.

In the past decade the fields of obstetrics, maternal fetal medicine, fetal imaging, and molecular diagnostics have exponentially increased the ability to provide fetal and maternal precision care. At the core of this ability to appropriately diagnose, manage, and initiate guided monitoring, therapies, and interventions in a prenatal or neonatal setting is a comprehensive testing option with a short turnaround time allowing for proper counseling, decision making, and treatment initiation. Prenatal GS represents a single comprehensive test that avoids the need for multiple sequential testing modalities, requires lower DNA concentration than sequential testing, and can be resulted in a shorter time frame than current standard of care (SOC) methodologies [11], thus creating an exciting opportunity for precision prenatal and maternal care, management, and application of available treatments.

HISTORY OF PRENATAL TESTING

Significant evolution in prenatal screening, imaging, and diagnostic testing methodologies have occurred since amniocentesis was first described in the late 1950s. Detailed history of the path to current prenatal testing methodologies has been described in depth elsewhere [12–14] and is summarized in Fig. 1. This historical foundation contextualizes the emergence of GS as a natural progression in prenatal diagnostics. Ultrasonography, analysis of maternal serum, or assessment of fetal DNA extracted from maternal blood are noninvasive methodologies used in prenatal screening, and invasive procedures including CVS (9–13 weeks of gestation) [15], amniocentesis (>15 weeks of gestation) [15], or sampling fetal tissues or products of conception are required for diagnostics.

Maternal serum screening was adopted in the 1970s with a single marker, alpha-fetoprotein, which when elevated can be associated with fetal neural tube defects [16]. Additional markers were progressively added including human chorionic gonadotropin, estriol, and inhibin-A which expanded the ability to simultaneously screen for increased risk of several autosomal trisomies [17]. Combining these analytes with early and midgestation ultrasonography increased sensitivity and specificity of screening.

Cell-free DNA (cfDNA) is non-nuclear, fragmented DNA found in circulation, and during gestation fetal cfDNA can be extracted and isolated from blood of the gestational carrier. In the early 2010s fetal cfDNA was first used for aneuploidy screening using massively parallel sequencing methodologies, termed noninvasive prenatal testing (NIPT) or noninvasive prenatal screening (NIPS) [18]. Ensuing studies demonstrated NIPS' improved sensitivity, specificity, and negative predictive values over previous aneuploidy screening workflows [19]. NIPS has since been routinely used for prenatal screening and is currently recommended in all pregnancies regardless of a-priori risk [20,21]. A positive screen with any screening methodology requires diagnostic confirmation in fetal DNA obtained by CVS, amniocentesis, or fetal tissues.

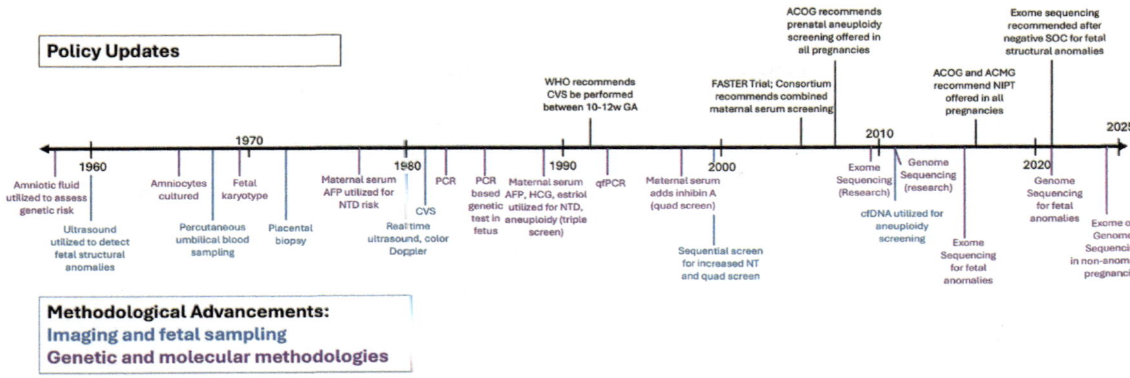

FIG. 1 General timeline of advancements in prenatal screening and diagnostics. Policy updates and guideline recommendations from professional societies and associations above the timeline. Relevant methodological advancements in fetal imaging and sampling techniques (*blue*) or genetic and molecular methodologies (*purple*) below. ACMG, American College of Medical Genetics and Genomics; ACOG, American College of Obstetrics and Gynecology; AFP, alpha-fetoprotein; CVS, chorionic villus sampling; FASTER, first- and second-trimester evaluation of risk; HCG, human chorionic gonadotropin; NTD, neural tube defect; PCR, polymerase chain reaction; qfPCR, quantitative real-time PCR; WHO, World Health Organization.

In the 1960s to 1970s amniocentesis and CVS were used to explore fetal risk and diagnose known familial genetic disorders [22,23], although with suboptimal positive and negative predictive values and higher maternal and fetal risk than present-day procedures [24,25]. Ensuing years led to rapid methodological progress in culturing of fetal cells, isolation of fetal DNA, and improvements in procedural techniques that significantly reduced fetal and maternal morbidity and mortality associated with invasive procedures. In parallel the collective expansion of knowledge on the genetic etiology of many fetal disorders and development of molecular methodologies including karyotype, fluorescent in situ hybridization (FISH), array comparative genomic hybridization (array CGH), and chromosomal microarray (CMA) led to improvement in fetal screening and diagnosis of large copy number variants or aneuploidies [12].

The pioneers in fetal genetic screening and diagnostic testing were historically focused on screening and detection of aneuploidies and large chromosomal aberrations because of their microscopic visibility with specific techniques, and current screening methodologies also target chromosomal aneuploidies. The development of molecular methodologies in the 1970s to 1980s enabled detection of smaller genetic variants for fetal diagnosis of familial monogenic disorders [26,27], and within the past decade the development of NGS methodologies, mostly driven by exome sequencing (ES), has broadened prenatal diagnostic capabilities to monogenic disorders of unknown etiology. NGS methodologies allow the analysis of genetic variation in thousands of genes simultaneously [13]. On the horizon of prenatal diagnostics is GS, which has emerged as the most comprehensive test currently available to diagnose the largest variety of genetic disorders *in utero*.

Background and Evolution Toward Genome Sequencing as a First-Tier Test

The evolution of prenatal genetic testing reflects a paradigm shift from cytogenetic techniques toward high-resolution, genome-wide analyses. Combining CMA and ES has improved diagnostic yields; however, these methodologies still leave significant gaps. GS fills these gaps by offering more comprehensive variant detection across the genome.

CMA has been considered the first-tier test for individuals with neurodevelopmental anomalies and in euploid pregnancies complicated by multiple congenital anomalies for more than a decade [28–30]. Karyotype with CMA is currently considered SOC testing in all pregnancies [29–31], as using both karyotype and CMA collectively detects copy number variants (CNVs), aneuploidies, and large balanced structural arrangements [32,33] (Table 1). Despite the diagnostic utility of karyotype and CMA, a large proportion of disease-causing genetic variation is not detectable by

TABLE 1
Summary of testing methodologies currently used in prenatal screening or diagnostics

	Karyotype	FISH	CMA	NIPS	NGS Gene Panel	ES	GS
Test Methodology							
General description of methodology	Whole chromosome preparation and fixation on slides Variety of staining techniques with G-banding most often used. Microscopy	Whole chromosome preparation and fixation Application of fluorescent oligonucleotide probes and microscopy	DNA fragmentation and hybridization to microarray chip. Variety of chips commercially available. Chip scanner and associated software calculate copy number at probes on chip	Fetal cfDNA extracted from plasma, massively parallel sequencing or other counting method screen for anomalies of chromosome copy number	ES or GS sequencing. Analysis restricted to in silico panel of preselected genes	DNA fragmentation, probe based capture, PCR amplification and sequencing. Bioinformatics analysis for variant calling, mapping of sequence reads, annotation	DNA fragmentation, library preparation, sequencing. Bioinformatics analysis for variant calling, mapping of sequence reads, annotation
Resolution	Depends on chromosome preparation, as low as 5–10 Mb	Not applicable. Analysis restricted to probe design and presence/absence/ number of fluorescent probes detected	Depends on chip used and probe density, as low as 20 kb	Depends on methodology and test - microduplications and microdeletions included in some NIPS	Single nucleotide	Single nucleotide	Single nucleotide
Turn around time	1–2 wk	3 d - 2 wk	2 wk	1–2 wk	2–3 wk	2–3 wk (rapid)	1–2 wk (rapid)
Current utilization in prenatal screening/ diagnostics	SOC testing	Confirmatory testing, often in parallel with karyotype	SOC testing	Recommended to be offered in all pregnancies	Broadly available, used after negative SOC testing	Broadly available, used for diagnosis of fetal structural anomalies after negative SOC testing	Increasing availability though not currently broadly available. Diagnosis of fetal structural anomalies
Variant Type and Detection by Methodology							
Aneuploidy	Yes	Yes, if chromosome specific probe utilized	Yes	Yes	No	No	Yes
Large CNVs (≥200kb)	Possibly, if ≥3-5 Mb depends on location	Yes, if CNV specific probe used	Yes	Depends if the CNV is covered by methodology/ testing limitations	Possibly, if multiplex ligation-dependent probe amplification (MLPA) or similar copy number calling method is used and the CNV includes gene on the panel	No	Yes
Small CNVs (<200kb)	No	No	Possibly, depending on size of CNV and probe coverage of chip in the region	No	Possibly, if MLPA or similar copy number calling method is used and the CNV includes gene on the panel	No	Yes

Balanced translocation	Yes	Possibly, but likely requires specific probe design	No	No	No	No	Possible, but limited by specific pipeline, variant calling algorithm(s), and mappability of breakpoint region(s)
Intrachromosome balanced structural variant	Depends on size and chromosome location	Possibly, but likely requires specific probe design	No	No	No	No	Possible, but limited by specific pipeline, variant calling algorithm(s), and mappability of breakpoint region(s)
Clinically relevant repeat expansions	No	No	No	No	No	No	Yes
Insertion-deletion variant	No	No	No	No	Yes, if gene included on panel	Yes	Yes
Single nucleotide variant	No	No	No	No	Yes, if gene included on panel	Yes	Yes
Mitochondrial DNA variant	No	No	No	No	Yes, if specific panel used	No	Yes
Mosaic CNV or aneuploidy	Yes	Yes, if specific probe used	Yes	Possibly, depends on fetal fraction and level of mosaicism	No	No	Yes
Mosaic SNV, indel	No	No	No	No	Yes, if gene included on panel	Yes	Yes
Uniparental disomy	No	No	Yes - isodisomy, if SNP probes used No - heterodisomy	No	No	Yes/no - regions of homozygosity can be identified potentially associated with isodisomy (coding regions) No - heterodisomy	Yes
Intronic variants outside of exon splice regions	No	No	No	No	Maybe - well known pathogenic variants can be specifically added to panels	No	Yes
Intergenic variants, variants in nonprotein coding genes	No	No	No	No	Not currently - could be added in future	No	Yes

Details regarding methodology at the top and types of variants detected and limitations for each methodology.

these methodologies including single nucleotide variants (SNVs), small insertion-deletion (indel) variants, and CNVs or structural variants below their limit of detection (see Table 1).

NGS methodologies are high-throughput DNA sequencing and variant detection techniques that further increase the diagnostic utility of prenatal testing by detecting genomic variants outside the limitations of karyotype and CMA. Although not yet recommended as a first-tier prenatal diagnostic test, NGS methodologies including ES or GS have been increasingly used for genetic diagnosis in pregnancies complicated by fetal anomalies, resulting in position statements from the International Society for Prenatal Diagnosis, the Society for Maternal Fetal Medicine, and the American College of Medical Genetics [34–36] regarding their use after negative SOC testing [35,36].

Initial studies on the utility of NGS methodologies used ES because of its availability, lower cost, and wide clinical utility. Many studies comparing the utility of ES with other diagnostic methodologies in prenatal, neonatal, and pediatric cohorts have demonstrated increased diagnostic yield for a large variety of indications [37–39]. In prenatal diagnostics, ES performed in structurally anomalous fetuses with normal SOC testing has an average incremental yield of 30% to 40%, and as high as 88.5% when selected for high likelihood of monogenic etiology [39–41]. Diagnostic rates for ES in prenatal samples is variable depending on the structural anomaly and if it is isolated or part of multiple congenital anomalies [38,39,42–44]. Although ES significantly improves diagnostic yield compared with SOC testing [38,39], methodological limitations including lower coverage in GC-rich regions, limitations to identification of copy number changes, structural variants, and inability to detect variation in intronic regions outside ±10 bp or in the noncoding genome are shortcomings of the methodology [45,46].

GS is a comprehensive test able to ameliorate many of the limitations of ES, CMA, and karyotype (see Table 1). GS reliably identifies aneuploidies and variants throughout the coding and noncoding genome including large and small copy number variants, unbalanced structural variants, and some balanced structural variants dependent on variant calling algorithms and mappability of breakpoint regions [47,48]. Uniparental isodisomy is detectable in all probands submitted for GS, and uniparental heterodisomy can be identified in trio analysis with parental samples; however, identification of uniparental disomy by GS requires methylation analysis for orthogonal confirmation [49]. GS also detects single nucleotide variants, small and large indels, mitochondrial DNA variants, mosaic variants with sensitivity similar to or better than other NGS methodologies [50,51].

As GS has become more readily available, increased diagnostic yield of GS over other NGS methodologies is becoming recognized [1,52–54], supporting GS as a first-tier comprehensive test effectively combining the diagnostic power of karyotype, CMA, and ES with additional variant detection capabilities. Unique to GS is its ability to reliably detect variants in nonprotein coding and intronic regions of the genome, as emerging evidence demonstrates the presence of disease-associated variation in these regions [55,56]. GS can also be completed with turnaround times less than or equal to SOC testing, and the comprehensive nature of GS reduces the need for sequential testing strategies that may delay diagnosis. GS is being increasingly used in prenatal testing, as it offers unmatched diagnostic breadth by capturing nearly all classes of variants detectable by prior technologies and additional variants not captured by other tests because of their methodological limitations.

Current Evidence of Diagnostic and Incremental Yield of Prenatal Genome Sequencing

Although in its relative infancy for prenatal diagnostics, GS is quickly demonstrating its utility in diagnosis of fetal structural anomalies. In 2024, a literature review and meta-analysis [11] compared diagnostic yields of GS to quantitative polymerase chain reaction (qPCR), CMA, ES, or a combination of these testing modalities. The article included 902 prenatal or neonatal cases with fetal structural anomalies across 18 studies. Meta-analysis demonstrated GS has increased diagnostic yield of 39% over qPCR/CMA, and 1% over ES with CMA. The authors noted that the direct comparison of GS with ES was underpowered because of the paucity of studies and suggested the incremental yield of GS would likely be higher in unscreened populations [11].

Another study [50] examined the utility of GS compared with karyotype, CMA, and/or ES in autism spectrum disorder (ASD) cohorts and fetuses with structural anomalies. In their benchmark cohorts, GS detected 100% of the variants that were reported by the 3 methodologies in the ASD cohort, and 100% of the reportable copy number, small indel, and SNVs in the prenatal cohort. GS additionally identified variants that were missed by other methodologies including SNVs, small indels, retrotransposon insertions, CNVs, uniparental disomy, and structural variants [50]. The authors combined their benchmarking data with historical data from unselected cohorts to conclude that GS likely has an incremental yield of 38.3% over ES, or 4.1% over ES with copy number calling [50], suggesting GS could be used as a comprehensive first-tier test.

Detecting disease associated variants *in utero* allows the family time to understand the implications and prognosis of the finding, plan for management, treatment, and allow for any available pregnancy and neonatal therapies. As prenatal GS becomes more readily available, clinicians will better understand the true incremental yield of this methodology and better appreciate the impact early diagnosis can make for precision care.

CHALLENGES OF PRENATAL GENOME SEQUENCING

Although its clinical utility is high, prenatal GS also presents distinct technical and interpretive challenges that require careful consideration in laboratory and clinical settings. Several key categories where these complexities are most apparent will be discussed.

Technical Challenges of Short-Read Genome Sequencing

Short-read GS technologies, although powerful, have known limitations in certain genomic regions. Some genes with clinical relevance in prenatal context (*CYP21A2, HBA1, HBA2, GBA1*) reside in areas with low mappability or have associated pseudogenes. These regions present sequencing challenges that may result in false-negative or false-positive variant calls. Platform-specific specialized callers are available for many of these complex regions, which increases sensitivity of GS for some of these genes [57,58]; however, variability from laboratory to laboratory remains a consideration. Detection of variants in genes within these regions requires gene-specific orthogonal confirmation, which potentially delays reporting. Similarly, short-read GS is currently underpowered to detect balanced translocations that depend on variant calling algorithms employed and mappability of associated breakpoints. Balanced structural variants with breakpoints in low complexity regions may be underrecognized by short-read GS [50].

Interpretation and Reporting Challenges

A major hurdle of prenatal testing is not unique to GS, but inherent to prenatal NGS in general. Interpreting variants in the prenatal setting is uniquely difficult because of undercharacterized fetal phenotypes and limited correlative data. Although the field has seen significant advances in prenatal imaging, screening, and more refined phenotyping, there remains room for elucidation of fetal phenotypes associated with most genetic disorders. Consequently, variants of uncertain significance (VUSs) are common and may not be classifiable as pathogenic or likely pathogenic in prenatal context. Although some VUSs may be reclassified as likely pathogenic postnatally with clearer phenotype delineation, imaging, biochemical testing, or additional orthogonal assays, their interim reporting can create anxiety and confusion, and complicate reporting and counseling.

Maternal Cell Contamination, Mosaicism, and Mitochondrial Heteroplasmy

Accurate prenatal analysis relies heavily on the purity of fetal DNA. Maternal cell contamination (MCC) is contamination of fetal DNA with maternal DNA caused by the invasive nature of obtaining fetal diagnostic samples. Significant levels of MCC can reduce sensitivity and specificity of prenatal diagnostic testing or lead to uninterpretable results [59]. Rigorous laboratory protocols and quantification methods must be in place to assess MCC levels before fetal diagnostic testing. Laboratory workflows should be established for MCC-positive samples that depend on sample type, specific diagnostic testing to be performed, availability of a cultured sample or ability to obtain a new sample, and the level of MCC detected.

Presence of MCC in a fetal sample also significantly reduces sensitivity to detect mosaicism. Mosaicism refers to the presence of 2 populations of cells; 1 population that has a genetic variant and a second population that is variant negative. Mosaicism is most often the result of a postzygotic mutation or trisomy rescue event in mosaic aneuploidies that is proliferated in dividing cells resulting in a variable proportion of variant-positive fetal cells [60,61]. Mosaicism can lead to highly variable phenotypes that depend on the variant allele fraction in the fetus and variant burden in specific tissues [60,61]. Identification of mosaicism in CVS samples is additionally complicated by the possibility that the variant represents confined placental mosaicism, requiring additional testing in amniotic fluid to determine true fetal mosaicism, which may delay diagnosis and increase anxiety [61]. Low-level mosaicism for any variant type, while detectable by GS, often requires confirmatory testing depending on variant allele fraction and prenatal tissue source.

Similar to mosaic variants in nuclear DNA, heteroplasmy for mitochondrial DNA (mtDNA) variants presents a reporting and counseling challenge in prenatal testing. Pathogenic mtDNA variants have highly variable phenotypes that depend on the specific variant, tissue-specific heteroplasmy, and other genetic and environmental factors with high inter- and intrafamilial variability noted in individuals with the same mtDNA variant [62]. Furthermore, few studies have examined correlation between mtDNA heteroplasmy in fetal samples and neonatal tissues, and although the available evidence suggests some correlation [63,64], this has not been confirmed, or established for most mtDNA variants, making reporting, counseling, and prognosis of mtDNA variants particularly difficult in a prenatal setting.

Counseling and Consent Complexity

As with all diagnostic testing, prenatal GS is intended to provide the family and medical teams with information that leads to anticipatory guidance, treatments, and prognosis, but should be balanced to minimize anxiety and uncertainty regarding the pregnancy for the family. To that end, it is essential to ensure patients understand the implications of test results including incidental and uncertain findings, and that variants reported comply with the desires of the family regarding these potential uncertainties.

Before initiation of prenatal GS testing, collaborative discussion between laboratories, clinicians, and the genetic counselors performing test counseling should reach consensus regarding the scope of prenatally reportable variants including incidental and uncertain findings. A clearly worded patient consent form should be developed containing clear explanations of potential GS results and any opt-in choices regarding incidental findings or uncertain results. The complexity of GS demands robust pre- and post-test counseling by a certified genetic counselor who can clearly explain the complexities of testing, and consent processes should be tailored to patient values and supported by clear documentation.

FUTURE DIRECTIONS

As GS technologies evolve, new methodologies and integrations are poised to enhance the diagnostic accuracy and clinical utility of prenatal testing.

Long-Read Sequencing

Long-read GS overcomes several limitations of short-read platforms, especially in repetitive or low-complexity regions. These technologies enhance detection of structural variants, complex rearrangements, and phasing of alleles. As costs decrease and platforms mature, long-read sequencing may become integrated into routine prenatal diagnostics [65].

Transcriptome Sequencing (RNA Sequencing)

Transcriptome sequencing adds a valuable layer to variant interpretation, especially for suspected splicing anomalies. Targeted RNA sequencing is increasingly used to resolve splice region or intronic variants, synonymous variants with potential splicing effects, and transcriptional alterations from variants in noncoding regions. In prenatal settings, it offers an orthogonal approach to interpret intronic or cryptic splice variants identified by GS. Although logistical and tissue-specific expression challenges remain, future integration of RNA sequencing into prenatal diagnostics could help resolve more VUSs and clarify uncertain findings [66].

Noninvasive Genome Sequencing via Cell-Free DNA

The possibility of performing GS on fetal cfDNA represents a paradigm shift toward noninvasive comprehensive diagnostics. Advances in analyzing fetal cfDNA may eventually enable noninvasive GS. Although currently limited to small gene panels or familial variants [67], improvements in enrichment, depth, and bioinformatics may expand this capability to genome-wide analysis. This could redefine prenatal screening paradigms.

DISCUSSION

Prenatal screening and diagnostics have seen rapid evolution and progression since the first analysis of amniotic fluid contents in the mid- 1900s with exponential expansion of methodologies that have increased sensitivity, specificity, and reduced turnaround times. The current SOC for prenatal testing in fetuses with anomalies is karyotype and CMA to detect aneuploidies or large CNVs, followed by ES in the event of negative SOC testing [29,35,36]. Although this approach collectively detects most disease-causing genetic variation, the sequential testing workflow increases the timeline for potential diagnosis and requires multiple testing modalities; and methodological limitations prevent the detection of some known disease-causing genetic variation [11,45–48,50].

GS is the most comprehensive genetic test currently available and is capable of detecting variants identified by karyotype, CMA, and ES, as well as variants in intronic and noncoding regions, disease-associated repeat expansions, and mtDNA variants that are not detectable by current SOC methodologies. Cumulatively, GS has the highest diagnostic yield of any single genetic test currently available and can be performed with turnaround times less than or equal to any other currently available diagnostic molecular test, making it a prime first-tier screening or diagnostic test in a prenatal setting.

Prenatal GS is increasingly salient as the field of prenatal, neonatal, and presymptomatic therapies is also rapidly expanding, many of which are gene- or disease-specific and significantly reduce morbidity and mortality compared to natural history of the disorder [8,9]. Even in the absence of gene specific therapy, a genetic diagnosis can lead to specific managements, specialty referrals, and reduced overall medical costs, inpatient hospitalizations, and unnecessary treatments or interventions [9,10].

With the steadily reducing cost and improvement in bioinformatic analysis pipelines, its implementation as a first-tier test for undiagnosed disease as well as prenatal diagnostics is potentially on the horizon as more diagnostic labs transition to GS platforms. Prenatal GS provides an exciting opportunity to revolutionize prenatal diagnosis, maternal fetal medicine, and precision care throughout prenatal and postnatal life.

SUMMARY

Rapid advances in prenatal imaging, screening, and diagnostics in the past years have provided an unprecedented opportunity for precision care in maternal-fetal medicine. The current ability to screen for and diagnose genetic conditions *in utero* is reshaping prenatal management, treatments, and therapies, and enabling more precise neonatal care. At the core of this is the ability to rapidly detect underlying genetic etiology of fetal anomalies and congenital conditions. GS is redefining prenatal genetic diagnostics by offering a comprehensive, single-test approach to detect a wide array of genetic variations. Compared with conventional methods like karyotyping, CMA, and ES, GS demonstrates higher diagnostic yield in pregnancies complicated by fetal anomalies, and is more rapid than sequential testing methodologies. GS is poised to become a first-tier diagnostic test in postnatal undiagnosed disease, and shows analogous utility in prenatal diagnostic testing. More routine utilization of GS in this setting may lead to a paradigm shift in the field of maternal fetal medicine toward GS as a first-tier test in prenatal diagnostics.

CLINICS CARE POINTS

- Prenatal GS is a comprehensive test able to detect variants typically identified by SOC testing, as well as a large variety of variants not detectable by those methodologies, reducing the need for sequential testing methodologies.
- Prenatal GS has turnaround times less than current SOC testing and requires lower DNA concentration that current sequential SOC testing methodologies.
- Availability of prenatal, neonatal, and presymptomatic therapies is exponentially increasing, and prenatal GS enables guided treatments and therapies for specific genetic disorders.
- Early studies demonstrate the diagnostic utility of prenatal GS in fetuses with structural anomalies and show an incremental yield over other testing methodologies, suggesting GS could become a first-tier test for fetal diagnostics.

DISCLOSURE

The authors have nothing to disclose.

REFERENCES

[1] Lionel AC, Costain G, Monfared N, et al. Improved diagnostic yield compared with targeted gene sequencing panels suggests a role for whole-genome sequencing as a first-tier genetic test. Genet Med 2018;20(4):435–43.

[2] Bowling KM, Thompson ML, Amaral MD, et al. Genomic diagnosis for children with intellectual disability and/or developmental delay. Genome Med 2017;9(1):43.

[3] Bonini KE, Thomas-Wilson A, Marathe PN, et al. Identification of copy number variants with genome sequencing: clinical experiences from the NYCKidSeq program. Clin Genet 2023;104(2):210–25.

[4] Odgis JA, Gallagher KM, Rehman AU, et al. Detection of mosaic variants using genome sequencing in a large pediatric cohort. Am J Med Genet 2023;191(3):699–710.

[5] Chen YS, He JF, Quan T, et al. Hydrocephalus and growth retardation: a Fetal RNU4ATAC-opathy missed by whole-exome sequencing. Mol Syndromol 2023;13(6):522–6.

[6] Liaqat K, Treat K, Mantcheva L, et al. Research-based whole genome sequencing identifies biallelic loss of function variants in DOCK3 gene causing DOCK3-related disorder: the end of a diagnostic journey for this family. Clin Genet 2025;108(1):109–11.

[7] Wen T, Boyden SE, Hocutt CM, et al. Identification of 2 novel noncoding variants in patients with Diamond-Blackfan anemia syndrome by whole genome sequencing. Blood Adv 2025;9(10):2443–52.

[8] Cohen JL, Duyzend M, Adelson SM, et al. Advancing precision care in pregnancy through a treatable fetal findings list. Am J Hum Genet 2025;112(6): 1251–69.
[9] Farnaes L, Hildreth A, Sweeney NM, et al. Rapid whole-genome sequencing decreases infant morbidity and cost of hospitalization. NPJ Genom Med 2018;3:10.
[10] Moore C, Arenchild M, Waldman B, et al. Rapid whole-genome sequencing as a first-line test is likely to significantly reduce the cost of acute care in a private payer system. J Appl Lab Med 2025;10(4): 833–42.
[11] Shreeve N, Sproule C, Choy KW, et al. Incremental yield of whole-genome sequencing over chromosomal microarray analysis and exome sequencing for congenital anomalies in prenatal period and infancy: systematic review and meta-analysis. Ultrasound Obstet Gynecol 2024;63(1):15–23.
[12] Levy B, Stosic M. Traditional prenatal diagnosis: past to present. Methods Mol Biol 2019;1885:3–22.
[13] Vora NL, Norton ME. Prenatal exome and genome sequencing for fetal structural abnormalities. Am J Obstet Gynecol 2023;228(2):140–9.
[14] Cuckle H, Maymon R. Development of prenatal screening–A historical overview. Semin Perinatol 2016; 40(1):12–22.
[15] American College of O. Gynecologists. ACOG practice bulletin no. 88, December 2007. Invasive prenatal testing for aneuploidy. Obstet Gynecol 2007;110(6): 1459–67.
[16] Wald NJ, Cuckle H, Brock JH, et al. Maternal serum-alpha-fetoprotein measurement in antenatal screening for anencephaly and spina bifida in early pregnancy. Report of U.K. collaborative study on alpha-fetoprotein in relation to neural-tube defects. Lancet 1977;1(8026): 1323–32.
[17] Malone FD, Canick JA, Ball RH, et al. First-trimester or second-trimester screening, or both, for Down's syndrome. N Engl J Med 2005;353(19):2001–11.
[18] Maktabi MA, Vossaert L, Van den Veyver IB. Cell-based Noninvasive Prenatal Testing (cbNIPT)-A review on the current developments and future prospects. Clin Obstet Gynecol 2023;66(3):636–48.
[19] Bianchi DW, Parker RL, Wentworth J, et al. DNA sequencing versus standard prenatal aneuploidy screening. N Engl J Med 2014;370(9):799–808.
[20] American College of O, Gynecologists' Committee on Practice B-O, Committee on G, Society for Maternal-Fetal M. Screening for Fetal Chromosomal Abnormalities. ACOG practice bulletin, number 226. Obstet Gynecol 2020;136(4):e48–69.
[21] Dungan JS, Klugman S, Darilek S, et al. Noninvasive prenatal screening (NIPS) for fetal chromosome abnormalities in a general-risk population: an evidence-based clinical guideline of the American College of Medical Genetics and Genomics (ACMG). Genet Med 2023; 25(2):100336.
[22] Burton BK, Gerbie AB, Nadler HL. Present status of intrauterine diagnosis of genetic defects. Am J Obstet Gynecol 1974;118(5):718–46.
[23] O'Brien JS, Okada S, Fillerup DL, et al. Tay-Sachs disease: prenatal diagnosis. Science 1971;172(3978):61–4.
[24] Alter BP, Modell CB, Fairweather D, et al. Prenatal diagnosis of hemoglobinopathies. A review of 15 cases. N Engl J Med 1976;295(26):1437–43.
[25] Manganiello PD, Byrd JR, Tho PT, et al. A report of the safety and accuracy of midtrimester amniocentesis at the Medical College of Georgia: eight and one half years' experience. Am J Obstet Gynecol 1979;134(8): 911–6.
[26] Kan YW, Dozy AM. Antenatal diagnosis of sickle-cell anaemia by D.N.A. analysis of amniotic-fluid cells. Lancet 1978;2(8096):910–2.
[27] Kogan SC, Doherty M, Gitschier J. An improved method for prenatal diagnosis of genetic diseases by analysis of amplified DNA sequences. Application to hemophilia A. N Engl J Med 1987;317(16):985–90.
[28] Miller DT, Adam MP, Aradhya S, et al. Consensus statement: chromosomal microarray is a first-tier clinical diagnostic test for individuals with developmental disabilities or congenital anomalies. Am J Hum Genet 2010;86(5):749–64.
[29] Committee on G, the Society for Maternal-Fetal M.. Committee opinion No.682: microarrays and next-generation sequencing technology: the use of advanced genetic diagnostic tools in obstetrics and gynecology. Obstet Gynecol 2016;128(6):e262–8.
[30] Manning M, Hudgins L, Professional P, et al. Array-based technology and recommendations for utilization in medical genetics practice for detection of chromosomal abnormalities. Genet Med 2010;12-(11):742–5.
[31] Practice bulletin No. 162 summary: prenatal diagnostic testing for genetic disorders. Obstet Gynecol 2016; 127(5):976–8.
[32] Wapner RJ, Martin CL, Levy B, et al. Chromosomal microarray versus karyotyping for prenatal diagnosis. N Engl J Med 2012;367(23):2175–84.
[33] Hillman SC, McMullan DJ, Hall G, et al. Use of prenatal chromosomal microarray: prospective cohort study and systematic review and meta-analysis. Ultrasound Obstet Gynecol 2013;41(6):610–20.
[34] International Society for Prenatal D, Society for M, Fetal M, Perinatal Quality F. Joint position statement from the international society for prenatal diagnosis (ISPD), the society for maternal fetal medicine (SMFM), and the perinatal quality foundation (PQF) on the use of genome-wide sequencing for fetal diagnosis. Prenat Diagn 2018;38(1):6–9.
[35] Van den Veyver IB, Chandler N, Wilkins-Haug LE, et al. International society for prenatal diagnosis updated position statement on the use of genome-wide sequencing for prenatal diagnosis. Prenat Diagn 2022;42(6): 796–803.

[36] Monaghan KG, Leach NT, Pekarek D, et al. The use of fetal exome sequencing in prenatal diagnosis: a points to consider document of the American College of Medical Genetics and Genomics (ACMG). Genet Med 2020; 22(4):675–80.
[37] Arduc A, De Vries JIP, M BT-S, et al. Perinatal genetic diagnostic yield in a population of fetuses with the phenotype arthrogryposis multiplex congenita: a cohort study 2007-2021. Eur J Hum Genet 2025. https://doi.org/10.1038/s41431-025-01848-3.
[38] Allen VM, Schollenberg E, Aberg E, et al. Use of clinically informed strategies and diagnostic yields of genetic testing for fetal structural anomalies following a non-diagnostic microarray result: a population-based cohort study. Prenat Diagn 2025;45(3):318–25.
[39] Mellis R, Oprych K, Scotchman E, et al. Diagnostic yield of exome sequencing for prenatal diagnosis of fetal structural anomalies: a systematic review and meta-analysis. Prenat Diagn 2022;42(6):662–85.
[40] Gabriel H, Korinth D, Ritthaler M, et al. Trio exome sequencing is highly relevant in prenatal diagnostics. Prenat Diagn 2022;42(7):845–51.
[41] Pauta M, Martinez-Portilla RJ, Borrell A. Diagnostic yield of exome sequencing in fetuses with multisystem malformations: systematic review and meta-analysis. Ultrasound Obstet Gynecol 2022;59(6):715–22.
[42] Moradi B, Ariaei A, Heidari-Foroozan M, et al. Diagnostic yield of prenatal exome sequencing in the genetic screening of fetuses with brain anomalies detected by MRI and ultrasonography: a systematic review and meta-analysis. BJOG 2024;131(11):1435–43.
[43] Qin L, Liu D, Wang X, et al. Application of whole-exome sequencing in the genetic diagnosis of prenatal ultrasound abnormalities. Br J Hosp Med 2024;85-(12):1–21.
[44] Petrovski S, Aggarwal V, Giordano JL, et al. Whole-exome sequencing in the evaluation of fetal structural anomalies: a prospective cohort study. Lancet 2019;393-(10173):758–67.
[45] Burdick KJ, Cogan JD, Rives LC, et al. Limitations of exome sequencing in detecting rare and undiagnosed diseases. Am J Med Genet 2020;182(6):1400–6.
[46] Clark MJ, Chen R, Lam HY, et al. Performance comparison of exome DNA sequencing technologies. Nat Biotechnol 2011;29(10):908–14.
[47] Yu MHC, Chau JFT, Au SLK, et al. Evaluating the clinical utility of genome sequencing for cytogenetically balanced chromosomal abnormalities in prenatal diagnosis. Front Genet 2020;11:620162.
[48] Wojcik MH, Lemire G, Berger E, et al. Genome sequencing for diagnosing rare diseases. N Engl J Med 2024;390(21):1985–97.
[49] Del Gaudio D, Shinawi M, Astbury C, et al. Diagnostic testing for uniparental disomy: a points to consider statement from the American College of Medical Genetics and Genomics (ACMG). Genet Med 2020;22(7): 1133–41.
[50] Lowther C, Valkanas E, Giordano JL, et al. Systematic evaluation of genome sequencing for the diagnostic assessment of autism spectrum disorder and fetal structural anomalies. Am J Hum Genet 2023;110(9): 1454–69.
[51] Souche E, Beltran S, Brosens E, et al. Recommendations for whole genome sequencing in diagnostics for rare diseases. Eur J Hum Genet 2022;30(9):1017–21.
[52] Taylor JC, Martin HC, Lise S, et al. Factors influencing success of clinical genome sequencing across a broad spectrum of disorders. Nat Genet 2015;47(7):717–26.
[53] Pandey R, Brennan NF, Trachana K, et al. A meta-analysis of diagnostic yield and clinical utility of genome and exome sequencing in pediatric rare and undiagnosed genetic diseases. Genet Med 2025;27(6): 101398.
[54] Abul-Husn NS, Marathe PN, Kelly NR, et al. Molecular diagnostic yield of genome sequencing versus targeted gene panel testing in racially and ethnically diverse pediatric patients. Genet Med 2023;25(9): 100880.
[55] Chen Y, Dawes R, Kim HC, et al. De novo variants in the RNU4-2 snRNA cause a frequent neurodevelopmental syndrome. Nature 2024;632(8026):832–40.
[56] Pitsava G, Hawley M, Auriga L, et al. Genome sequencing reveals the impact of non-canonical exon inclusions in rare genetic disease. medRxiv 2024. https://doi.org/10.1101/2024.12.21.24318325.
[57] Behera S, Catreux S, Rossi M, et al. Comprehensive genome analysis and variant detection at scale using DRAGEN. Nat Biotechnol 2024. https://doi.org/10.1038/s41587-024-02382-1.
[58] Rojahn S, Hambuch T, Adrian J, et al. Scalable detection of technically challenging variants through modified next-generation sequencing. Mol Genet Genomic Med 2022;10(12):e2072.
[59] Nagan N, Faulkner NE, Curtis C, et al, Committee MCCGWGotAfMPCP. Laboratory guidelines for detection, interpretation, and reporting of maternal cell contamination in prenatal analyses a report of the association for molecular pathology. J Mol Diagn 2011; 13(1):7–11.
[60] Thorpe J, Osei-Owusu IA, Avigdor BE, et al. Mosaicism in human health and disease. Annu Rev Genet 2020; 54:487–510.
[61] Levy B, Hoffmann ER, McCoy RC, et al. Chromosomal mosaicism: origins and clinical implications in preimplantation and prenatal diagnosis. Prenat Diagn 2021; 41(5):631–41.
[62] Gorman GS, Chinnery PF, DiMauro S, et al. Mitochondrial diseases. Nat Rev Dis Primers 2016;2:16080.
[63] Steffann J, Monnot S, Magen M, et al. A retrospective study on the efficacy of prenatal diagnosis for pregnancies at risk of mitochondrial DNA disorders. Genet Med 2021;23(4):720–31.
[64] Monnot S, Gigarel N, Samuels DC, et al. Segregation of mtDNA throughout human embryofetal development:

m.3243A>G as a model system. Hum Mutat 2011; 32(1):116–25.

[65] Eisfeldt J, Ek M, Nordenskjold M, et al. Toward clinical long-read genome sequencing for rare diseases. Nat Genet 2025;57(6):1334–43.

[66] Marquez J, Cech JN, Paschal CR, et al. Clinical RNA sequencing clarifies variants of uncertain significance identified by prior testing. Genet Med Open 2024;2: 101886.

[67] Vora NL, Langlois S, Chitty LS. Current controversy in prenatal diagnosis: the use of cfDNA to screen for monogenic conditions in low risk populations is ready for clinical use. Prenat Diagn 2024;44(4): 389–97.

SECTION: HEMATOPATHOLOGY

Advances in Molecular Pathology 8 (2025) 27–39
ADVANCES IN MOLECULAR PATHOLOGY

Role of Long-read Sequencing in Comprehensive Genomic Profiling of Hematolymphoid Malignancies

Lauren M. Wainman, PhD[a], Liam L. Donnelly, MD[b], Prabhjot Kaur, MD[c], Parth S. Shah, MD[b], Jeremiah Karrs, DO[b,*]

[a]Department of Pathology and Laboratory Medicine, Dartmouth Hitchcock Medical Center, Geisel School of Medicine, Lebanon, NH, USA; [b]Dartmouth Hitchcock Medical Center, Geisel School of Medicine, Lebanon, NH, USA; [c]Department of Pathology, Dartmouth Hitchcock Medical Center, Geisel School of Medicine, Lebanon, NH, USA

KEYWORDS

• Long-read sequencing • Hematolymphoid • Phasing • Epigenetics • Structural variants

KEY POINTS

- Long-read sequencing has specific advantages compared to short-read sequencing for evaluating hematolymphoid malignancies.
- These advantages include sequencing through repetitive regions, structural variant detection, haplotype phasing, and direct epigenetic marker determination.
- Utilizing these advantages can provide more comprehensive genomic profiling to resolve complex cases.

INTRODUCTION

Hematolymphoid neoplasms represent a diverse group of malignancies arising from hematopoietic and lymphoid tissues, characterized by complex genetic alterations that drive pathogenesis and influence clinical behavior [1,2]. Accurate molecular characterization of these alterations is critical for proper classification, prognostication, and therapeutic decision-making in the current era of precision medicine. Traditional approaches for genomic analysis in hematolymphoid neoplasms have included conventional cytogenetics, fluorescence in situ hybridization (FISH), microarrays, and, more recently, next-generation sequencing based on short-read technology [3].

Incorporating short-read sequencing (SRS) platforms, which typically generate reads of 100 to 300 base pairs, into clinical use has reconfigured classification systems and our understanding of the mutational landscape in hematologic malignancies [1,2,4]. However, SRS has inherent limitations in fully eliciting genomic alterations particularly relevant in hematolymphoid neoplasms, including complex structural variants (SVs), gene fusions, repetitive regions, epigenetic modifications, allele resolution, and distant phased variants [5,6].

Long-read sequencing (LRS) technologies can generate reads from several kilobases to megabases in length and thus have the potential to address many of these limitations [7,8]. LRS platforms, which at present include those from Pacific Biosciences (PacBio) and Oxford Nanopore Technologies (ONT), offer new opportunities for the comprehensive characterization of complex genomic alterations in hematolymphoid neoplasms [9,10]. By spanning sequencing gaps, these technologies enable the detection of complex SVs, resolution of repetitive regions, the identification of novel fusion

*Corresponding author. 1 Medical Center Drive, Lebanon, NH 03756. *E-mail address:* jeremiah.x.karrs@hitchcock.org

https://doi.org/10.1016/j.yamp.2025.05.002 www.advancesinmolecularpathology.com
2589-4080/25/ © 2025 Elsevier Inc. All rights are reserved, including those for text and data mining, AI training, and similar technologies.

ABBREVIATIONS

5 mC	5-methylcytosine
5hmC	5-hydroxymethylcytosine
6 mA	N6-methyladenine
AML	acute myeloid leukemia
B-ALL	B-cell acute lymphoblastic leukemia
CLL	chronic lymphocytic leukemia
FISH	fluorescence in situ hybridization
HiFi	High-Fidelity
IGH	immunoglobulin heavy chain
ITDs	internal tandem duplications
LRS	long-read sequencing
MDS	myelodysplastic syndromes
MPNs	myeloproliferative neoplasms
ONT	Oxford Nanopore Technologies
PacBio	Pacific Biosciences
PCR	polymerase chain reaction
SMRT	Single Molecule Real-Time
SNVs	single-nucleotide variants
SRS	short-read sequencing
SVs	structural variants

transcripts, and haplotype phasing that are generally unable to be resolved with short-read approaches [11,12].

In this review, we examine the principles of LRS technology, specific applications in hematolymphoid neoplasms, potential clinical implementations, and future directions. We focus on how LRS complements existing molecular diagnostic approaches and addresses challenges in characterizing leukemias, lymphomas, and other hematologic malignancies [13,14]. As LRS evolves and becomes more accessible, understanding capabilities, limitations, and appropriate applications will be essential for molecular pathologists and hematopathologists seeking to implement this technology in clinical practice.

FUNDAMENTALS OF LONG-READ SEQUENCING TECHNOLOGIES

Technical principles and platforms

LRS technologies are distinguished by their ability to generate significantly longer sequence reads compared to conventional short-read platforms [7,15]. Currently, 2 main commercial companies' technologies are utilized in the LRS landscape: PacBio (Menlo Park, CA) and ONT (Edmund Halley Road, Oxford). Each employs distinct sequencing mechanisms that contribute to their unique advantages and limitations.

PacBio has pioneered single molecule real-time (SMRT) sequencing, which utilizes zero-mode waveguides containing immobilized DNA polymerases [16,17]. In this approach, as the polymerase incorporates fluorescently labeled nucleotides into the growing DNA strand, light pulses are detected in real-time, allowing for direct observation of sequencing. The most recent PacBio systems (Sequel II and Sequel IIe) routinely generate average read lengths of 10 to 30 kb, with some reads exceeding 100 kb. This technology has evolved to offer 2 main sequencing modalities that balance accuracy and read length. High-Fidelity (HiFi) sequencing involves circular consensus sequencing where the same DNA molecule is read multiple times to generate highly accurate consensus sequences, achieving greater than 99.9% accuracy [18]. Alternatively, continuous long-read sequencing produces longer reads but with lower accuracy in the range of 85% to 90%, offering a trade-off that may be beneficial for certain applications.

In contrast, ONT employs a fundamentally different approach with nanopore sequencing, which utilizes protein nanopores embedded in electrically resistant membranes [19]. As DNA molecules pass through these nanopores, they cause characteristic disruptions in ionic current that are measured and translated into nucleotide sequences. This approach allows for exceptional read lengths, with ONT platforms including MinION, GridION, and PromethION generating reads that typically average 10 to 100 kb, with some exceeding 2 Mb. While ONT sequencing was historically challenged by higher error rates (typically 85%–95% accuracy), recent advances in chemistry (particularly the R10.4 flow cells) and improvements in base-calling algorithms have substantially enhanced accuracy, making nanopore sequencing increasingly viable for clinical applications [20].

Comparative advantages and limitations of long-read sequencing versus short-read sequencing

LRS offers several distinct advantages over SRS that are particularly relevant for the genomic characterization of hematolymphoid neoplasms (summarized in Table 1). Arguably, the most significant advantage is LRS's superior capability in structural variant detection. These technologies excel at identifying translocations, inversions, duplications, and complex rearrangements that serve as common drivers in hematologic malignancies [21,22]. Many such variants, especially those with breakpoints occurring in repetitive regions, may be missed entirely by short-read approaches, leading

TABLE 1
Advantages and limitations of long-read sequencing relative to current methods

Category	Advantages	Limitations
Technical aspects	• Read lengths *1 kb – 2+ Mb* (vs. SRS: 50–300 bp) • Resolves complex genomic regions (repeats, structural variants)	• Higher error rates (*0.1% PacBio HiFi, 0.4%–5% Oxford Nanopore*) vs SRS (<0.1%) • Lower throughput than Illumina platforms
Variant detection	• Superior for *large SVs*, *haplotype phasing*, and *isoform sequencing* • Captures full-length transcripts without assembly	• Less accurate for *SNVs* and small indels • Requires higher coverage for confident calls
Implementation	• *PCR-free library prep* • Direct detection of base modifications (eg, 5 mC and 6 mA)	• *Computationally intensive* • Fewer standardized pipelines than Illumina
Clinical use	• Higher diagnostic yield for complex variants (ie, *cancer structural variants*) • Rapid pathogen identification (Nanopore real-time sequencing)	• Limited *FDA-approved clinical assays* (most LRS is research-use-only) • Challenges with degraded formalin fixed paraffin embedded (FFPE) samples
Epigenetics	• *Simultaneous genetic + epigenetic profiling* • No bisulfite conversion needed (Nanopore)	• Fewer analysis tools than bisulfite sequencing whole genome bisulfite sequencing (WGBS) • Lower resolution for methylation quantitation

to incomplete characterization of complex cases at the genomic level [23].

The ability to resolve repetitive regions represents another notable advantage of long-read technologies. Many clinically relevant genes in hematolymphoid neoplasms contain repetitive elements that pose significant challenges for SRS [24]. By generating reads that can span these repetitive regions entirely, LRS enables a more complete characterization of these complex genomic areas [25]. Similarly, haplotype phasing—determining whether multiple variants occur on the same chromosomal copy (ie, cis) or different copies (ie, trans)—becomes feasible with long reads that span distant variants. This phasing information may have important functional implications for gene expression and protein function in the context of hematolymphoid malignancies [26].

In transcript analysis, long-read RNA sequencing can directly sequence full-length transcripts, thereby enabling unambiguous identification of fusion genes without requiring complex bioinformatic reconstruction that may introduce errors or ambiguities [27,28]. Additionally, both PacBio and ONT platforms offer the unique capability to detect DNA epigenetic modifications during the sequencing process without additional sample preparation steps. This feature allows for simultaneous analysis of genetic and epigenetic alterations, which may be particularly relevant in myeloid malignancies where epigenetic dysregulation has been found to play a significant role [29,30].

Despite these advantages, LRS also presents specific challenges that must be carefully considered when implementing these technologies in clinical settings. Error rates, while continuously improving, generally remain slightly higher for certain LRS technologies compared to high-quality short-read data [31]. This limitation potentially impacts variant calling accuracy, particularly for detecting single-nucleotide variants (SNVs) and small insertions/deletions [32]. Throughput considerations and cost-effectiveness also factor into implementation decisions, as LRS generally offers lower throughput and higher per-base cost compared to short-read approaches. However, technological advancements continue to narrow this gap [33].

The analysis of long-read data introduces additional complexities, requiring specialized bioinformatic pipelines that differ significantly from those established for SRS [34]. Furthermore, LRS often requires high-quality, high-molecular-weight DNA input, which may present challenges when working with certain clinical specimens, particularly those with formalin fixation or limited quantity [35].

These trade-offs must be carefully evaluated when selecting appropriate sequencing approaches to characterize hematolymphoid neoplasms comprehensively. In many cases, particularly for diagnostically challenging cases, the complementary use of both short-read and long-read technologies may provide the most complete genomic characterization, leveraging the strengths of each approach while mitigating their respective limitations [36].

Implementation and wet laboratory considerations

LRS allows for investigating complex variation, such as homologous regions of the genome [37–40]. For example, *CYP2D6* and *HLA* genes contain homologous regions in which LRS would be advantageous to detect potential variants. In addition, LRS allows for detecting structural variation, especially large-scale variants (ie, variants >50 bp) and complex variants in a single read that would be unclear with SRS.

An important consideration for implementation is sample type, which is determined by what you want to detect. Sample type can guide the selection of the extraction technique, library preparation kit, and sequencing platform best suited for the assay. Another important consideration is whether samples will be multiplexed. Multiplexing needs and the sequencing depth required to detect the variant(s) of interest can also inform the library prep kit and sequencing platform selection.

The 2 aforementioned well-developed LRS platforms currently available are provided by PacBio and ONT. These 2 technologies offer library preparation kits that do not require amplification or fragmentation and are truly polymerase chain reaction (PCR)-free. Each sequencing platform has its pros and cons (Fig. 1). For example, ONT can sequence long reads (<100 kb) and ultra-long read DNA (>5 Mb), while PacBio can generate long reads up to greater than 30 kb. In addition, both platforms allow for the direct sequencing of native molecules to detect epigenetic changes in DNA and RNA (ie, methylation status). While both platforms can detect 5-methylcytosine (5 mC) status, ONT can also detect other methylation modifications that play a role in gene regulation or genomic imprinting (ie, 5-hydroxymethylcytosine [5hmC] and N6-methyladenine [6 mA]). Each platform has different costs and may require additional resources to be purchased for implementation. For example, ONT offers several sequencers with varying throughput capabilities, but specific compute power is needed to process the data.

Bioinformatic pipelines and packages for variant detection

Bioinformatic pipelines and packages used for variant detection can be similar between both platforms (see Fig. 1). The first step of long-read data processing is base calling. As mentioned earlier, PacBio produces a light signal while ONT detects a change in the electrical current, both converted into a nucleic acid sequence. Currently, PacBio sequencers perform base calling directly on the instrument, outputting unaligned binary alignment map (BAM) files. In contrast, ONT sequencers require a separate computer with a graphics processing unit (GPU) for base calling. After base calling, sequences are aligned to the reference genome using a mapping tool (eg, *minimap2*). There are several reference genomes (ie, hg19, hg38, and T2T) available for mapping and selecting which reference genome to use will depend on the purpose of the clinical test. Reference genome selection may depend on the need for a gap-free sequence and genetic diversity in the research setting, but in the clinical setting, this decision will also depend on available annotation tools, databases, historical data, and other tools often used in variant curation.

Next, variant calling is performed to detect variants that can fall into 2 categories: small variants (<50 bp) and large variants (>50 bp). Several packages have been developed to detect SVs such as cuteSV, Delly, NanoVar, pbsv, Sniffles2, and structural variant identification using mapped long reads (SVIM) to name a few [41]. PacBio has developed a package called pbsv, a suite of tools to call and analyze SVs from PacBio SMRT reads in diploid genomes. It is important to note that some of these variant callers require informatics knowledge to become operational and may need to be retrained on user data and following updates. Lastly, an annotation package needs to be used to annotate the variants. Overall, the level of informatics knowledge needed to process and analyze LRS data is generally higher than SRS, regardless of the sequencing platform.

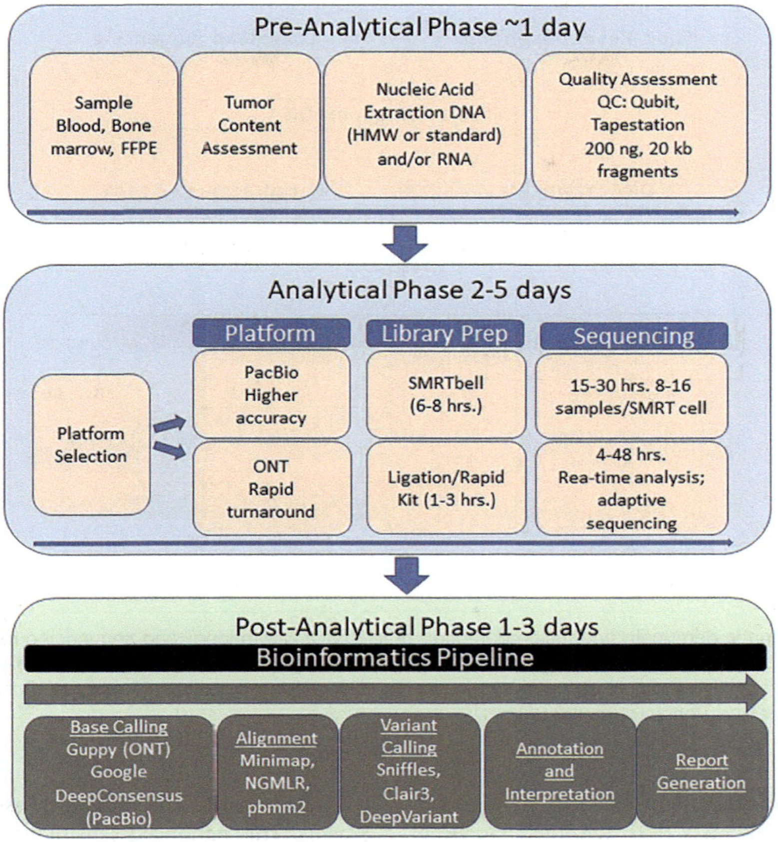

FIG. 1 Comparison of workflows for long-read sequencing versus short-read sequencing.

APPLICATIONS OF LONG-READ SEQUENCING IN HEMATOLYMPHOID NEOPLASMS

Detection of structural variants and gene fusions

SVs, including gene fusions, represent critical drivers and diagnostic markers in many hematolymphoid neoplasms, influencing disease classification, prognostication, and therapeutic decision-making [42,43]. LRS has demonstrated particular utility in characterizing these complex genomic alterations across a spectrum of hematologic malignancies [44–46].

In chronic myeloid leukemia, the defining *BCR*::*ABL1* fusion typically results from the standard t(9;22) translocation, but variant and complex rearrangements are observed in approximately 5% to 10% of cases [47]. LRS can precisely characterize the exact breakpoints and identify atypical *BCR*::*ABL1* fusions that might be missed by standard diagnostic approaches such as FISH or multiplex PCR [47–49]. This capability is particularly valuable in cryptic translocations or complex rearrangements involving additional chromosomes beyond the standard Philadelphia chromosome, where accurate characterization may have therapeutic implications.

KMT2A (formerly *MLL*) represents another clinically significant locus where LRS offers distinct advantages. With over 80 reported fusion partners in acute leukemias, *KMT2A* rearrangements present considerable challenges for standard diagnostic techniques [50,51]. Long-read approaches can identify novel or complex *KMT2A* rearrangements, including those partial tandem duplications and rearrangements involving multiple partner genes or cryptic insertions that may be missed by FISH or SRS [44]. Precisely characterizing these fusions can have significant implications for

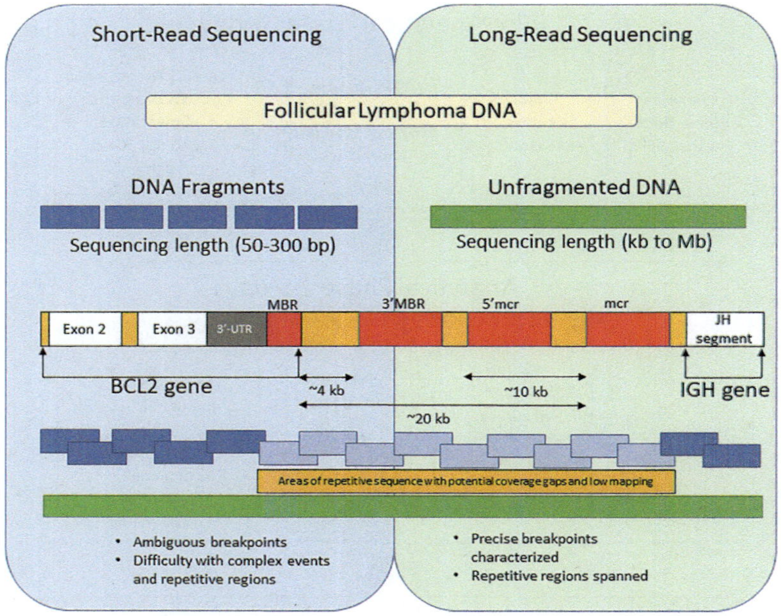

FIG. 2 Schematic demonstrating fusion detection of *IGH::BCL2* with long-read sequencing in comparison to short-read sequencing. Dark blue boxes: SRS fragments in general regions, light blue boxes: SRS fragments in repetitive regions, and dark green boxes: LRS uniform coverage. (*Adapted from* van Dongen and colleagues and Panjan et al. [92,93].)

risk stratification and treatment selection, particularly in pediatric acute leukemias [52]. Recently, targeting Menin-KMT2A has shown promise in clinical trials leading to its approval for targeted therapy [53].

B-cell malignancies frequently harbor rearrangements involving immunoglobulin heavy chain (IGH) and light chain genes, which serve as key diagnostic and prognostic markers [54,55] (Fig. 2). These genomic regions are notoriously difficult to analyze with short-read technologies due to their highly repetitive and polymorphic nature [56]. LRS can effectively span these complex regions to identify partner genes and precise breakpoints, providing a more comprehensive characterization of B-cell lymphomas and leukemias [57,58]. This improved detection capability may reveal cryptic rearrangements in cases previously classified as negative by standard approaches.

In B-cell acute lymphoblastic leukemia (B-ALL), rearrangements involving CRLF2, including *P2RY8::CRLF2* and *IGH::CRLF2*, are important prognostic markers associated with poor outcomes, particularly in certain patient populations [59]. LRS can detect structural alterations in B-ALL more reliably than short-read approaches, which could be utilized as a complementary or stand-alone assay for these neoplasms. This enhanced sensitivity has been shown to identify SVs, including cryptic fusions and large deletions overlooked by clinical tests [60].

Myeloid neoplasms, including myelodysplastic syndromes (MDS) and acute myeloid leukemia (AML), often harbor complex karyotypes with multiple structural rearrangements that present significant challenges for comprehensive characterization [61,62]. LRS can resolve these complex events and identify cryptic abnormalities that conventional cytogenetics or targeted approaches miss. Au and colleagues [45] demonstrated resolution of an AML with complex karyotype with multiple translocations unresolved by other techniques. This comprehensive genomic profiling may reveal previously unrecognized driver events or therapeutic targets in cases with complex genomic landscapes.

Analysis of repetitive regions and difficult-to-sequence genes

Genetic variants in hematolymphoid neoplasms include several clinically significant genes containing repetitive elements, homopolymer regions, or other complex sequence contexts that present technical challenges for SRS technologies. LRS offers important advantages for these difficult-to-sequence regions, enabling more accurate and comprehensive characterization of diagnostically and prognostically relevant alterations.

FLT3 internal tandem duplications (ITDs) represent one of the most clinically significant examples where LRS demonstrates clear advantages. These duplications, which occur in approximately 20% to 30% of AML cases, vary considerably in size (from a few nucleotides to over 100 base pairs) and precise sequence composition [63,64]. The accurate characterization of *FLT3*-ITDs, including their exact size, location, and allelic ratio, has important prognostic and therapeutic implications, particularly with the advent of *FLT3* inhibitors [63,65]. LRS can span the entire duplicated region, allowing for precise characterization that may be challenging or impossible with fragmented short reads, especially for larger ITDs or those occurring in complex structural alterations [66].

Similarly, the *CEBPA* gene, which encodes a critical transcription factor frequently mutated in AML, presents technical challenges due to its highly GC-rich nature (approximately 80% GC content in some regions) [67]. This high GC content often results in poor amplification and uneven coverage with short-read technologies, potentially leading to false negatives or inaccurate variant calling. LRS can provide more uniform coverage across these problematic regions, improving the detection of both the N-terminal frameshift mutations and C-terminal in-frame insertions/deletions that characterize *CEBPA*-mutated AML, a distinct entity with a generally favorable prognosis [2].

NPM1 insertions in exon 12, which define a specific genetic subtype of AML, are generally detectable by short-read methods but can occasionally present challenges, particularly for atypical variants [68]. While standard 4 base pair insertions are usually well-characterized by conventional approaches, LRS can provide additional confidence in cases with unusual insertion patterns or complex genomic contexts, ensuring accurate classification of these prognostically relevant alterations.

ASXL1 contains homopolymer regions, mainly G-rich stretches, prone to sequencing errors with short-read technologies, potentially leading to false-positive variant calls [69]. The high accuracy of PacBio HiFi reads or carefully optimized nanopore sequencing can improve the specificity of variant detection in these regions, reducing false-positive calls that might otherwise lead to the misclassification of myeloid neoplasms. This improved accuracy is crucial given the adverse prognostic significance of *ASXL1* mutations in various myeloid malignancies [70].

Haplotype phasing and compound heterozygosity

Whether multiple mutations occur on the same chromosome (cis configuration) or different chromosomes (trans configuration) can have profound functional and clinical implications in hematolymphoid neoplasms [71]. Traditional SRS approaches typically cannot resolve the phase of variants separated by distances greater than individual read lengths, creating limitations in understanding complex mutational landscapes. LRS addresses this limitation by generating reads spanning distant variants, enabling direct phasing without statistical inference or family studies [72].

In chronic lymphocytic leukemia (CLL) and other hematolymphoid neoplasms, biallelic inactivation of *TP53* through various mechanisms (mutation plus deletion or compound heterozygous mutations) confers an inferior prognosis. It may predict resistance to conventional chemoimmunotherapy regimens [73,74]. While both a *TP53* mutation and a 17p deletion strongly suggest biallelic inactivation, the situation becomes more complex when multiple *TP53* mutations are detected without an accompanying deletion. LRS could directly determine the phase of these mutations, distinguishing between compound heterozygosity (affecting both alleles) and multiple mutations affecting the same allele, which may have different functional and prognostic implications. Black and colleagues [46] utilized LRS for CLL, distinguishing different bruton tyrosine kinase (BTK)-mutant clones rather than being on different haplotypes within the cells of a single subclone.

Similarly, in myeloproliferative neoplasms (MPNs), the relationship between co-occurring driver mutations, such as *JAK2* V617F and *CALR* mutations, can significantly influence disease phenotype and progression. Through haplotype phasing, LRS can determine whether these mutations occur in the same or different clones, providing insights into clonal architecture that may inform prognosis and therapeutic decisions. This information may be particularly valuable in complex cases with features overlapping multiple MPN subtypes or those transforming into acute leukemia. Additionally, Jones and colleagues [75] demonstrated a specific *JAK2* haplotype, designated 46/1, predisposed to the development of *JAK2* V617F, providing additional utility for haplotype testing for MPNs.

For patients with an inherited predisposition to hematologic malignancies, such as those with germline mutations in *GATA2* or *RUNX1*, long-read sequencing can clarify inheritance patterns and phase relationships between variants. This information may be critical for accurate genetic counseling and family testing, particularly in complex genotypes involving multiple variants of uncertain significance [76]. Additionally, in the setting of somatic mutations arising in the context of germline predisposition, LRS can determine whether the somatic event affects the wild-type or already mutated allele, which may have implications for the mechanism of leukemogenesis [77].

Full-length transcript analysis

Analyzing full-length transcripts represents another domain where LRS offers significant advantages over conventional approaches. LRS of cDNA (Iso-Seq for PacBio or direct cDNA/RNA sequencing for ONT) enables comprehensive transcript diversity and structure characterization, providing unique insights into transcriptome complexity that may be particularly relevant in hematolymphoid neoplasms.

Aberrant splicing has emerged as an essential pathogenic mechanism in hematologic malignancies, particularly in MDS and certain leukemias harboring mutations in key splicing factors such as *SF3B1*, *SRSF2*, and *U2AF1* [78]. These splicing factor mutations can generate novel isoforms with diverse functional consequences, but the comprehensive characterization of their effects requires technologies capable of sequencing entire transcripts. Short-read RNA sequencing, while powerful for quantitative expression analysis, often struggles to resolve complex splicing patterns unambiguously due to the fragmented nature of the reads [79]. In contrast, long-read approaches can sequence full-length transcripts from 5′ to 3′, enabling unambiguous identification of all splice variants produced, including novel or cryptic splice sites induced by splicing factor mutations. This comprehensive characterization may reveal previously unrecognized disease mechanisms or therapeutic vulnerabilities. Pacholewska and colleagues [80] utilized LRS full transcript abilities to study molecular mechanisms of *SF3B1* in CLL and MDS and revealed shared splicing alterations, novel isoforms, and constrained 3' splice site dynamics.

For fusion transcripts, familiar drivers in many hematolymphoid neoplasms, LRS offers the unique ability to determine the resulting chimeric transcripts' precise exon composition and structure. While standard diagnostic approaches can identify the presence of specific gene fusions, they typically provide limited information about the exact exons involved or additional complexities, such as alternative splicing of the fusion transcript. LRS can capture the complete fusion transcript, revealing details about the protein domains in the chimeric protein, which may have significant implications for protein structure, function, and sensitivity to targeted therapies. For example, in Philadelphia chromosome-positive leukemias, different *BCR::ABL1* transcript variants may exhibit varying sensitivities to tyrosine kinase inhibitors, information that could guide therapeutic decision-making [81,82].

Beyond characterizing individual transcript structures, LRS enables the quantification of specific transcript isoforms that may be difficult to resolve with short-read approaches. This capability is particularly valuable in hematolymphoid neoplasms where specific isoforms may have distinct functional properties or therapeutic vulnerabilities. For instance, alternative splicing of genes involved in apoptosis, cell cycle regulation, or drug metabolism may generate isoforms with different functional properties that influence disease biology or treatment response. By accurately quantifying these specific isoforms, long-read approaches have the potential to identify novel biomarkers or therapeutic targets not evident from gene-level expression analysis.

Epigenetic marker analysis

Epigenetic dysregulation is a common finding of many hematolymphoid neoplasms, particularly myeloid malignancies, where mutations in epigenetic regulators are frequent drivers of disease pathogenesis [83,84]. Studying DNA methylation and other epigenetic modifications has traditionally required specialized techniques such as bisulfite sequencing, chromatin immunoprecipitation sequencing, or array-based approaches. However, LRS offers the unique capability to directly detect DNA modifications during the sequencing process itself, without the need for additional sample preparation steps that may introduce biases or artifacts [85].

Both major long-read platforms provide distinct approaches to epigenetic profiling. Oxford Nanopore sequencing can directly detect 5 mC, 5hmC, and other modified bases through characteristic alterations in the electrical signal as DNA molecules traverse the nanopore [86]. Recent advances in base-calling algorithms have significantly improved the accuracy of these modification calls, enabling genome-wide methylation profiling from the same sequencing run used for structural variant and sequence variant detection [87]. This capability is particularly valuable in hematolymphoid neoplasms, where integrated genetic and epigenetic analysis may provide more comprehensive insights into disease biology and potential therapeutic vulnerabilities.

PacBio SMRT sequencing similarly enables the detection of DNA modifications through systematic variations in polymerase kinetics as modified nucleotides are incorporated [88]. Both platforms allow for the analysis of native DNA, avoiding the chemical conversion steps required for bisulfite sequencing, which can lead to DNA degradation and biased amplification.

The clinical applications of epigenetic profiling using LRS in hematolymphoid neoplasms are rapidly expanding. In AML, distinct DNA methylation patterns have been associated with specific genetic subtypes and have demonstrated prognostic significance independent of genetic features [89,90]. LRS can characterize these methylation patterns across larger genomic regions than traditional approaches, potentially revealing epigenetic signatures that predict disease behavior or treatment response more accurately. Additionally, in MDS, where hypermethylation of promoter regions contributes to aberrant gene silencing, comprehensive methylation profiling may identify patients most likely to benefit from hypomethylating agents such as azacitidine or decitabine [30].

Beyond DNA methylation, LRS is increasingly applied to analyzing chromatin structure and histone modifications through techniques such as assay for transposase-accessible chromatin using sequencing with long reads. This approach can provide insights into the relationship between chromatin accessibility, transcription factor binding, and gene expression in hematolymphoid neoplasms [91]. The ability to span entire regulatory elements with single reads offers advantages over short-read approaches, particularly for complex enhancers or regions with multiple regulatory elements that may be difficult to resolve with fragmented reads.

As analytical methods mature, integrating genetic and epigenetic data from the same LRS will likely become increasingly valuable in the comprehensive molecular characterization of hematolymphoid neoplasms. This integrated approach may reveal complex relationships between genetic alterations and epigenetic reprogramming that drive disease pathogenesis and influence treatment response, ultimately leading to more precise diagnostic, prognostic, and therapeutic strategies.

SUMMARY

LRS represents a robust and rapidly evolving approach to the genomic analysis of hematolymphoid neoplasms. Its unique capabilities in detecting SVs, resolving repetitive regions, analyzing full-length transcripts, and phasing variants address essential limitations of conventional molecular and cytogenetic techniques. While challenges remain regarding bioinformatic analysis, validation, and cost-effectiveness, the potential clinical benefits of more comprehensive genomic characterization are substantial.

As LRS technologies advance in accuracy, throughput, and cost-efficiency, they will become increasingly integrated into routine clinical practice for hematolymphoid neoplasms. The complementary use of long-read and SRS, along with conventional cytogenetic approaches, offers the most comprehensive strategy for genomic characterization in the near term.

For molecular pathology laboratories considering the implementation of LRS, careful attention to validation, quality control, bioinformatics analysis, and integration with existing workflows is essential. Collaboration among pathologists, hematologists, cytogeneticists, molecular biologists, and bioinformaticians will be critical for the successful clinical implementation and reporting of LRS results.

In the rapidly evolving landscape of precision medicine for hematolymphoid neoplasms, LRS represents a significant technological advance that will continue to enhance our ability to provide accurate diagnosis, prognostication, and therapeutic guidance for patients with these complex diseases.

CLINICS CARE POINTS

- Complex structural variants are common in hematolymphoid malignancies and can be better characterized by long read sequencing compared to short read sequencing.
- The ability to sequence through repetitive regions with long read sequencing allows better haplotype reconstruction.
- Methylation detection performed as a byproduct of long sequencing provides further information which can be leveraged as epigenetic marker for classification, prognostication and therapeutic decisions.

DECLARATION OF ARTIFICIAL INTELLIGENCE AND ARTIFICIAL INTELLIGENCE-ASSISTED TECHNOLOGIES IN THE WRITING PROCESS

During the preparation of this article, the author(s) used Grammarly, Claude 3.7 Sonnet, DeepSeek for outlining structure, text editing, searching additional references, and refining verbiage. After using this tool/service, the author(s) reviewed and edited the content as needed and take(s) full responsibility for the content of the publication.

REFERENCES

[1] Arber DA, Orazi A, Hasserjian R, et al. The 2016 revision to the World Health Organization classification of myeloid neoplasms and acute leukemia. Blood 2016; 127(20):2391–405.

[2] Swerdlow SH, Campo E, Pileri SA, et al. The 2016 revision of the World Health Organization classification of lymphoid neoplasms. Blood 2016;127(20): 2375–90.

[3] Merker JD, Valouev A, Gotlib J. Next-generation sequencing in hematologic malignancies: what will be the dividends? Ther Adv Hematol 2012;3(6):333–9.

[4] Mardis ER. The impact of next-generation sequencing technology on genetics. Trends Genet 2008;24(3):133–41.

[5] Alkan C, Coe BP, Eichler EE. Genome structural variation discovery and genotyping. Nat Rev Genet 2011; 12(5):363–76.

[6] Sedlazeck FJ, Lee H, Darby CA, et al. Piercing the dark matter: bioinformatics of long-range sequencing and mapping. Nat Rev Genet 2018;19(6):329–46.

[7] Mantere T, Kersten S, Hoischen A. Long-read sequencing emerging in medical genetics. Front Genet 2019;10:426.

[8] Amarasinghe SL, Su S, Dong X, et al. Opportunities and challenges in long-read sequencing data analysis. Genome Biol 2020;21(1):30.

[9] Ardui S, Ameur A, Vermeesch JR, et al. Single molecule real-time (SMRT) sequencing comes of age: applications and utilities for medical diagnostics. Nucleic Acids Res 2018;46(5):2159–68.

[10] Jain M, Olsen HE, Paten B, et al. The Oxford Nanopore MinION: delivery of nanopore sequencing to the genomics community. Genome Biol 2016;17(1). https://doi.org/10.1186/s13059-016-1103-0.

[11] Chaisson MJP, Sanders AD, Zhao X, et al. Multi-platform discovery of haplotype-resolved structural variation in human genomes. Nat Commun 2019;10(1): 1784.

[12] Seo JS, Rhie A, Kim J, et al. De novo assembly and phasing of a Korean human genome. Nature 2016;538-(7624):243–7.

[13] Duncavage EJ, Schroeder MC, O'Laughlin M, et al. Genome sequencing as an alternative to cytogenetic analysis in myeloid cancers. N Engl J Med 2021;384-(10):924–35.

[14] Arindrarto W, Borràs DM, de Groen RAL, et al. Comprehensive diagnostics of acute myeloid leukemia by whole transcriptome RNA sequencing. Leukemia 2021;35(1): 47–61.

[15] Sedlazeck FJ, Rescheneder P, Smolka M, et al. Accurate detection of complex structural variations using single-molecule sequencing. Nat Methods 2018;15(6):461–8.

[16] Eid J, Fehr A, Gray J, et al. Real-time DNA sequencing from single polymerase molecules. Science 2009;323-(5910):133–8.

[17] Travers KJ, Chin CS, Rank DR, et al. A flexible and efficient template format for circular consensus sequencing and SNP detection. Nucleic Acids Res 2010;38(15): e159.

[18] Wenger AM, Peluso P, Rowell WJ, et al. Accurate circular consensus long-read sequencing improves variant detection and assembly of a human genome. Nat Biotechnol 2019;37(10):1155–62.

[19] Deamer D, Akeson M, Branton D. Three decades of nanopore sequencing. Nat Biotechnol 2016;34(5): 518–24.

[20] Rang FJ, Kloosterman WP, de Ridder J. From squiggle to basepair: computational approaches for improving nanopore sequencing read accuracy. Genome Biol 2018;19(1):90.

[21] Huddleston J, Chaisson MJP, Steinberg KM, et al. Discovery and genotyping of structural variation from long-read haploid genome sequence data. Genome Res 2017;27(5):677–85.

[22] Cretu SM, van Roosmalen MJ, Renkens I, et al. Mapping and phasing of structural variation in patient genomes using nanopore sequencing. Nat Commun 2017;8(1): 1326.

[23] Hiatt SM, Lawlor JMJ, Handley LH, et al. Long-read genome sequencing for the molecular diagnosis of neurodevelopmental disorders. HGG Adv 2021;2(2). https://doi.org/10.1016/j.xhgg.2021.100023.

[24] Treangen TJ, Salzberg SL. Repetitive DNA and next-generation sequencing: computational challenges and solutions. Nat Rev Genet 2011;13(1):36–46.

[25] Miga KH, Koren S, Rhie A, et al. Telomere-to-telomere assembly of a complete human X chromosome. Nature 2020;585(7823):79–84.

[26] Edge P, Bafna V, Bansal V. HapCUT2: robust and accurate haplotype assembly for diverse sequencing technologies. Genome Res 2017;27(5):801–12.

[27] Minervini CF, Cumbo C, Orsini P, et al. Nanopore sequencing in blood diseases: a wide range of opportunities. Front Genet 2020;11:76.

[28] Gong L, Wong CH, Cheng WC, et al. Picky comprehensively detects high-resolution structural variants in nanopore long reads. Nat Methods 2018;15(6):455–60.

[29] Simpson JT, Workman RE, Zuzarte PC, et al. Detecting DNA cytosine methylation using nanopore sequencing. Nat Methods 2017;14(4):407–10.

[30] Issa JP. The myelodysplastic syndrome as a prototypical epigenetic disease. Blood 2013;121(19):3811–7.

[31] Mahmoud M, Huang Y, Garimella K, et al. Utility of long-read sequencing for all of us Nat Commun 2024;15(1):837.

[32] Salk JJ, Schmitt MW, Loeb LA. Enhancing the accuracy of next-generation sequencing for detecting rare and subclonal mutations. Nat Rev Genet 2018;19(5): 269–85.

[33] Logsdon GA, Vollger MR, Eichler EE. Long-read human genome sequencing and its applications. Nat Rev Genet 2020;21(10):597–614.

[34] De Coster W, De Rijk P, De Roeck A, et al. Structural variants identified by Oxford Nanopore PromethION sequencing of the human genome. Genome Res 2019; 29(7):1178–87.

[35] Branton D, Deamer DW, Marziali A, et al. The potential and challenges of nanopore sequencing. Nat Biotechnol 2008;26(10):1146–53.

[36] Mahmoud M, Gobet N, Cruz-Dvalos DI, et al. Structural variant calling: the long and the short of it. Genome Biol 2019;20(1):246.

[37] Merker JD, Wenger AM, Sneddon T, et al. Long-read genome sequencing identifies causal structural variation in a Mendelian disease. Genet Med 2018;20(1): 159–63.

[38] Yuan N, Jia P. Comprehensive assessment of long-read sequencing platforms and calling algorithms for detection of copy number variation. Brief Bioinform 2024; 25(5). https://doi.org/10.1093/bib/bbae441.

[39] Cuber P, Chooneea D, Geeves C, et al. Comparing the accuracy and efficiency of third generation sequencing technologies, Oxford Nanopore Technologies, and Pacific Biosciences, for DNA barcode sequencing applications. Ecol Genet Genom 2023;28:100181.

[40] Zeng S, Zhang MY, Wang XJ, et al. Long-read sequencing identified intronic repeat expansions in SAMD12 from Chinese pedigrees affected with familial cortical myoclonic tremor with epilepsy. J Med Genet 2019; 56(4):265–70.

[41] Wang Y, Zhao Y, Bollas A, et al. Nanopore sequencing technology, bioinformatics and applications. Nat Biotechnol 2021;39(11):1348–65.

[42] Bullinger L, Dhner K, Dhner H. Genomics of acute myeloid leukemia diagnosis and pathways. J Clin Oncol 2017;35(9):934–46.

[43] Meyer C, Burmeister T, Grger D, et al. The MLL recombinome of acute leukemias in 2017. Leukemia 2018; 32(2):273–84.

[44] Todd J, Hogg G, Holden K, et al. Detection of KMT2A partial tandem duplication in myeloid samples by Pacbio® long read sequencing. Blood 2024;144-(Supplement 1):1551.

[45] Au CH, Ho DN, Ip BBK, et al. Rapid detection of chromosomal translocation and precise breakpoint characterization in acute myeloid leukemia by nanopore long-read sequencing. Cancer Genet 2019;239:22–5.

[46] Black G, Huang X, Qiao Y, et al. Single-cell long-read sequencing enables the dissection of BTK subclonal dynamics in CLL treatment. Blood 2023;142(Supplement 1):1893.

[47] Cumbo C, Impera L, Minervini CF, et al. Genomic BCR-ABL1 breakpoint characterization by a multi-strategy approach for "personalized monitoring" of residual disease in chronic myeloid leukemia patients. Oncotarget 2018;9:10978–86. Available at: www.impactjournals.com/oncotarget.

[48] Primo D, Tabernero MD, Rasillo A, et al. Pattern of BCR/ABL gene rearrangements by interphase fluorescence in situ hybridization (FISH) in BCR/ABL+ leukemias: incidence and underlying genetic abnormalities. Leukemia 2003;17(6):1124–9.

[49] Zhao H, Chen Y, Shen C, et al. Breakpoint mapping of a t(9;22;12) chronic myeloid leukaemia patient with e14a3 BCR-ABL1 transcript using Nanopore sequencing. J Gene Med 2021;23(1). https://doi.org/10.1002/jgm.3276.

[50] Meyer C, Hofmann J, Burmeister T, et al. The MLL recombinome of acute leukemias in 2013. Leukemia 2013;27(11):2165–76.

[51] De Braekeleer E, Douet-Guilbert N, De Braekeleer M. FISH analysis in hematological malignancies: from the molecular detection of chromosome abnormalities to the screening for specific genomic alterations. Expert Rev Mol Diagn 2015;15(5):657–72.

[52] Guarnera L, D'Addona M, Bravo-Perez C, et al. KMT2A rearrangements in leukemias: molecular aspects and therapeutic perspectives. Int J Mol Sci 2024;25(16). https://doi.org/10.3390/ijms25169023.

[53] Issa GC, Aldoss I, Thirman MJ, et al. Menin inhibition with revumenib for KMT2A-rearranged relapsed or refractory acute leukemia (AUGMENT-101). J Clin Oncol 2025;43(1):75–84.

[54] Nadeu F, Diaz-Navarro A, Delgado J, et al. Genomic and epigenomic insights into the origin, pathogenesis, and clinical behavior of mantle cell lymphoma subtypes. Blood 2020;136(12):1419–32.

[55] Rabkin CS, Hirt C, Janz S, et al. t(14;18) Translocations and risk of follicular lymphoma. J Natl Cancer Inst Monogr 2008;39:48–51.

[56] Thomson AJ, Rehn JA, Heatley SL, et al. Reproducible bioinformatics analysis workflows for detecting IGH gene fusions in B-cell acute lymphoblastic leukaemia patients. Cancers (Basel) 2023;15(19). https://doi.org/10.3390/cancers15194731.

[57] Tian L, Shao Y, Nance S, et al. Long-read sequencing unveils IGH-DUX4 translocation into the silenced IGH allele in B-cell acute lymphoblastic leukemia. Nat Commun 2019;10(1):2789.

[58] Liszt K, von der Linde M, Schinnerl D, et al. Nanopore Cas9-targeted long-read sequencing - a fast and flexible diagnostic tool for the identification of B-cell acute lymphoblastic leukemia associated gene rearrangements. Blood 2023;142(Supplement 1):2984.

[59] Reshmi SC, Harvey RC, Roberts KG, et al. Targetable kinase gene fusions in high-risk B-ALL: a study from the Children's Oncology Group. Blood 2017;129(25):3352–61.
[60] Kato S, Sato-Otsubo A, Nakamura W, et al. Genome profiling with targeted adaptive sampling long-read sequencing for pediatric leukemia. Blood Cancer J 2024;14(1):145.
[61] Papaemmanuil E, Gerstung M, Bullinger L, et al. Genomic classification and prognosis in acute myeloid leukemia. N Engl J Med 2016;374(23):2209–21.
[62] Haferlach T, Nagata Y, Grossmann V, et al. Landscape of genetic lesions in 944 patients with myelodysplastic syndromes. Leukemia 2014;28(2):241–7.
[63] Kiyoi H, Kawashima N, Ishikawa Y. FLT3 mutations in acute myeloid leukemia: therapeutic paradigm beyond inhibitor development. Cancer Sci 2020;111(2):312–22.
[64] Tao S, Wang C, Chen Y, et al. Prognosis and outcome of patients with acute myeloid leukemia based on FLT3-ITD mutation with or without additional abnormal cytogenetics. Oncol Lett 2019;18(6):6766–74.
[65] Larson RA, Mandrekar SJ, Huebner LJ, et al. Midostaurin reduces relapse in FLT3-mutant acute myeloid leukemia: the Alliance CALGB 10603/RATIFY trial. Leukemia 2021;35(9):2539–51.
[66] Tung JK, Suarez CJ, Chiang T, et al. Accurate detection and quantification of FLT3 internal tandem duplications in clinical hybrid capture next-generation sequencing data. J Mol Diagn 2021;23(10):1404–13.
[67] Grossmann V, Schnittger S, Schindela S, et al. Strategy for robust detection of insertions, deletions, and point mutations in CEBPA, a GC-rich content gene, using 454 next-generation deep-sequencing technology. J Mol Diagn 2011;13(2):129–36.
[68] Martelli MP, Rossi R, Venanzi A, et al. Novel NPM1 exon 5 mutations and gene fusions leading to aberrant cytoplasmic nucleophosmin in AML. Blood 2021;138(25): 2696–701.
[69] Alberti MO, Srivatsan SN, Shao J, et al. Discriminating a common somatic ASXL1 mutation (c.1934dup; p. G646Wfs*12) from artifact in myeloid malignancies using NGS. Leukemia 2018;32(8):1874–8.
[70] Thol F, Friesen I, Damm F, et al. Prognostic significance of *ASXL1* mutations in patients with myelodysplastic syndromes. J Clin Oncol 2011;29(18):2499–506.
[71] Bernard E, Nannya Y, Hasserjian RP, et al. Implications of TP53 allelic state for genome stability, clinical presentation and outcomes in myelodysplastic syndromes. Nat Med 2020;26(10):1549–56.
[72] Maestri S, Maturo MG, Cosentino E, et al. A long-read sequencing approach for direct haplotype phasing in clinical settings. Int J Mol Sci 2020;21(23). https://doi.org/10.3390/ijms21239177.
[73] Malcikova J, Smardova J, Rocnova L, et al. Monoallelic and biallelic inactivation of TP53 gene in chronic lymphocytic leukemia: selection, impact on survival, and response to DNA damage. Blood 2009;114(26): 5307–14.
[74] Al-Sawaf O, Fischer K. TP53 mutations in CLL: does frequency matter? Blood 2021;138(25):2600–1.
[75] Jones AV, Chase A, Silver RT, et al. JAK2 haplotype is a major risk factor for the development of myeloproliferative neoplasms. Nat Genet 2009;41(4):446–9.
[76] Tewhey R, Bansal V, Torkamani A, et al. The importance of phase information for human genomics. Nat Rev Genet 2011;12(3):215–23.
[77] Calvo KR, Hickstein DD. The spectrum of GATA2 deficiency syndrome. Blood 2023;141(13):1524–32.
[78] Tseng C-C, Obeng EA. RNA splicing as a therapeutic target in myelodysplastic syndromes. Semin Hematol 2024;61(6):431–41.
[79] Su T, Hollas MAR, Fellers RT, et al. Identification of splice variants and isoforms in transcriptomics and proteomics. Annu Rev Biomed Data Sci 2023;6:357–76.
[80] Pacholewska A, Lienhard M, Bŗggemann M, et al. Long-read transcriptome sequencing of CLL and MDS patients uncovers molecular effects of SF3B1 mutations. Genome Res 2024;34(11):1832–48.
[81] Chen K, Ruan Y, Tian K, et al. Impact of BCR-ABL1 transcript type on outcome in chronic myeloid leukemia patients treated with tyrosine kinase inhibitors: a pairwise and bayesian network meta-analysis. Front Oncol 2022; 12:841546. https://doi.org/10.3389/fonc.2022.841546.
[82] Simone C, Jane FA, Robert Peter G, et al. E14a2 BCR-ABL1 transcript is associated with a higher rate of treatment-free remission in individuals with chronic myeloid leukemia after stopping tyrosine kinase inhibitor therapy. Haematologica (Roma) 2017;102(8): e297–9.
[83] Figueroa ME, Lugthart S, Li Y, et al. DNA methylation signatures identify biologically distinct subtypes in acute myeloid leukemia. Cancer Cell 2010;17(1):13–27.
[84] Corces MR, Chang HY, Majeti R. Preleukemic hematopoietic stem cells in human acute myeloid leukemia. Front Oncol 2017;7:263.
[85] Flusberg BA, Webster DR, Lee JH, et al. Direct detection of DNA methylation during single-molecule, real-time sequencing. Nat Methods 2010;7(6):461–5.
[86] Liu Q, Fang L, Yu G, et al. Detection of DNA base modifications by deep recurrent neural network on Oxford Nanopore sequencing data. Nat Commun 2019;10(1): 2449.
[87] Yuen ZW, Srivastava A, Daniel R, et al. Systematic benchmarking of tools for CpG methylation detection from nanopore sequencing. Nat Commun 2021;12(1): 3438.
[88] Feng Z, Fang G, Korlach J, et al. Detecting DNA modifications from SMRT sequencing data by modeling sequence context dependence of polymerase kinetic. PLoS Comput Biol 2013;9(3):e1002935.
[89] Glass JL, Hassane D, Wouters BJ, et al. Epigenetic identity in AML depends on disruption of nonpromoter regulatory elements and is affected by antagonistic effects of mutations in epigenetic modifiers. Cancer Discov 2017;7(8):868–83.

[90] Qu X, Othus M, Davison J, et al. Prognostic methylation markers for overall survival in cytogenetically normal patients with acute myeloid leukemia treated on SWOG trials. Cancer 2017;123(13):2472–81.

[91] Corces MR, Buenrostro JD, Wu B, et al. Lineage-specific and single-cell chromatin accessibility charts human hematopoiesis and leukemia evolution. Nat Genet 2016; 48(10):1193–203.

[92] van Dongen JJ, Langerak AW, Brüggemann M, et al. Design and standardization of PCR primers and protocols for detection of clonal immunoglobulin and T-cell receptor gene recombinations in suspect lymphoproliferations: report of the BIOMED-2 Concerted Action BMH4-CT98-3936. Leukemia 2003;17(12): 2257–317.

[93] Panjan M, Boltezar L, Novakovic S, et al. Correlation of t (14;18) translocation breakpoint site with clinical characteristics in follicular lymphoma. Radiol Oncol 2023; 57(4):487–92.

Advances in Molecular Pathology 8 (2025) 41–52
ADVANCES IN MOLECULAR PATHOLOGY

DNA Methylation-Based Profiling in Mature B-cell Neoplasms

Julia Wang, MD, PhD[a], Annapurna Saksena, MBBS, MD[b,*]
[a]Hospital of the University of Pennsylvania, Philadelphia, PA, USA; [b]Division of Hematopathology, Department of Pathology and Laboratory Medicine, Hospital of the University of Pennsylvania, Philadelphia, PA, USA

KEYWORDS
• Methylation • Epigenetics • Lymphoma • DNA-Methylation • B-cell lymphoma

KEY POINTS

- Epigenetic modifications like DNA methylation regulate gene expression without changing the DNA sequence, playing a key role in cell differentiation and cancer development.
- B-cell lymphomas exhibit distinct DNA methylation profiles that can be linked to their cellular origin and may serve as biomarkers for tumor classification and prognosis.
- DNA methylation profiling in B-cell lymphomas could help identify targets and contribute to improving patient stratification and treatment strategies.

INTRODUCTION

Epigenetic modifications refer to inheritable changes in DNA chemistry that do not alter the actual nucleotide sequence. These changes can also affect the structure of proteins that form chromatin. The primary goal of these modifications is to establish and maintain a stable, global gene expression program, which fine-tunes gene expression and responses to external signals. The overall pattern of epigenetic modifications acts like the *software* that determines the specific roles of a particular cell type, and disruptions to this system are a key feature of neoplasia [1].

Numerous epigenetic modifications work in concert to regulate both normal and abnormal gene behavior. This article specifically focuses on DNA methylation (5' -methylcytosine, 5 mC), the most extensively studied epigenetic modification in B-cell tumors. In mammals, DNA methylation primarily occurs at cytosine-guanine dinucleotides (CpG). Its regulation is controlled by a various enzymes, including DNA methyltransferases (*writers*), 5 mC binding proteins (*readers*), and enzymes involved in demethylation processes, such as ten-eleven translocation methylcytosine dioxygenase (TET) and thymine-DNA glycosylase (*erasers*) [1]. Cytosine demethylation can also occur passively when new DNA is not methylated during cell replication.

Typically, DNA methylation levels are linked to the CpG content in DNA, with lower levels found in CpG-rich regions (CpG islands) and higher levels elsewhere. Studies have shown that DNA methylation at promoter regions is generally inversely correlated with gene expression [2]. However, recent genome-wide studies suggest that this relationship is more complex than initially thought [1]. DNA methylation can serve different roles depending on its genomic context, such as at promoters, enhancers, gene bodies, and repetitive elements within heterochromatin.

*Corresponding author. Department of Pathology and Laboratory Medicine, Division of Hematopathology Hospital of the University of Pennsylvania, Perelman School of Medicine at the University of Pennsylvania, 7 East Gates 7.010, 3400 Spruce Street, Philadelphia, PA 19104. *E-mail address:* annapurna.saksena@pennmedicine.upenn.edu

https://doi.org/10.1016/j.yamp.2025.05.003 www.advancesinmolecularpathology.com
2589-4080/25/ © 2025 Elsevier Inc. All rights are reserved, including those for text and data mining, AI training, and similar technologies.

ABBREVIATIONS

5 mC	5'-methylcytosine
ABC	activated B cells
aSHM	aberrant somatic hypermutation
B-ALL	B-cell acute lymphoblastic leukemia
BCR	B-cell receptor
CLL	chronic lymphocytic leukemia
cMCL	conventional mantle cell lymphoma
CpG	cytosine-guanine dinucleotides
DLBCL	diffuse large B-cell lymphoma
DLBCL	diffuse large B-cell lymphoma
epiCMIT	epigenetically determined cumulative mitoses
FL	follicular lymphoma
GC	germinal center
GCB	germinal center B cells
i-CLL	intermediate CLL
IGHV	immunoglobulin heavy-chain locus
MCL	mantle cell lymphoma
M-CLL	mutated CLL
m-CLL	memory B-cell-like CLL
MGUS	monoclonal gammopathy of undetermined significance
MM	multiple myeloma
MP	methylation patterns
n-CLL	naïve B-cell like CLL
nnMCL	non-nodal mantle cell lymphoma
OS	overall survival
TET	ten-eleven translocation methylcytosine dioxygenase
TFs	transcription factors
TTFT	time to treatment failure
U-CLL	unmutated CLL
WM	Waldenström's Macroglobulinemia

Epigenetic changes are influenced by a range of cellular processes, including polycomb-mediated silencing, transcription, signaling pathways, and the activity of transcription factors [3]. B-cell-specific processes like activation-induced cytidine deaminase activity and germinal center-specific events also play critical roles. By deepening our understanding of the epigenetic events occurring during B-cell differentiation, we can more accurately identify tumor-specific epigenetic abnormalities and leverage this knowledge to develop targeted therapies. These insights also hold promise for improving tumor classification and understanding tumor-specific mechanisms, potentially guiding the development of both epigenetic and nonepigenetic cancer treatments [1].

In recent years, there has been growing interest in studying epigenetic modifications, including DNA methylation, in hematolymphoid neoplasms. This article summarizes our current understanding of DNA methylation profiling in mature B-cell lymphomas.

A key principle in classifying lymphoid neoplasms is that each B-cell tumor can be linked to a specific maturation stage, based on the assumption that it reflects the normal cellular origin from which the tumor developed [4,5]. For instance, B-cell acute lymphoblastic leukemia (B-ALL) is classified as a precursor B-cell neoplasm, multiple myeloma (MM) is a plasma cell-derived cancer, and diffuse large B-cell lymphoma (DLBCL) is subclassified into activated B cells (ABC) or germinal center B cells (GCB) based on transcriptional similarities to these normal cellular states [6]. From an epigenetic standpoint, normal B cell maturation involves significant DNA methylation changes—both gains and losses—that accumulate as differentiation progresses, with substantial epigenetic programming occurring during the germinal center (GC) reaction [7,8]. Furthermore, each B cell type is associated with a distinct DNA methylation signature [7] and DNA methylation serves as a powerful molecular marker for identifying the potential normal counterpart of tumors [9] (52).

In addition to the DNA methylation signatures linked to their cellular origin, tumor methylation profiles also comprise specific de novo alterations that may be informative about their underlying pathogenic mechanisms. For example, the binding sites of certain transcription factors (TFs) implicated in B-cell tumor pathogenesis undergo demethylation [10], which aligns with the observed DNA methylation loss in regulatory regions upon TF binding [11,12].

With increasing interest in B-cell lymphoma biology, a large body of data generated in past years on somatic mutations and epigenetic changes in mature B-cell neoplasms raises questions about how these events are interrelated. This article summarizes recent DNA-based methylation profiling studies in B-cell lymphomas focusing on epigenetic subtypes and their clinicopathological and genetic characteristics.

Most B-cell malignancies investigated to date show an overall global reduction in DNA methylation, except for acute lymphocytic leukemia [7,13,14]. Interestingly, the overall extent of global hypomethylation in B-cell tumors correlates with the methylation patterns of the tumor's presumed originating normal cell type.

For example, B-ALL arising from pre-B cells and the most phenotypically immature, shows the least hypomethylation, while MM displays the highest levels of hypomethylation, a feature that aligns with the naturally low methylation levels of plasma cells. The observed decrease in global methylation in tumors, compared to normal cells, is likely a consequence of increased cell proliferation following the transformation process.

Chronic Lymphocytic Leukemia/Small Lymphocytic Lymphoma

Chronic lymphocytic leukemia (CLL) is traditionally classified into 2 subtypes based on the degree of somatic hypermutation (SHM) in the the variable region of the immunoglobulin heavy chain (IGHV) gene. Patients with unmutated CLL (U-CLL) either has few or no mutations in their IGHV genes and generally experience poorer clinical outcomes, while those with mutated CLL (M-CLL) exhibit a higher mutational load in their IGHV genes and tend to have a more favorable prognosis [15].

Studies analyzing the DNA methylomes of M-CLL and U-CLL cases have identified that most of the differences are associated with CpGs whose methylation status is influenced by the differentiation of B cells from pregerminal center (GC to post-GC stages, such as naive B cells versus memory B cells) [13]. Subsequent research described 3 CLL methylation epitypes/subgroups which differ in IGHV mutational load, VH usage, and proportions of somatic mutations in NOTCH1 and SF3B1 [16]. The naïve B-cell like CLL (n-CLL) subgroup exhibits an epigenetic signature of pre-GC B-cells and the memory B-cell-like CLL (m-CLL) of post-GC B- cells, overlapping with U-CLL and M-CLL respectively. The third subgroup, intermediate CLL (i-CLL) showed moderately mutated IGHV, specific VH usage (VH3-23 and VH1-18), and higher SF3B1 mutation incidence suggesting that i-CLL represented a distinct clinicopathologic group. The cell of origin of i-CLL is not definitively established and while based on IGHV mutational status, it would also classify as m-CLL, it showed a worse clinical behavior than m-CLL. These findings showed that the 3 epigenetic subgroups may offer a more accurate prognosis for CLL than the traditional classification based on IGHV mutational status, and this new epigenetic classification may pave the way for the development of targeted therapies tailored to specific patient subgroups [16]. However, subsequent studies indicated that the previously observed intermediate prognosis for the intermediate epitype can be further refined based on the presence of the IGLV3-21R110 mutation. These studies showed that i-CLL, previously linked to an intermediate prognosis between m-CLL and n-CLL, could be further divided into 2 subgroups with distinct genomic and transcriptomic profiles and contrasting clinical outcomes based on IGLV3-21R110 mutation. The i-CLLs without the IGLV3-21R110 mutation were not stereotyped, exhibited a higher IGHV mutational load, frequently had rearranged IGLV3-25 and IGKV1-8 genes, and lacked SF3B1 and ATM mutations but carried MYD88 mutations and phenotypically resembled m-CLL/M-IGHV tumors. The i-CLL cases with the IGLV3-21R110 mutation exhibited an aggressive disease course, characterized by shorter time to treatment failure (TTFT) and overall survival (OS), resembling n-CLL. In contrast, i-CLL cases without IGLV3-21R110 showed a more indolent disease progression, with longer TTFT and OS, like m-CLL. Thus, it may be more clinically appropriate to classify patients into 2 categories: those with worse prognosis naive-like CLLs (primarily U-CLLs) and intermediate CLLs carrying the IGLV3-21R110 mutation, and those with better prognosis memory-like CLLs (mainly M-CLLs) and intermediate CLLs without the IGLV3-21R110 mutation [17].

Interestingly, recent studies using consensus clustering approach have identified two robust clusters based on epigenetic signatures, which are associated with significantly different clinical outcomes, which primarily, though not exclusively, encompass IGHV mutational status, epitypes, stereotypes and IGLV3-21R110 [18]. These findings highlight the potential for DNA methylation classifiers to more accurately identify clinically relevant CLL subgroups [19].

In addition to subclassification, methylation pattern may also provide insights into the pathogenic mechanisms of CLL. CLL is one of the lymphoid malignancies with a well-characterized DNA methylome [13,19–23] with studies having shown that U-CLL exhibits more DNA methylation changes than M-CLL, particularly affecting genes such as ZAP70 [24].

Mantle Cell Lymphoma

In mantle cell lymphoma (MCL), 2 distinct subtypes are recognized with distinct clinicopathological and biological features [25]. Conventional MCL (cMCL) cases are more aggressive, exhibit low or absent SHM in the IGHV genes, and often express the SOX11 oncogene. In contrast, leukemic non-nodal MCL (nnMCL) cases typically have a more favorable prognosis, show higher levels of IGHV SHM, and are generally SOX11-negative.

Methylation profiling studies identified 2 MCL methylation subgroups/epitypes with distinct characteristics [26]. The unmutated MCLs(C1) lack the GC epigenetic signature, suggesting that they originate from GC-inexperienced cells, likely pre-GC B-cells. These cases often carry the t(11;14) translocation and show absence to low levels of IGHV SHM [27]. Early during transformation, these cells show expression of SOX11 (which prevents these cells entering the germinal center) [28] and acquire mutations and extensive methylation changes with an aggressive course. In contrast, mutated MCLs(C2) show a clear epigenetic mark of the GC reaction, indicating that these cases likely originate from GC-experienced B cells. They also carry the t(11;14) but unlike C1, they lack SOX11 expression and show high levels of IGHV somatic hypermutation. C2 cases lack oncogenic mutations and acquire few epigenetic changes with an indolent clinical course. These epigenetic findings align with a transcriptional profiling study that associates cMCL with pre-GC B-cells/naive B cells and nnMCL with GC-experienced B-cells/memory B cells [27].

In addition to determining the cell of origin, DNA methylation also plays a significant role in MCL tumorigenesis, and it has been identified as a dynamic process that can be disrupted during neoplastic transformation [29]. In MCL cells, a higher DNA methylation burden, which corresponds to the accumulation of methylation changes in tumor cells, is linked to poorer clinical outcomes and an increased number of driver mutations [26]. The magnitude of these de novo hypermethylation and hypomethylation changes in cMCL is 10 times larger than in nnMCL, likely reflecting their more aggressive clinical behavior [19]. Furthermore, genomic analyses of MCL have shown that epigenetic regulators are frequently altered. The most mutated epigenetic modifier in MCL is KMT2D (17%–23%), a key regulator of transcriptional and posttranslational processes, whose mutations in this gene can affect patient prognosis [30]. Mutations in the catalytic domain of NSD2 have also been observed in cMCL, where they are associated with the overexpression of genes related to cell proliferation and the cell cycle, as well as with global chromatin methylation changes that promote oncogenic reprogramming in other lymphoid tumors [31,32]. Recently, NSD2 has been found to mediate the dimethylation of PTEN, helping recruit it to DNA-damage sites, which aids in the repair of DNA double strand breaks [33]. Additionally, alterations in SWI-SNF chromatin remodeling complexes, such as mutations in SMARCA4 (5%–12%) or deletions involving SMARCA2 (9p24) or ARID2 (12q12), have been shown to confer resistance to treatments like Ibrutinib and Venetoclax [34]. Other dysregulated epigenetic modifiers in MCL include KMT2C (5%–16%), BMI1 (6%–12%), and TET2 (5%–12%). Lastly, mutations affecting transcriptional regulators like MEF2B (3%–7%) or the posttranscriptional regulator UBR5 (7%–18%) are also recurrently found in MCL [35,36].

Waldenström's Macroglobulinemia

DNA methylome profiling of Waldenström's Macroglobulinemia (WM) has provided crucial insights into its cellular origins and the heterogeneity, revealing 2 subtypes based on the methylation signatures of memory B-cells (MBC) and plasma cells [37].

The memory B-cell (MBC) like WM subgroup shows a notable enrichment in genetic alterations such as CXCR4 mutations and 13q deletions, as well as clinical features like splenomegaly and thrombocytopenia. On the other hand, the plasma-cell(PC)-like WM subgroup is characterized by 6q deletions and 6p gains, higher usage of IGHV3 genes, increased CD38 expression, and more pronounced plasmacytic differentiation.

A comparative analysis of DNA methylation changes in normal development and WM progression revealed tumor-specific alterations, highlighting a selective reprogramming of enhancer regions in the MBC-like WM subtype and repressed and heterochromatic regions in the PC-like WM subtype. MBC-like WM exhibited hypomethylation in motifs belonging to transcription factors PU.1, TCF3, and OCT2, which involved elevated MYD88/TLR pathway activity. In contrast, PC-like WM displayed significant global hypomethylation and a selective overexpression of histone genes [37].

Follicular Lymphoma

Previous studies have suggested that follicular lymphoma (FL) may be more susceptible to methylation changes than other B-cell lymphomas [38–40]. Unsupervised hierarchical clustering showed FL separated from benign lymph node as distinct groups, and within the FL, 2 clusters were identified based on change in beta value relative to controls. However, there were no significant differences in the demographics or clinical outcome of patients including age, grade of malignancy, stage, progression free or OS between these groups. However, the study reiterated frequent aberrant tumor-specific methylation in FL in support of ongoing clinical trials of demethylating agents in FL and noted the similarities in the methylation patterns found in sequential FL and transformed-FL biopsies, along with the overrepresentation of genes targeted for epigenetic repression by PRC2 in stem cells within the hypermethylated gene set, suggesting that this widespread methylation could be an early occurrence in the development of lymphoma [41].

A recent study by Glaser and colleagues examining DNA methylation patterns (MP) in FL and diffuse large B-cell lymphoma (DLBCL) identified 2 main clusters (MP1 and MP2), predominantly composed of FL cases [42]. MP2 was characterized by an older age at diagnosis, a higher proliferation history based on the mitotic clock epigenetically determined cumulative mitoses (epiCMIT), and a greater mutational load of single nucleotide variants compared to MP1. Despite these clinical differences, both MP1 and MP2 exhibited a high frequency of BCL2 rearrangements and a predominance of the GCB subtype. Interestingly, while distinct methylation patterns were observed between MP1 and MP2, with clinical differences, RNA expression profiles were not reflective of these variations. A third cluster, MP3, which included a mix of FL, DLBCL, and FL-DLBCL, was distinguished by fewer cases with BCL2 rearrangements compared to MP1 and MP2, though it maintained a similar predominance of the GCB subtype [42].

Diffuse Large B-cell Lymphoma

In DLBCL, hypermethylation is associated with polycomb regions with no significant differences between systemic cases and those with primary central nervous system involvement [43,44]. Many studies on DLBCL have focused on the heterogeneity of its DNA methylome, as the GC acts as an (epi) mutagenic environment, leading to intense epigenetic programming [7]. This heterogeneity appears to be partly driven by the activity of AICDA [45] and is linked to poor outcomes and clonal selection during relapse [46,47]. Additionally, the degree of epigenetic variability has led to the identification of 6 distinct DLBCL epigenetic subtypes [47], though their relationship to the recently classified genetic subtypes of DLBCL [48,49] remains to be fully investigated.

One study found overall low hypermethylation in DLBCL, and DNA methylation patterns could not be used to distinguish between GCB and non-GCB DLBCL cases [50]. A recent study by Glaser and colleagues correlated MPs with the recently published epidemiologic, histopathological, transcriptomic, and genetic characteristics of FL and DLBCL [42]. The study identified 2 MPs related to FL (MP1 and MP2) and 1 intermediate MP (MP3), as previously discussed, along with 4 MPs predominantly associated with DLBCL. Among these, MP4 and MP5 primarily included cases of the GCB subtype, while MP6 and MP7 were mainly composed of ABC subtype cases. Additionally, MP4 showed the highest proportion of cases within the PIM1-like mutational cluster. MP6 was enriched for cases with MYD88 and CD79 B mutations, reflecting the C5/MCD subgroup [49,51], alongside the ABC subtype enrichment and the absence of BCL2 rearrangement. No significant differences in clinical parameters, such as stage or International Prognostic Index, were observed between the MPs, likely due to the limited power of the analysis, based on small sample sizes [42].

Burkitt Lymphoma

A study comparing FL and Burkitt lymphoma (BL) showed BL carries hypomethylation and upregulation of dark-zone specific genes, whereas FL instead shows a hypermethylation and silencing of those genes, which supports the view that BL is mostly frozen in the dark-zone state and FL in the light-zone state. The study also found negatively correlated differential methylation and gene expression in pathways associated with inflammation and immunity in BL, and with cell cycle regulation and DNA repair in FL [52].

Thomas and colleagues recently elucidated key mechanisms underlying BL pathogenesis and demonstrated that DNA methylation-based BL epitypes exhibit distinct molecular and clinical features [53]. Clustering analysis identified 2 epigenetic subgroups, termed hyperBL (cluster 1) and hypoBL (cluster 2). Principal component analysis revealed that hyperBL is positioned further along the trajectory of B-cell differentiation, suggesting a more terminally differentiated B-cell state. HyperBL exhibited greater hypermethylation, a higher prevalence of Epstein-Barr virus (EBV)-positive tumors, and significantly elevated mitotic clock estimates based on DNA methylation (epiCMIT), indicating a more extensive proliferative history. To further explore the molecular basis for these epitypes, they studied gene expression differences and distinct driver mutation patterns. The genomes of hyperBL tumors displayed an overall greater mutation burden and significantly higher mutation burden within regions affected by aberrant somatic hypermutation (aSHM), which was associated with a higher frequency of mutations attributed to the SBS9 mutational signature. Gene expression differences illustrated hypoBL tumors have upregulation of *IRF4* induced pathways. Furthermore, on survival analysis, hyperBL samples showed significantly inferior progression free survival.

These findings suggest that epigenetic changes in BL offer potential therapeutic targets [53].

Multiple Myeloma

DNA methylome analysis of MM revealed a heterogenous methylation pattern globally characterized by regional DNA hypermethylation embedded in extensive hypomethylation [54]. Unlike the well-established DNA hypermethylation of promoter-associated CpG islands (CGIs) observed in various cancers, hypermethylated regions in MM were found outside of CpG islands and, surprisingly, were linked to intronic enhancer regions typically identified in normal B cells and plasma cells. These hypermethylated enhancer regions coincided with binding sites for B cell-specific TFs, and the extent of enhancer methylation showed an inverse relationship with the expression levels of these TFs in MM. Additionally, the hypermethylated regions in MM were also methylated in stem cells and gradually underwent demethylation as B cells differentiated, suggesting that MM cells either reacquire epigenetic traits of less differentiated cells or preserve an epigenetic signature characteristic of a potential myeloma stem cell progenitor [54].

The well-defined MM cytogenetic subtypes partially show differential DNA methylation patterns, taking place in the context of a globally hypomethylated methylome [54–56]. The global DNA methylation loss increases from monoclonal gammopathy of undetermined significance (MGUS) to overt MM. Hyperdiploidy and translocations involving the immunoglobulin heavy locus appear to be associated with the highest number of DNA methylation changes, with the t(4;14) showing a specific hypermethylation signature affecting genes such as *APC*, *PAX1*, *SOC2*, or *CDKN2A* [19]. Additionally, the inactivation of tumor suppressor genes by promoter methylation is also present in MM, with hypermethylation of *GPX3*, *RBP1*, *SPARC*, and *TGFBI* associated with adverse outcomes [57].

Interestingly, MM also exhibits remethylation of B cell–specific enhancers, which may reflect the typical downregulation of the B cell–specific phenotype seen in plasma cells. This epigenetic alteration is absent in normal plasma cells but is already present in the premalignant MGUS stage [54]. Interestingly, a similar phenomenon has also been observed in classical Hodgkin lymphoma cell lines [58] and more recently in certain DLBCL patients [18], suggesting that MM may not be the only lymphoid malignancy to experience a loss of epigenetic B cell identity.

POTENTIAL OF DNA METHYLATION-BASED PROFILING AS A MITOTIC CLOCK

Initially, hypermethylation and global hypomethylation of low-CpG regions were considered nongenetic mechanisms for silencing of tumor suppressor genes [59] and chromosomal instability in cancer [60], respectively. However, subsequent research and integration with other epigenetic modifications have prompted a reevaluation of these mechanisms [61–63].

Early studies on histone modifications in stem cells revealed polycomb-repressed and bivalent chromatin domains [64], which were later associated with genes that undergo hypermethylation in cancer. This suggested a stem cell-like chromatin pattern is present, supporting the stem cell hypothesis in cancer [65–67]. A similar pattern was also observed in lymphomas, suggesting a potential link between lymphomagenesis and stem cells [68]. In these studies, polycomb-associated hypermethylation was not connected to de novo gene silencing. Instead, it was proposed that this hypermethylation reduces the epigenetic flexibility of cancer cells by replacing reversible histone modification-based repression with irreversible silencing via DNA methylation [69]. Additional findings indicated that hypermethylation in lymphomas corresponded to polycomb-repressed regions already present in normal B cells [58]. Further research demonstrated that the degree of DNA hypermethylation in CpG-rich polycomb regions was associated with cell mitosis [70], which led to the concept of using these methylation changes as a mitotic clock [71–73]. Consequently, it is not surprising that proliferating cancer cells and normal cells with extensive proliferative histories, such as postgerminal center B cells, exhibit hypermethylation of polycomb-repressed regions [7]. This hypermethylation is likely a reflection of cumulative cell proliferation, which occurs in both normal and pathologic contexts.

Concerning hypomethylation, earlier models linked it to chromosomal instability (8), but later findings suggested that DNA methylation loss in late-replicating regions accumulates progressively with cell division [74,75]. In B cells, this process occurs without chromatin instability, as cells with extensive proliferative histories—such as healthy memory B cells or plasma cells—remain hypomethylated but do not display genomic instability [7]. This global hypomethylation of late-replicating regions manifests as partially methylated domains, independent of gene expression changes. This phenomenon has been consistently observed across various cancer types, leading to the hypothesis of a hypomethylation-based mitotic clock [76,77].

A specialized mitotic clock that incorporates both DNA methylation gains and losses during cell division has been developed for normal and neoplastic B cells [10]. This mitotic clock called epiCMIT was initially developed using Illumina DNA methylation arrays and later adapted to sequencing technologies, including reduced-representation and whole-genome bisulfite sequencing [78]. This method was created by integrating both DNA methylation data and chromatin immunoprecipitation sequencing (ChIP-seq) data. Specifically, CpG sites were selected based on significant changes in their methylation levels during B cell maturation and their mapping to regions that are constitutively polycomb-repressed and heterochromatic. Two separate scores were then calculated—one reflecting hypermethylation and the other hypomethylation. These scores showed a strong correlation in normal B cells, as well as in MCL, CLL, and DLBCL [19]. This observation corroborated an earlier study in colorectal cancer, which indicated a correlation between the degree of hypermethylation and hypomethylation [79].

This finding may imply that the DNA methylation increases in polycomb-repressed regions and decreases in heterochromatin typically occur simultaneously during cell division. However, the authors noted that this pattern may not be universal. For example, in B-ALL, hypermethylation predominantly occurs in polycomb-repressed regions, while in MM, hypomethylation is more common in heterochromatic regions [10]. The precise mechanisms behind this difference remain unclear, but it suggests that the stage of tumor cell maturation may influence whether DNA methylation gains or losses happen during cell division. To address this variability, the authors developed a single epiCMIT score by selecting the higher of the 2 values (hypermethylation or hypomethylation). Unlike static markers such as Ki67, which reflect current proliferation status, this mitotic clock provides a cumulative readout of all factors—both intrinsic (eg, genetic changes) and extrinsic (eg, environmental influences)—that drive cell proliferation.

During normal B cell maturation, epiCMIT increases as the cells mature, correlating with known bursts of proliferation at specific stages. For instance, it sharply rises in GCBs and reaches its peak in terminally differentiated plasma cells, which, while nonproliferative, retain the entire proliferative history of the B-cell lineage within their DNA methylome. In cancer cells, the epiCMIT reflects both the proliferative history of the original cell and the additional proliferation related to malignant transformation and tumor progression. In B-ALL, which originates from precursor B cells with minimal prior proliferation, epiCMIT primarily represents leukemic proliferation. In contrast, mature lymphoid tumors like CLL or MM show a significant contribution from the proliferation history of the normal precursor cells. Specifically, in CLL, naive-like/low-programmed CLLs display a lower epiCMIT than memory-like/high-programmed CLLs, indicating their less mature origin. Notably, epiCMIT is linked to disease progression, showing an increase from precursor stages to overt cancer, such as from monoclonal B cell lymphocytosis to CLL, or from MGUS to MM, and from diagnosis to progression, relapses, and high-grade transformation (eg, Richter's transformation, RT) [10,80]. Thus, when the cell of origin is constant, the epiCMIT serves as a robust and independent prognostic factor for clinical outcomes in B-ALL, CLL, and MCL [10,78,80]. These results suggest that the proliferative history of cancer cells could be used to predict future cell proliferation and patient outcomes. Importantly, the epiCMIT mitotic clock has recently been validated in a variety of normal and cancerous cell types [77], supporting its broader applicability beyond the hematopoietic system.

DNA METHYLATION-BASED CLASSIFICATION OF MATURE B-CELL NEOPLASMS

From a diagnostic standpoint, several studies have developed accurate DNA methylation-based classifiers for various B-cell tumor types and their subtypes, achieving mean sensitivities greater than 90%, which surpasses sensitivities reported for other molecular alterations [19]. In small B-cell lymphomas, a set of only 26 CpGs can accurately differentiate between CLL, MCL, FL, and marginal zone lymphoma [81]. Another study analyzing over 2,000 DNA methylomes from different B-cell tumors created and validated a 2-step classifier using 56 CpGs. The first step classifies major B cell tumor types, including B-ALL, MCL, DLBCL, CLL, and MM, while the second step identifies subtypes within these entities, ultimately categorizing 14 different B-cell tumor subtypes in a single assay [10]. Furthermore, with the use of unsupervised nonnegative matrix factorization methods a recent study identified 300 CpGs in DNA from cryopreserved FL and DLBCL that categorize these lymphomas into subgroups and shows that the selected CpG modules and DNA methylation profiles also have the potential to differentiate others, like BL and nonmalignant B-cell populations [42].

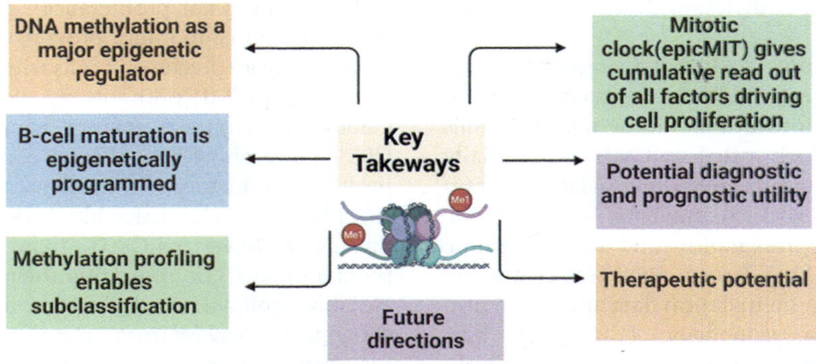

FIG. 1 Overview of key insights into DNA methylation-based profiling in B-cell lymphomas presented herein (*Created in* BioRender. Desai, P. (2025) https://BioRender.com/d365x4y.)

POTENTIAL ADVANTAGES OF DNA METHYLATION-BASED CLASSIFICATION

Employing DNA methylation-based categorization offers highly attractive features. The detection of specific methylation patterns in mature B-cell neoplasms may be of particular interest, especially for those that lack a pathognomonic genetic alteration. DNA methylation patterns of a tumor are relatively stable throughout tumor progression compared to some other *omics* technologies like gene expression profiling making it a promising tool for tumor classification and identification. While there is some evidence suggesting some changes in tumor progression [82], experience with methylation classifiers show high concordances between matched primary-recurrent tumor pairs in the same patient [83].

Moreover, DNA methylation is a robust technique that can be performed on DNA extracted from formalin-fixed paraffin-embedded tissues, which are commonly available in clinical settings. A variety of specimens including surgical excisions and/or core biopsies can be used for DNA methylation profiling, if sufficient DNA is obtainable. Additionally, since the DNA methylome remains stable in circulating free DNA [84,85], it opens up the possibility of using epigenetic biomarkers for liquid biopsies to diagnose and monitor lymphoid tumors, including those without leukemic presentations [86].

Furthermore, the digital nature of methylation data facilitates easy data exchange and the aggregation of large tumor libraries. This could pave the way for multi-institutional collaborations, advancing our understanding of tumor biology and enabling the identification of exceptionally rare tumor types that may only be recognized through the aggregation of individual cases across multiple institutions.

POTENTIAL CLINICAL APPLICATIONS OF DNA METHYLATION-BASED PROFILING IN MATURE B-CELL NEOPLASMS

While DNA methylation-based classification has already entered clinical practice for several solid tumor types [87,88], its application in hematolymphoid neoplasms is still in the emerging stages. Genome wide methylation-based classification represents a novel and promising method for tumor classification with the potential to complement genetic classifications in prognostic models, particularly for tumor types with low frequencies of recurrent mutations [1].Future studies, leveraging artificial intelligence and machine learning could follow a similar roadmap to those established for solid tumors to enhance DNA methylation-based classification in hematolymphoid tumors.

Notably, various B-cell cancers exhibit frequent genetic alterations in key components of the epigenetic machinery, such as critical histone acetyltransferases and methyltransferases [89]. These tumor-specific epigenetic patterns could serve to complement genetic data, facilitating the development of epigenetic therapies. In the future, epigenetic information may be used for individualized therapy [1]. For example, CLL patients who maintain stronger B-cell receptor (BCR) signaling tend to respond better to BCR inhibition [90]. These patients exhibit a DNA methylation pattern indicative of hyperactivity of Nuclear factor of activated T-cells (NFAT) transription factor family [20], suggesting that identifying this signature in other B-cell malignancies could help identify those likely to benefit from similar treatments. Additionally, the extensive epigenetic changes observed in MCL suggest that patients could benefit from epigenetic therapies [91]. However, the observed epigenetic heterogeneity in MCL may affect therapeutic efficacy, and this could be considered when stratifying patients [26]. Recently, a range of new therapies have been approved or are under investigation for WM. Many of these therapies show promise for other B-cell lymphomas and MM, including proteasome inhibitors, immunomodulatory drugs, histone deacetylase inhibitors, anti-CD38 monoclonal antibodies, and other novel agents [37].The MBC-like WM subtype exhibits an elevated MYD88-associated gene expression signature, suggesting that targeting the TLR pathway, potentially using JAK/STAT or IRAK-specific inhibition [92], may show added benefit in MBC-like WM.

SUMMARY AND FUTURE DIRECTIONS

In all, epigenetics, including DNA methylation in mature B-cell neoplasms, offers a wide array of clinical applications, from powerful diagnostic and prognostic biomarkers to novel therapeutic targets (Fig. 1). Beyond DNA methylation, there is an increasing focus on mapping other epigenetic markers, such as histone modifications, chromatin accessibility, and the three-dimensional structure of chromatin [19,93]. Furthermore, studying intratumor epigenetic variability and subclonal architecture using single-cell technologies may offer valuable insights for prognosis and treatment monitoring [1]. Combining these approaches is expected to enhance our understanding of B-cell neoplasms' biology and pave the way for new clinical applications.

CLINICS CARE POINTS

- DNA methylation profiling in mature B-cell neoplasms offers key insights into their cell of origin, pathogenic drivers, and paths of evolution.
- Epigenetic signatures and biomarkers show promise to serve as robust diagnostic and prognostic tools, with the potential to complement genetic studies in clinical hematopathology.
- DNA methylation-based profiling in mature B-cell neoplasms deepens our understanding of tumor biology and facilitates the development of novel clinical applications that exploit tumor-specific epigenetic features.

DISCLOSURES

The authors have nothing to disclose.

REFERENCES

[1] Oakes CC, Martin-Subero JI. Insight into origins, mechanisms, and utility of DNA methylation in B-cell malignancies. Blood 2018;132(10):999–1006.
[2] Jones PA, Baylin SB. The fundamental role of epigenetic events in cancer. Nat Rev Genet 2002;3(6):415–28.
[3] Laisń M, Lupien M, Vallot C. Epigenomic heterogeneity as a source of tumour evolution. Nat Rev Cancer 2025; 25(1):7–26.
[4] Alaggio R, Amador C, Anagnostopoulos I, et al. The 5th edition of the world health organization classification of haematolymphoid tumours: lymphoid neoplasms. Leukemia 2022;36(7):1720–48.
[5] Campo E, Jaffe ES, Cook JR, et al. The international consensus classification of mature lymphoid neoplasms: a report from the clinical advisory committee. Blood 2022;140(11):1229–53.
[6] Alizadeh AA, Eisen MB, Davis RE, et al. Distinct types of diffuse large B-cell lymphoma identified by gene expression profiling. Nature 2000;403(6769):503–11.
[7] Kulis M, Merkel A, Heath S, et al. Whole-genome fingerprint of the DNA methylome during human B cell differentiation. Nat Genet 2015;47(7):746–56.
[8] Martin-Subero JI, Oakes CC. Charting the dynamic epigenome during B-cell development. Semin Cancer Biol 2018;51:139–48.
[9] Hoadley KA, Yau C, Hinoue T, et al. Cell-of-Origin patterns dominate the molecular classification of 10,000 tumors from 33 types of cancer. Cell 2018;173(2): 291–304.e6.
[10] Duran-Ferrer M, Clot G, Nadeu F, et al. The proliferative history shapes the DNA methylome of B-cell tumors and predicts clinical outcome. Nat Cancer 2020;1(11): 1066–81.
[11] Stadler MB, Murr R, Burger L, et al. DNA-binding factors shape the mouse methylome at distal regulatory regions. Nature 2011;480(7378):490–5.
[12] Kreibich E, Kleinendorst R, Barzaghi G, et al. Single-molecule footprinting identifies context-dependent regulation of enhancers by DNA methylation. Mol Cell 2023;83(5):787–802.e9.
[13] Kulis M, Heath S, Bibikova M, et al. Epigenomic analysis detects widespread gene-body DNA hypomethylation in chronic lymphocytic leukemia. Nat Genet 2012;44(11): 1236–42.
[14] Wedge E, Hansen JW, Garde C, et al. Global hypomethylation is an independent prognostic factor in diffuse large B cell lymphoma. Am J Hematol 2017;92(7): 689–94.
[15] Kipps TJ, Stevenson FK, Wu CJ, et al. Chronic lymphocytic leukaemia. Nat Rev Dis Primers 2017;3:16096. https://doi.org/10.1038/nrdp.2016.96.
[16] Queiros AC, Villamor N, Clot G, et al. A B-cell epigenetic signature defines three biologic subgroups of chronic lymphocytic leukemia with clinical impact. Leukemia 2015;29(3):598–605.

[17] Nadeu F, Royo R, Clot G, et al. IGLV3-21R110 identifies an aggressive biological subtype of chronic lymphocytic leukemia with intermediate epigenetics. Blood 2021; 137(21):2935–46.
[18] Duran-Ferrer M, Mansouri L, Nadeu F, et al. A comprehensive DNA methylome analysis of stereotyped and non-stereotyped CLL reveals an epigenetic signature with strong clinical impact encompassing IGHV status, stereotypes and IGLV3-21r110. Blood 2022;140:1800–2.
[19] Duran-Ferrer M, Martín-Subero JI. Epigenomic characterization of lymphoid neoplasms. Annu Rev Pathol 2024;19:371–96.
[20] Oakes CC, Seifert M, Assenov Y, et al. DNA methylation dynamics during B cell maturation underlie a continuum of disease phenotypes in chronic lymphocytic leukemia. Nat Genet 2016;48(3):253–64.
[21] Tsagiopoulou M, Papakonstantinou N, Moysiadis T, et al. DNA methylation profiles in chronic lymphocytic leukemia patients treated with chemoimmunotherapy. Clin Epigenetics 2019;11(1):177.
[22] Cahill N, Bergh AC, Kanduri M, et al. 450K-array analysis of chronic lymphocytic leukemia cells reveals global DNA methylation to be relatively stable over time and similar in resting and proliferative compartments. Leukemia 2013;27(1):150–8.
[23] Landau DA, Clement K, Ziller MJ, et al. Locally disordered methylation forms the basis of intratumor methylome variation in chronic lymphocytic leukemia. Cancer Cell 2014;26(6):813–25.
[24] Claus R, Lucas DM, Stilgenbauer S, et al. Quantitative DNA methylation analysis identifies a single CpG dinucleotide important for ZAP-70 expression and predictive of prognosis in chronic lymphocytic leukemia. J Clin Oncol 2012;30(20):2483–91.
[25] Navarro A, Bè S, Jares P, et al. Molecular pathogenesis of mantle cell lymphoma. Hematol Oncol Clin North Am 2020;34(5):795–807.
[26] Queirs AC, Beekman R, Vilarrasa-Blasi R, et al. Decoding the DNA methylome of mantle cell lymphoma in the light of the entire B cell lineage. Cancer Cell 2016; 30(5):806–21.
[27] Navarro A, Clot G, Royo C, et al. Molecular subsets of mantle cell lymphoma defined by the IGHV mutational status and SOX11 expression have distinct biologic and clinical features. Cancer Res 2012;72(20):5307–16.
[28] Palomero J, Vegliante MC, Eguileor A, et al. SOX11 defines two different subtypes of mantle cell lymphoma through transcriptional regulation of BCL6. Leukemia 2016;30(7):1596–9.
[29] Rane SU, Shet T, Sridhar E, et al. Interobserver variation is a significant limitation in the diagnosis of Burkitt lymphoma. Indian J Med Paediatr Oncol 2014;35(1): 44–53.
[30] Ferrero S, Rossi D, Rinaldi A, et al. KMT2D mutations and TP53 disruptions are poor prognostic biomarkers in mantle cell lymphoma receiving high-dose therapy: a FIL study. Haematologica 2020;105(6):1604–12.
[31] Oyer JA, Huang X, Zheng Y, et al. Point mutation E1099K in MMSET/NSD2 enhances its methyltranferase activity and leads to altered global chromatin methylation in lymphoid malignancies. Leukemia 2014; 28(1):198–201.
[32] Valds-Mas R, Bea S, Puente DA, et al. Estimation of copy number alterations from exome sequencing data. PLoS One 2012;7(12):e51422. https://doi.org/10.1371/journal.pone.0051422.
[33] Zhang J, Lee YR, Dang F, et al. PTEN methylation by NSD2 controls cellular sensitivity to DNA damage. Cancer Discov 2019;9(9):1306–23.
[34] Agarwal R, Chan YC, Tam CS, et al. Dynamic molecular monitoring reveals that SWI-SNF mutations mediate resistance to ibrutinib plus venetoclax in mantle cell lymphoma. Nat Med 2019;25(1):119–29.
[35] Bè S, Valds-Mas R, Navarro A, et al. Landscape of somatic mutations and clonal evolution in mantle cell lymphoma. Proc Natl Acad Sci U S A 2013;110(45):18250–5.
[36] Meissner B, Kridel R, Lim RS, et al. The E3 ubiquitin ligase UBR5 is recurrently mutated in mantle cell lymphoma. Blood 2013;121(16):3161–4.
[37] Roos-Weil D, Giacopelli B, Armand M, et al. Identification of 2 DNA methylation subtypes of Waldenström macroglobulinemia with plasma and memory B-cell features. Blood 2020;136(5):585–95.
[38] Guo J, Burger M, Nimmrich I, et al. Differential DNA methylation of gene promoters in small B-cell lymphomas. Am J Clin Pathol 2005;124(3):430–9.
[39] Rahmatpanah FB, Carstens S, Guo J, et al. Differential DNA methylation patterns of small B-cell lymphoma subclasses with different clinical behavior. Leukemia 2006;20(10):1855–62.
[40] Taylor KH, Kramer RS, Davis JW, et al. Ultradeep bisulfite sequencing analysis of DNA methylation patterns in multiple gene promoters by 454 sequencing. Cancer Res 2007;67(18):8511–8.
[41] O'Riain C, O'Shea DM, Yang Y, et al. Array-based DNA methylation profiling in follicular lymphoma. Leukemia 2009;23(10):1858–66.
[42] Glaser S, Fischer A, Martínez-Manjn JE, et al. Subgrouping germinal center-derived B-cell lymphomas based on machine learning-deduced DNA methylation modules. Leukemia 2025. https://doi.org/10.1038/s41375-025-02533-6.
[43] Vogt J, Wagener R, Montesinos-Rongen M, et al. Array-based profiling of the lymphoma cell DNA methylome does not unequivocally distinguish primary lymphomas of the central nervous system from non-CNS diffuse large B-cell lymphomas. Genes Chromosomes Cancer 2019;58(1):66–9.
[44] Richter J, Ammerpohl O, Martín-Subero JI, et al. Array-based DNA methylation profiling of primary lymphomas of the central nervous system. BMC Cancer 2009;9:455.
[45] Teater M, Dominguez PM, Redmond D, et al. AICDA drives epigenetic heterogeneity and accelerates germinal

center-derived lymphomagenesis. Nat Commun 2018; 9(1):222.
[46] Pan H, Jiang Y, Boi M, et al. Epigenomic evolution in diffuse large B-cell lymphomas. Nat Commun 2015;6: 6921.
[47] Chambwe N, Kormaksson M, Geng H, et al. Variability in DNA methylation defines novel epigenetic subgroups of DLBCL associated with different clinical outcomes. Blood 2014;123(11):1699–708.
[48] Wright GW, Huang DW, Phelan JD, et al. A probabilistic classification tool for genetic subtypes of diffuse large B cell lymphoma with therapeutic implications. Cancer Cell 2020;37(4):551–68.e14.
[49] Chapuy B, Stewart C, Dunford AJ, et al. Molecular subtypes of diffuse large B cell lymphoma are associated with distinct pathogenic mechanisms and outcomes. Nat Med 2018;24(5):679–90.
[50] Carlund O, Thörn E, Osterman P, et al. Semimethylation is a feature of diffuse large B-cell lymphoma, and subgroups with poor prognosis are characterized by global hypomethylation and short telomere length. Clin Epigenetics 2024;16(1):68.
[51] Schmitz R, Wright GW, Huang DW, et al. Genetics and pathogenesis of diffuse large B-cell lymphoma. N Engl J Med 2018;378(15):1396–407.
[52] Kretzmer H, Bernhart SH, Wang W, et al. DNA methylome analysis in Burkitt and follicular lymphomas identifies differentially methylated regions linked to somatic mutation and transcriptional control. Nat Genet 2015; 47(11):1316–25.
[53] Thomas ND, Harris NL, Irvin JD, et al. DNA methylation-based Burkitt lymphoma epitypes have distinct molecular and clinical features. Blood 2022; 140:1734–6.
[54] Agirre X, Castellano G, Pascual M, et al. Whole-epigenome analysis in multiple myeloma reveals DNA hypermethylation of B cell-specific enhancers. Genome Res 2015;25(4):478–87.
[55] Walker BA, Wardell CP, Chiecchio L, et al. Aberrant global methylation patterns affect the molecular pathogenesis and prognosis of multiple myeloma. Blood 2011;117(2):553–62.
[56] Choudhury SR, Ashby C, Tytarenko R, et al. The functional epigenetic landscape of aberrant gene expression in molecular subgroups of newly diagnosed multiple myeloma. J Hematol Oncol 2020;13(1):108.
[57] Kaiser MF, Johnson DC, Wu P, et al. Global methylation analysis identifies prognostically important epigenetically inactivated tumor suppressor genes in multiple myeloma. Blood 2013;122(2):219–26
[58] Ammerpohl O, Haake A, Pellissery S, et al. Array-based DNA methylation analysis in classical Hodgkin lymphoma reveals new insights into the mechanisms underlying silencing of B cell-specific genes Leukemia 2012; 26(1):185–8.
[59] Esteller M. Epigenetics in cancer. N Engl J Med 2008; 358(11):1148–59.
[60] Eden A, Gaudet F, Waghmare A, et al. Chromosomal instability and tumors promoted by DNA hypomethylation. Science 2003;300(5618):455.
[61] Luo C, Hajkova P, Ecker JR. Dynamic DNA methylation: in the right place at the right time. Science 2018;361(6409):1336–40.
[62] Jones PA. Functions of DNA methylation: islands, start sites, gene bodies and beyond. Nat Rev Genet 2012; 13(7):484–92.
[63] Mattei AL, Bailly N, Meissner A. DNA methylation: a historical perspective. Trends Genet 2022;38(7):676–707.
[64] Lee TI, Jenner RG, Boyer LA, et al. Control of developmental regulators by Polycomb in human embryonic stem cells. Cell 2006;125(2):301–13.
[65] Schlesinger Y, Straussman R, Keshet I, et al. Polycomb-mediated methylation on Lys27 of histone H3 pre-marks genes for de novo methylation in cancer. Nat Genet 2007;39(2):232–6.
[66] Widschwendter M, Fiegl H, Egle D, et al. Epigenetic stem cell signature in cancer. Nat Genet 2007;39(2):157–8.
[67] Ohm JE, McGarvey KM, Yu X, et al. A stem cell-like chromatin pattern may predispose tumor suppressor genes to DNA hypermethylation and heritable silencing. Nat Genet 2007;39(2):237–42.
[68] Martín-Subero JI, Kreuz M, Bibikova M, et al. New insights into the biology and origin of mature aggressive B-cell lymphomas by combined epigenomic, genomic, and transcriptional profiling. Blood 2009;113(11): 2488–97.
[69] Gal-Yam EN, Egger G, Iniguez L, et al. Frequent switching of Polycomb repressive marks and DNA hypermethylation in the PC3 prostate cancer cell line. Proc Natl Acad Sci U S A 2008;105(35):12979–84.
[70] Beerman I, Bock C, Garrison BS, et al. Proliferation-dependent alterations of the DNA methylation landscape underlie hematopoietic stem cell aging. Cell Stem Cell 2013;12(4):413–25.
[71] Teschendorff AE. A comparison of epigenetic mitotic-like clocks for cancer risk prediction. Genome Med 2020;12(1):56.
[72] Yang Z, Wong A, Kuh D, et al. Correlation of an epigenetic mitotic clock with cancer risk. Genome Biol 2016;17(1):205.
[73] Youn A, Wang S. The MiAge Calculator: a DNA methylation-based mitotic age calculator of human tissue types. Epigenetics 2018;13(2):192–206.
[74] Landan G, Cohen NM, Mukamel Z, et al. Epigenetic polymorphism and the stochastic formation of differentially methylated regions in normal and cancerous tissues. Nat Genet 2012;44(11):1207–14.
[75] Aran D, Toperoff G, Rosenberg M, et al. Replication timing-related and gene body-specific methylation of active human genes. Hum Mol Genet 2011;20(4): 670–80.
[76] Zhou W, Dinh HQ, Ramjan Z, et al. DNA methylation loss in late-replicating domains is linked to mitotic cell division. Nat Genet 2018;50(4):591–602.

[77] Endicott JL, Nolte PA, Shen H, et al. Cell division drives DNA methylation loss in late-replicating domains in primary human cells. Nat Commun 2022;13(1):6659.
[78] Knisbacher BA, Lin Z, Hahn CK, et al. Molecular map of chronic lymphocytic leukemia and its impact on outcome. Nat Genet 2022;54(11):1664–74.
[79] Berman BP, Weisenberger DJ, Aman JF, et al. Regions of focal DNA hypermethylation and long-range hypomethylation in colorectal cancer coincide with nuclear lamina-associated domains. Nat Genet 2011;44(1):40–6.
[80] Nadeu F, Royo R, Massoni-Badosa R, et al. Detection of early seeding of Richter transformation in chronic lymphocytic leukemia. Nat Med 2022;28(8):1662–71.
[81] Xia D, Leon AJ, Yan J, et al. DNA methylation-based classification of small B-cell lymphomas: a proof-of-principle study. J Mol Diagn 2021;23(12):1774–86.
[82] Li S, Garrett-Bakelman FE, Chung SS, et al. Distinct evolution and dynamics of epigenetic and genetic heterogeneity in acute myeloid leukemia. Nat Med 2016;22(7):792–9.
[83] Pajtler KW, Witt H, Sill M, et al. Molecular classification of Ependymal tumors across all CNS compartments, histopathological grades, and age groups. Cancer Cell 2015;27(5):728–43.
[84] Shen SY, Singhania R, Fehringer G, et al. Sensitive tumour detection and classification using plasma cell-free DNA methylomes. Nature 2018;563(7732):579–83.
[85] Moss J, Magenheim J, Neiman D, et al. Comprehensive human cell-type methylation atlas reveals origins of circulating cell-free DNA in health and disease. Nat Commun 2018;9(1):5068.
[86] Roschewski M, Rossi D, Kurtz DM, et al. Circulating tumor DNA in lymphoma: principles and future directions. Blood Cancer Discov 2022;3(1):5–15.
[87] Capper D, Jones DTW, Sill M, et al. DNA methylation-based classification of central nervous system tumours. Nature 2018;555(7697):469–74.
[88] Koelsche C, Schrimpf D, Stichel D, et al. Sarcoma classification by DNA methylation profiling. Nat Commun 2021;12(1):498.
[89] Lunning MA, Green MR. Mutation of chromatin modifiers; an emerging hallmark of germinal center B-cell lymphomas. Blood Cancer J 2015;5(10):e361. https://doi.org/10.1038/bcj.2015.89.
[90] Byrd JC, Furman RR, Coutre SE, et al. Targeting BTK with ibrutinib in relapsed chronic lymphocytic leukemia. N Engl J Med 2013;369(1):32–42.
[91] Fiskus W, Rao R, Balusu R, et al. Superior efficacy of a combined epigenetic therapy against human mantle cell lymphoma cells. Clin Cancer Res 2012;18(22):6227–38.
[92] Ni H, Shirazi F, Baladandayuthapani V, et al. Targeting myddosome signaling in Waldenström's macroglobulinemia with the interleukin-1 receptor-associated kinase 1/4 inhibitor R191. Clin Cancer Res 2018;24(24):6408–20.
[93] Beekman R, Chapaprieta V, Russiñol N, et al. The reference epigenome and regulatory chromatin landscape of chronic lymphocytic leukemia. Nat Med 2018;24(6):868–80.

SECTION: SOLID TUMORS

Advances in Molecular Pathology 8 (2025) 53–68
ADVANCES IN MOLECULAR PATHOLOGY

Emerging Biomarkers in Non–small Cell Lung Cancer

ERBB2 and *MET* Amplifications

Benjamin A. Bleiberg, MD[a], Melina E. Marmarelis, MD[a], Salvatore F. Priore, MD, PhD[b,*]
[a]Division of Hematology-Oncology, Department of Internal Medicine, Hospital of the University of Pennsylvania, Philadelphia, PA, USA; [b]Division of Precision and Computational Diagnostics, Department of Pathology and Laboratory Medicine, Hospital of the University of Pennsylvania, Philadelphia, PA, USA

KEYWORDS
• Gene amplification • Targeted therapy • Non–small cell lung cancer • ERBB2 • MET

KEY POINTS

- Multiple techniques exist to assess gene copy number gain (immunohistochemistry, fluorescence in situ hybridization (FISH), and next-generation sequencing), each with advantages and limitations relevant to interpreting patient results.
- Clinically relevant gene amplification does not have a universal definition and is based on clinical trial data demonstrating meaningful prognostic or therapeutic benefits.
- FISH remains the gold standard for identifying clinically relevant *ERBB2* and *MET* gene amplifications.
- Patients with progression on targeted therapy can benefit from repeat molecular profiling to evaluate for emergent copy number gain in genes such as *ERBB2* and *MET*.
- Ongoing trials of combinations of tyrosine kinase inhibitors, bispecific antibodies, and antibody drug conjugates are underway to improve clinical outcomes for patients with ERBB2 and *MET* amplifications.

INTRODUCTION

The accumulation of extra copies of genes above the usual diploid complement in a cell is a common occurrence in cancer and is mediated by multiple complex biological processes. This phenomenon is referred to as gene copy number gains (CNG), which is often used interchangeably with the term gene amplification. However, there are many important caveats to consider when defining exactly what constitutes a clinically significant gene amplification. This review article will review the concept of gene CNG, the diagnostic techniques available to assess them, and the implications of gene amplifications in the treatment of non–small cell lung cancer (NSCLC).

CNG can occur in either a chromosomal (chrDNA) or extrachromosomal (ecDNA) context (Fig. 1). Polysomy occurs when the gene and the chromosome where the gene is located duplicate together to maintain a 1:1 ratio of the gene and the corresponding centromere. A gene can also duplicate in a tandem fashion on a single chromosome, resulting in variable copies of the gene tied to a single corresponding centromere. Repetitive tandem duplications can form a homogeneously staining region (HSR). ecDNA are small circular pieces of

*Corresponding author. Division of Precision and Computational Diagnostics, Department of Pathology and Laboratory Medicine, Hospital of the University of Pennsylvania, 3400 Spruce Street, Philadelphia, PA 19104-4238. *E-mail address:* Salvatore.priore@pennmedicine.upenn.edu

https://doi.org/10.1016/j.yamp.2025.07.003 www.advancesinmolecularpathology.com
2589-4080/25/ © 2025 Elsevier Inc. All rights are reserved, including those for text and data mining, AI training, and similar technologies.

ABBREVIATIONS

chrDNA	chromosomal DNA
CNG	copy number gain
DCR	disease control rate
ecDNA	extrachromosomal DNA
ERBB	erythroblastic leukemia oncogene B
FFPE	formalin fixed paraffin embedded
FISH	fluorescence in situ hybridization
HER	human epidermal growth factor receptor
HSR	homogeneous staining region
IHC	immunohistochemistry
mDOR	median duration of response
MET	MET proto-oncogene
mOS	median overall survival
mPFS	median progression-free survival
NGS	next-generation sequencing
NSCLC	non–small cell lung cancer
ORR	objective response rate
OS	overall survival
TKI	tyrosine kinase inhibitor

DNA that contain the target gene but not a centromere. ecDNA may undergo autonomous replication and multiply to create hundreds of copies within a cell [1,2].

chrDNA gene amplification will replicate along with the chromosome and distribute into daughter cells during mitosis by disjunction. ecDNA sequences are centromere-independent and will distribute into daughter cells in a heterogenous fashion during mitosis. Diagnostically, it is important to appreciate how these different mechanisms create dramatically different conditions within each cell as well as the uniformity of CNG across the tumor cell population. The following sections will address different techniques for assessing CNG and discuss how the underlying biology can affect detection and interpretation of test results.

Techniques for Assessing Gene Copy Number Gains

Multiple techniques are available to detect gene CNG. Fluorescence in situ hybridization (FISH) works by using large fluorescently labeled DNA probes that are complementary to the gene sequence of interest. In

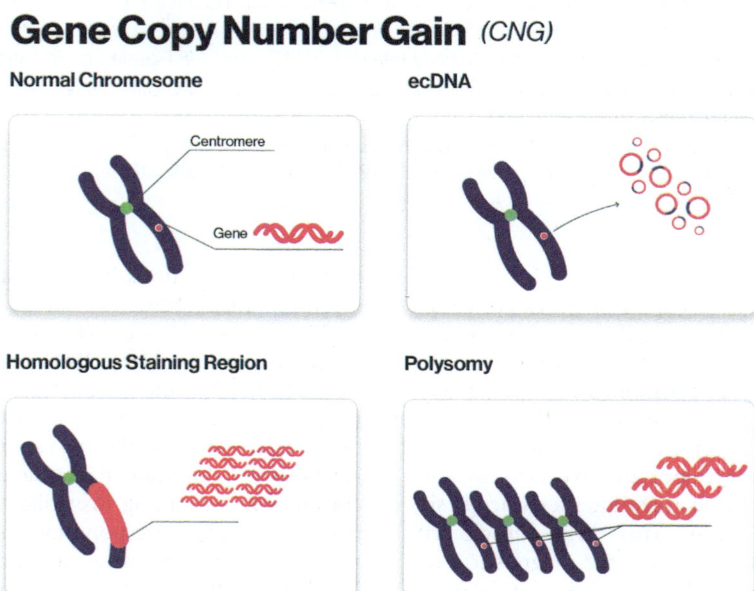

FIG. 1 The biology of CNG is complex and a very simplified overview is provided here. A normal metaphase chromosome has one unique copy of a gene and is associated with the centromere of its chromosome. As the cell divides, the gene travels in conjunction with the rest of the chromosome. Chromosomes can increase the copies of a gene as polysomy, with replication of the whole chromosome, or just the gene and surrounding regions, forming a homologous staining region. When extra copies of a gene are acquired outside of a chromosome, the gene and variable amounts of nearby sequence are copied and circularized as ecDNA, which replicate and segregate independently of chromosomes during cell division.

addition, using a different colored probe, FISH can also highlight the centromere of a chromosome of interest in the same reaction. In this way, both the total copies and the ratio of a gene to centromere can be assessed, providing an indication of the underlying mechanism of the CNG (Fig. 2). Polysomy would maintain the 1:1 ratio of centromeres to gene signals. Amorphous or widely dispersed staining for the gene may indicate ecDNA CNG. HSR are usually more discrete areas of staining, often forming signal clusters. Both ecDNA and HSR maintain an uneven and variable number of genes to centromere signals compared to polysomy [3,4].

Genomic tests using next-generation sequencing (NGS) typically detect DNA sequence changes like single nucleotides variants, insertions, and deletions. However, CNG can be detected as well if the test is designed for this purpose. For an NGS test that is run with stable performance capabilities (number of read generating samples, identical flow cell capacity, etc) the typical depth of sequencing at any given genomic locus is predictable with some amount of variation. For example, let's say that running DNA from a normal population of cells yields 100 sequencing reads at a given genomic position α. This cell population has 2 copies of genomic position α (1 on each chromosome) that contribute to the 100 reads. If we then sequence a tumor cell population that has 3 copies of genomic position α, we reasonably expect a total sequencing death of 150 reads in that sample (Fig. 3). This increase in sequencing reads above the normal baseline can be converted to a copy number estimate for the tumor sample [5].

Finally, immunohistochemistry (IHC) is a surrogate for CNG by assessing the expression of a specific gene product. Formalin fixed tissue slides are treated with conjugated antibodies to a specific protein and then treated with a special dye that highlights the bound antibody complex. The intensity of the staining can indicate the level of protein expression in each cell. The location of the staining (nuclear, cytoplasmic, membranous) is also important information that is conveyed by IHC staining (Fig. 4). IHC is used as a surrogate for *ERBB2* amplification, and has well-established rules for interpretation [6].

While RNA expression profiling is also a potential method to assess gene amplification, it is not widely used in the clinical laboratory setting currently.

Advantages and Limitations of Testing Methods

NGS is a useful technology that can provide mutational profiling and copy number changes in cancer in a single test. However, not all NGS tests are built the same and some do no assess CNG or only assess it for a limited set of genes. There are general guidelines for

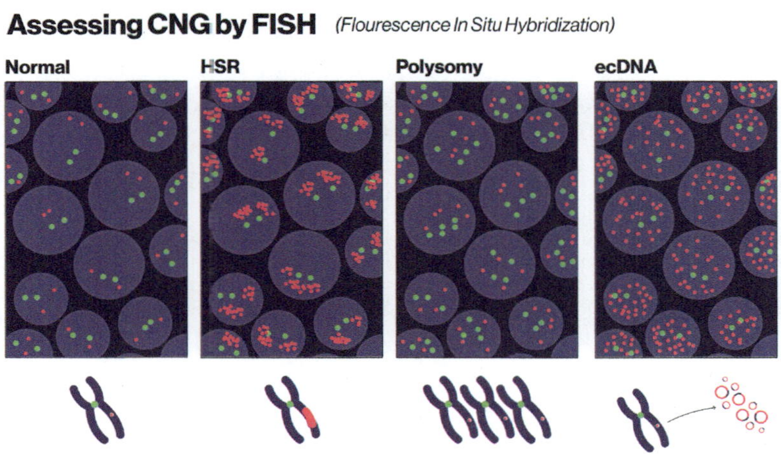

FIG. 2 Interphase FISH for CNG is commonly assessed on interphase cells using a fluorescent probe designed to target a gene (*red color*) and its corresponding chromosome's centromere (*green color*). A normal diploid cell will have 2 gene signals and 2 centromere signals. An HSR typically shows large well-formed clusters of gene staining. Polysomy will acquire gene signals in direct portion to centromere signals. Finally, ecDNA will show dispersed signals throughout the cell. The type of staining pattern, the actual numbers of gene signals, and the ratio of gene to centromere signals will vary between different tumor samples.

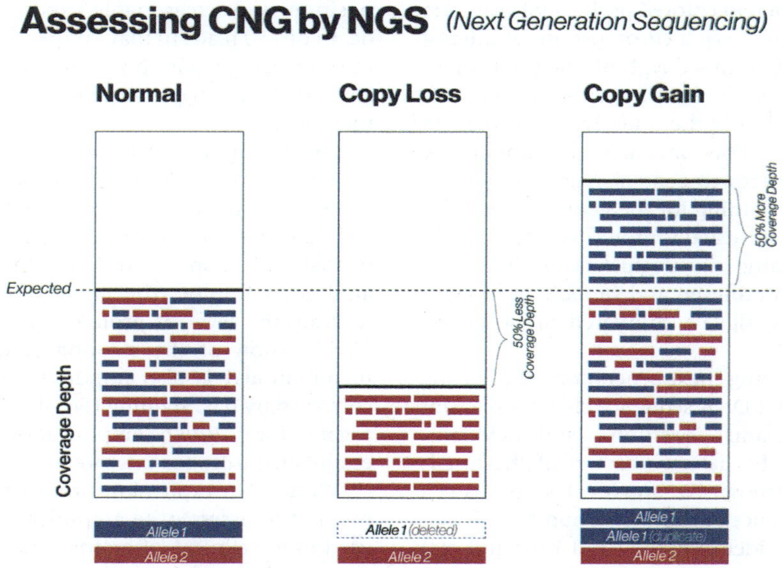

FIG. 3 A common technique to assess CNG by NGS is through read depth normalization. In a normal sample, each genomic locus has 2 alleles contributing to the total number of sequencing reads. In a tumor that loses or gains a copy of a gene, depicted here as a loss or gain of a single allele, you would expect a proportionate decrease and increase in the total number of sequencing reads, respectively. An NGS test needs to be specifically designed and validated for this specialized type of variant calling.

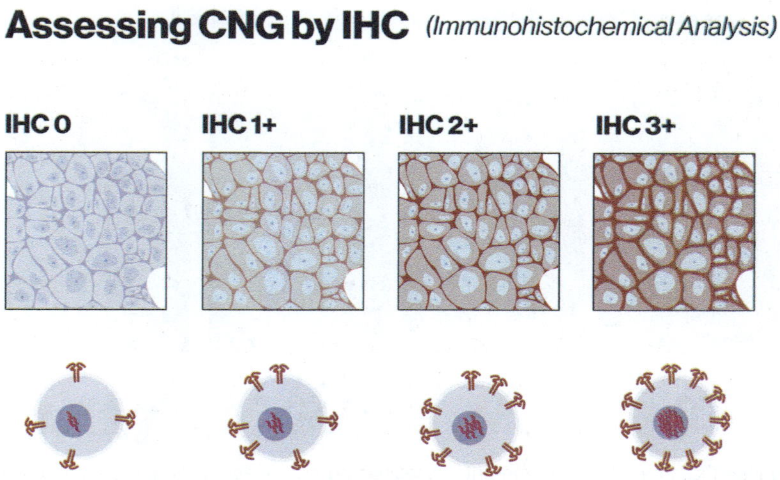

FIG. 4 IHC is commonly used as a surrogate for gene CNG by assessing the expression of the protein it encodes. A normal cell population with little or no protein expression will show minimal staining. As the amount of protein expression increases, the intensity of IHC staining increases. Certain genes, like *ERBB2*, have well established criteria for grading IHC staining that correlate well with clinical response to targeted therapies. The location of staining (eg, membranous for receptor tyrosine kinases like ERBB2) is an important part of the evaluation of IHC patterns.

the validation of NGS tests, but variability in how CNG detection is implemented and interpreted in different NGS tests is common [7,8]. While some tests may specifically label CNG as amplifications, it is critical that clinical providers understand how the test infers CNG and what validated cutoff they use to make a call of a gene amplification. These cutoffs and methods may differ substantially from what is clinically actionable based on clinical trial data, as described in this review for lung cancer. An individual tests cutoff may be based on literature for a specific tumor type (eg, breast cancer), may vary by gene, or apply tumor agnostic or universal cutoffs. Consult with your local laboratory molecular professionals, if available, to understand the characteristics of the test they offer and how you can best interpret results for your specific patient population. Reference laboratories can also be consulted, although the amount of detail they are willing to share about proprietary assays may be more limited.

In addition to technical considerations, biological properties of the tumor specimen are important including quality and tumor purity, especially when assessing a negative gene amplification result. NGS samples are almost always a mixture of normal and tumor cells in variable proportions. As noted above, the degree of amplification and the distribution of amplification across the tumor population can be quite heterogeneous (Fig. 5A). Since most clinical NGS is an ensemble technique this level of detail is not ascertainable from the data. However, as a rule, the lower the tumor percentage, the higher the likelihood of a false negative gene amplification result. Again, understanding the validated limits of a test is critical as some NGS tests will not even assess CNG if the tumor is reported to have less than a certain percentage of tumor cells (Fig. 5B). Some NGS tests will also try to adjust for tumor percentage when making copy number calls. At lower tumor percentages, this may increase the number of true positives but also may increase the number of false positives. Tests that employ tumor percentage corrections can also be subject to errors if the imputed percentage is not representative of the true tumor percentage [9].

FISH allows for a more detailed assessment of gene amplification since the gene and centromere signals can be specifically enumerated. While FISH has the advantage of being a single-cell technique, it requires a specialized skill set to analyze the fluorescent signal patterns and distinguish tumor cells from normal cells to ensure that an adequate number of tumor cells have been assessed. Interpretation of FISH results can also vary, and it is important to understand what cutoffs a particular laboratory may use for calling amplification. For example, if a FISH laboratory simply reports amplification as detected or not detected and does not provide a centromere to gene copy number ratio, you may have to specifically discuss the results with the laboratory to ensure that the cutoffs employed are relevant to your patient population (ie, lung cancer vs breast cancer for *ERBB2* FISH). There are technical issues that can contribute to false positive and false negative results when using FISH. Formalin fixed paraffin embedded (FFPE) tissue can suffer from DNA degradation and cut artifacts, which can lead to erroneous signals. The amount of background signal for a FISH probe will determine whether a specific sample has enough tumor cellularity to appreciate a true positive result. Fresh cell preparations can provide an alternative to FFPE but must be carefully validated as degradation of cells can lead to false positive results [10].

Finally, IHC can be one of the more challenging methods for assessing gene amplification. Since protein expression and stability can be influenced by many factors, including cold ischemia time (ie, time from procurement to fixation), under and over fixation in formalin, and excessive variations in environmental factors like temperature. IHC uses antibodies directed at specific protein epitopes, and different clones are available for the same protein that target different epitopes [11]. Thus, an understanding of variation in results and interpretation for a given probe is critical. Differences in IHC antibodies from laboratory to laboratory should be noted when comparing results. Even under optimal conditions, the interpretation of IHC staining is subjective and can suffer from problems of intraobserver variability. Careful attention must be given to having adequate control tissue for IHC staining efficiency and training for assessing IHC preparations in a consistent manner. Finally, as this surrogate has worked well for some targets (eg, *ERBB2*), it has proven not to be a robust clinical correlate to therapy response for other targets, including the *MET* proto-oncogene [12].

Thus far, we have provided an overview of CNG and associated testing methodologies. The rest of the article will discuss the major completed and ongoing clinical trials in NSCLC that are targeting gene amplifications along with the methods and cutoffs employed, and a summary of how gene amplifications impact patient management and prognosis.

Gene Amplification in Non–small Cell Lung Cancer

Clinical case

A 53-year-old man who presents with back pain, found to have metastatic nonsquamous NSCLC with disease in

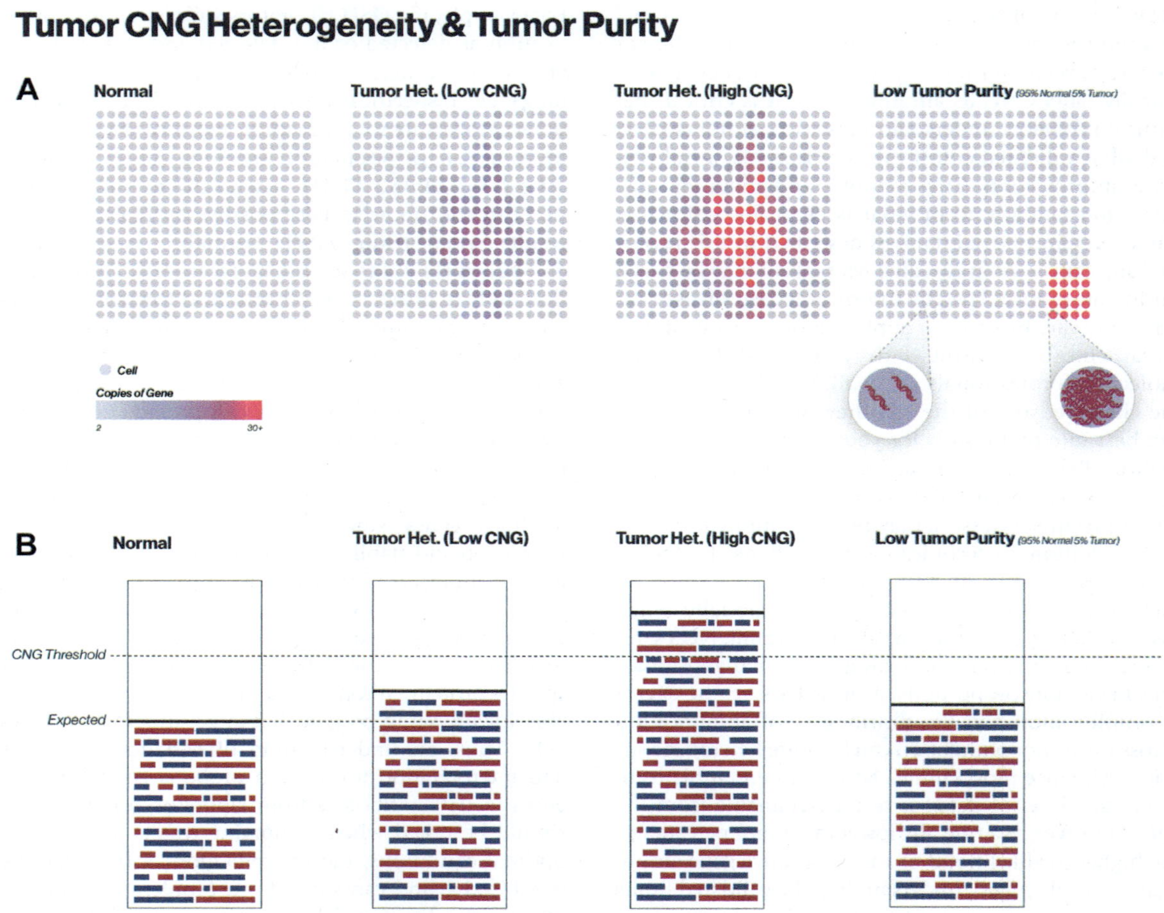

FIG. 5 (*A*) A normal cell population has 2 copies of a gene per cell at any given locus. When extra copies of genes are accumulated, this can occur in a very heterogenous fashion. The 2 examples shown here depict how even extensive CNG throughout a cell population can be modest (low CNG) versus more extensive (high CNG). Even when CNG is high, the mixture of tumor and normal cells can vary between tumor samples. (*B*) When using ensemble techniques, like NGS, for evaluating CNG, both tumor heterogeneity and tumor purity can influence detection rates. For any validated CNG threshold for an NGS test, tumors with low CNG heterogeneity or low tumor purity are more likely to give false negative results.

his lung, lymph nodes and bone. Tumor profiling by NGS on tissue at the time of diagnosis revealed no actionable alterations. PDL1 level was 90%. He was started on single-agent pembrolizumab with good response to therapy. Unfortunately, he developed pneumonitis after 10 months on treatment requiring steroids and cessation of immunotherapy. He remained off anticancer treatment for 4 months before he experienced disease progression in the lung. Rebiopsy of the growing area in the lung again revealed no actionable molecular alterations by NGS, but human epidermal growth factor receptor 2 (HER2) IHC staining was 3+. He was started on a HER2 antibody drug conjugate as second-line treatment.

ERBB2 alteration background and detection

The *ERBB* family of genes, encodes the HER family of transmembrane tyrosine kinases that are associated with tumorigenesis. Alterations in this family of genes can lead to constitutive cell proliferation [13,14]. Originally discovered in the 1980s, Slamon and colleagues [15] (1987) appreciated significant HER2 overexpression in 30% of breast cancer pathology samples. Overexpression was associated with lower patient survival time and shorter time to relapse. These alterations are highly prevalent in metastatic breast cancer with 20% to 30% of patients in both clinical trials and real-world registries testing positive for HER2 overexpression by IHC [16]. A greater understanding of HER2 signaling has demonstrated that HER2 signaling alterations can be triggered both by gene amplifications and somatic activating mutations [2,17]. Targeted therapies directed against HER2 alterations have been a breakthrough in the management of advanced breast, gastrointestinal, and ovarian cancers, leading to some of the most efficacious therapies available to patients with these malignancies. The initial studies of HER2-directed therapies such as the monoclonal antibody trastuzumab included patients based on IHC expression levels. IHC is scored from 0 to 3 by subjective grading of the degree of staining of the tumor-cell membrane [18]. Initial trials of HER2 directed therapies selected patients based on IHC 2+ or 3+ scoring [19]. However, subsequent studies demonstrated the efficacy of HER2 directed therapies even in patients with lower levels of IHC expression. FISH identification of *ERBB2* amplifications was used as an adjunctive pathologic marker to predict responsiveness to HER2-directed targeted therapy in patients with lower HER2 IHC staining levels [20]. Recent studies have identified a preserved response to treatment in breast cancer even in HER2 *ultra-low* cases where there is IHC >0 and <1+ membrane staining, suggesting that HER2 expression levels measured by IHC alone do not adequately predict the likelihood of response to HER2-directed therapy [21].

ERBB2 in non–small cell lung cancer

HER2 overexpression can be present at diagnosis or emerge as a resistance mechanism to other therapies in NSCLC [22]. Given the limited options available to patients with advanced NSCLC who progress beyond first-line targeted and chemo-immunotherapies, trastuzumab was studied as a possible second-line agent. However, multiple phase 2 trials of trastuzumab in advanced NSCLC failed to demonstrate a clinical benefit compared to or in combination with chemotherapy, even in patients with IHC 2+ and 3+ confirmed evidence of HER2 overexpression [23–25]. Future studies demonstrated that identifying *ERBB2* amplification and activating mutations, which can be detected by FISH or NGS, better predicted responses to HER2-directed therapy for NSCLC patients. However, the definition of clinically significant amplifications is variable and often trial dependent. Additionally, gene amplification identified by FISH does not always correlate with HER2 IHC expression and FISH is considered more sensitive than NGS for detecting amplifications, particularly when biopsy samples contain low tumor content (<20% viable tumor) [14]. *ERBB2* amplifications are identified in approximately 3% to 4% of treatment-naïve patients with nonsquamous NSCLC, but account for up to 10% of acquired resistance mutations to tyrosine kinase inhibitors (TKIs) used for the targeted therapy of other actionable genetic alterations [26]. Treatment emergent *ERBB2* amplifications are estimated to be responsible for up 2% of progression events for patients treated with third generation *EGFR* inhibitors [27].

Targeted therapies for ERBB2 amplifications

Despite the limitations of IHC in predicting response to HER2-directed therapies in NSCLC, the greatest recent breakthrough in HER2 targeted therapies was identified in the phase 2 DESTINY-PanTumor02 study. This trial demonstrated a clinical benefit of trastuzumab deruxtecan across a range of solid malignancies (including NSCLC) for patients with HER2 overexpression on IHC [28]. A sample of 75 patients with a heterogeneous mix of solid tumors and 3+ HER2 IHC treated with trastuzumab deruxtecan experienced a 61.3% objective response rate (ORR) with a median progression-free survival (mPFS) of 11.9 months and median overall survival (mOS) of 21.1 months [28]. This finding led to a tumor agnostic approval for trastuzumab deruxtecan in patients with HER2 IHC of 3+, reintroducing the clinical relevance of HER2 IHC in evaluating therapeutic options for patients with NSCLC.

While gene amplifications and activating mutations are both associated with tumorigenesis, they are associated with varying responses to HER2-directed therapies [2,17]. A phase 2 trial of the antibody drug conjugate trastuzumab emtansine identified patients by HER2 IHC 2+ or 3+ with NSCLC after progression on first line systemic therapy [29]. Only 4 patients of 49 participants enrolled, experienced a partial response (20% of the IHC 3+ cohort) and mPFS and mOS even in the IHC 3+ subgroup was only 2.6 months and 15.3 months, respectively. However, FISH testing of the 4 partial responders identified that 3 had *ERBB2* amplifications (defined by an *ERBB2*/CEP17 gene ratio ≥2) and NGS testing identified that 2 had a CNG greater than or equal to 5 [29]. This data provided further support for pursuing studies that selected patients based on *ERBB2* amplifications and activating mutations.

Evolving understanding of the importance of *ERBB2* activating mutations and amplifications in predicting response to HER2 directed therapies in NSCLC led to the international, open-label, single-arm, phase 2 DESTINY-Lung01 trial [30]. This trial enrolled patients with advanced NSCLC refractory to standard first-line treatment and with activating *ERBB2* mutations or gene amplifications and overexpression [30]. Responses to single-agent trastuzumab-deruxtecan, an antibody drug conjugate linking a *HER2* directed monoclonal antibody with a topoisomerase inhibitor chemotherapy payload, were robust considering the pretreated population. Primary and secondary endpoints of the trial included an ORR of 55% (95% CI 44%–65%), mPFS of 8.2 months (95% CI 6.0–11.9 months) and mOS of 17.8 months (95% CI 13.8–22.1 months) [30]. A subset analysis of 22 patients specifically with *ERBB2* amplifications identified by FISH (*ERBB2/CEP17* ratio ≥2.0) was reported to have preserved antitumor activity in the second line setting, but specific outcomes data were not published [30]. While future research is needed to determine the role for HER2 directed antibody drug conjugates in the first-line management of patients with *ERBB2* amplifications, this trial demonstrated their efficacy in the second line and later management of patients with advanced NSCLC [30].

Oral agents targeting HER2 alterations are currently being evaluated in clinical trials. The phase 1 Beamion-LUNG-1 trial evaluated the efficacy of Zongertinib, an oral HER2-directed TKI in pretreated patients with HER2 overexpression by IHC (2+/3+), activating *ERBB2* amplifications or activating mutations by NGS [31]. Preliminary data from a cohort of 24 patients with *ERBB2* amplifications, or overexpression without activating mutations, demonstrated an ORR of 33% and disease control rate (DCR) of 83%. A 36 patient cohort including patients with *ERBB2* activating mutations had a median duration of response (mDOR) of 12.7 months and a mPFS of 8.7 months, representing a potential oral targeted therapy for NSCLC with *ERBB2* alterations [31,32]. However, the phase 3 follow-up trial Beamion-LUNG-2 includes only patients with activating *ERBB2* alterations [33]. The phase 3 SOHO-02 trial assessing the efficacy of an oral reversible HER2 directed TKI in the first line setting for patients with advanced NSCLC also only includes patients with activating *ERBB2* alterations [34]. It remains to be seen if these TKIs will play a role in the treatment of patients with *ERBB2* amplifications.

Clinical case

A 55-year-old woman who presented with persistent cough, found to have metastatic nonsquamous NSCLC with disease in the lungs bilaterally. Liquid biopsy revealed an *EGFR* exon 19 deletion without other actionable alterations. MRI of the brain was negative for intracranial disease. She was started on osimertinib 80 mg daily and achieved an excellent partial response. After 12 months on osimertinib she experienced multifocal disease progression in the lung and chemotherapy was added. One year later, she experienced disease progression again in the lung. Bronchoscopic biopsy revealed lung adenocarcinoma, and molecular testing showed the same EGFR exon 19 deletion. Tissue-based NGS revealed *MET* CNG of 14 and *MET* FISH showed innumerable copies of *MET* with 4 to 15 copies of CEP7 in 90 of 100 cells evaluated (nuc ish(D7Z1x4-15,MET amp)[90/100]). Capmatinib at half dose was added to osimertinib, and she achieved a partial response that continues after 1.5 years of additional follow up.

MET alteration background and detection

The *MET* factor receptor or the MNNG HOS transforming gene on chromosome 7 encodes the c-MET protein, which is a receptor tyrosine kinase involved in tumor angiogenesis and metastasis. The primary actionable genetic alterations appreciated in patients with *MET*-dysregulated NSCLC are *MET* exon 14 skipping mutations and *MET* amplifications, which cooccur in 7.6% to 13.8% of cases [35]. Early studies of MET-directed TKIs identified de novo gene amplifications in 1% to 6% of cases [36,37]. FISH remains the reference standard technique for the detection of *MET* amplifications though other techniques including next-generation sequencing (NGS) and quantitative real-time polymerase chain reaction have been utilized. High-level *MET* amplifications have classically been defined by the Cappuzzo criteria as a CNG greater than or equal to 5 [38]. Clinical trials have generally defined MET amplification as *MET*/CEP7 ratio greater than or equal to 2 or CNG per cell greater than or equal to 5 to 6 by FISH, though there is notable variation between trials [39,40]. A series of 37 patients with *MET* dysregulations identified by FISH (CNG ≥6) found that the identification of FISH positive *MET* alterations was associated with a response to MET-directed TKIs in 82% of cases [41]. Further, the TATTON trial comparing identification of *MET* amplifications with FISH to tissue NGS demonstrated a negative-percent agreement of 98%, but a positive-percent agreement of 88% [42]. Xiang and colleagues [43] (2024) assessed 130 cases of *MET* amplification positive NSCLC identified by FISH and 101 negative controls study and using cutoffs of CNG greater than or equal to 5 and *MET*/CEP7 greater than or equal to 2 and found 79.2% concordance of *MET* amplification identification between NGS and FISH. These combined results cemented FISH as the gold standard for identifying *MET* amplifications and predicting responsiveness to MET-directed therapies. However, in clinical practice, the authors of several of these studies recommended ongoing use of FISH, IHC, and NGS for the evaluation of actionable genetic alterations in NSCLC patients, both to rule out cooccurring alterations and to optimize the likelihood of detecting a clinically relevant *MET* alteration [42].

Targeted therapies in de novo MET amplifications

Trials evaluating MET-directed therapies in *MET* amplified NSCLC have had mixed results, partially due to inconsistent definitions of MET amplification and differing methods of detection (FISH, IHC, NGS). The landmark phase 2, GEOMETRY mono-1 trial evaluated the efficacy of capmatinib, a selective MET TKI for patients with advanced NSCLC and *MET* alterations [37]. High-level *MET* amplifications were defined by a CNG greater than or equal to 10. Patients with *MET* amplifications experienced modest responses (ORR = 7% and mPFS = 4.1 and 4.2 months for previously treated and treatment naïve patients respectively). Though this trial led to the FDA approval of capmatinib for patients with *MET* exon 14 skipping mutations, the *MET* amplification arm was closed due to an ORR below the prespecified threshold for clinical activity on interim analysis (Wolf and colleagues, 2024) [37]. The PROFILE 1001 trial of crizotinib, identified a sub-group of patients with *MET* amplifications determined by FISH (MET/CEP7 $\geq$1.8, with CNG $\geq$4 considered high level amplification) [44]. Patients with high-level *MET* amplifications demonstrated a 38.1% ORR, mDOR of 5.2 months, and mPFS or 6.7 months [44]. However, the trial again demonstrated a diminished response to TKIs for patients with *MET* amplifications identified by FISH compared to those with *MET* exon 14 skipping mutations and sparked efforts to utilize novel therapeutics including bispecific antibodies and antibody drug conjugates to achieve better clinical outcomes.

Amivantamab , an EGFR-MET bispecific antibody, was shown in preclinical studies to block ligand-receptor binding in cell lines with *MET* amplifications [45]. The phase 1 CHRYSALIS trial demonstrated a promising ORR of 33% and mPFS of 6.7 months in a largely pretreated cohort of patients with *MET* exon 14 skipping mutations [45]. However, the results from the planned *MET* amplification cohort have not been reported, leaving the only published evidence of clinical efficacy of amivantamab in this context limited to case reports [46,47]. The phase 2 LUMINOSITY trial evaluated the clinical efficacy of telisotuzumab vedotin, a MET-directed antibody drug conjugate with a tubulin inhibitor chemotherapy payload in patients with non-squamous NSCLC with c-MET overexpression and *EGFR* wild-type status, including those with *MET* amplifications [48]. Patients were included based on IHC greater than or equal to 25% of tumor cells with membrane staining at 3+ intensity and less than or equal to 2 lines of previous systemic therapy. Telisotuzumab vedotin yielded an ORR of 28.6%, mPFS of 5.7 months, and mOS of 14.5 months and was not approved by the FDA [48]. Phase 1 data from the LUMINOSITY trial demonstrated an ORR of 80% in a 10-patient subgroup with *MET* amplifications identified by FISH (*MET*/CEP7 $\geq$1.8), but a planned phase 2 expansion trial of patients with *MET* amplifications identified by FISH enrolled only 9 of a planned 70 patients and results have not been presented [49]. The ongoing METalmark trial of amivantamab and capmatinib for patients with NSCLC and *MET* amplifications or exon 14 skipping mutations is currently undergoing safety and dose-escalation testing and is so far well-tolerated in phase 1b testing [50]. This combination represents a promising future therapeutic option for patients with *MET* amplifications backed by strong preclinical data [45].

Targeted therapies for treatment-emergent MET amplifications

While the previously noted studies have established the challenges of utilizing targeted therapies for the management of de novo *MET* amplifications, research has demonstrated that *MET* amplifications are a key driver of resistance to EGFR-directed TKIs. An estimated 6% to 22% of patients who progress following treatment with third-generation EGFR-directed TKIs are found to have treatment emergent *MET* amplifications. [40,51]. The ORCHARD trial by Yu and colleagues [52] in 2021 and FLAURA trial by Ramalingan and colleagues [53] in 2022 identified *MET* amplifications by NGS in 16% and 15%, respectively, of patients with *EGFR* mutant, advanced NSCLC who progressed on first-line osimertinib. Therefore, targeting *MET* by TKI or bispecific antibody is of great interest in this patient population.

The phase 2 INSIGHT trial evaluated the clinical efficacy of adding tepotinib, a MET-targeting TKI, versus transitioning to chemotherapy for patients with *EGFR*-mutant p.T790 M negative NSCLC who

GENE AMPLIFICATION TRIAL SUMMARY TABLE

Author (Year)	Cohort (Phase)	Trial Identifier – Line of Therapy	Study Population (*ERBB2* Amplification Subgroup)	*ERBB2* Amplification Criteria	Intervention and Comparator	Endpoints	Findings
HER2-directed trials							
Lara et al, [23] 2004	Phase 2	2L+	13 (2 with centrally confirmed amplifications)	*IHC:* 2+/3+	Trastuzumab ± Docetaxel	1° ORR 2° EFS, OS	ORR trastuzumab alone: 0% EFS: 4.3 mo OS: 5.7 mo
Zinner et al, [25] 2004	Phase 2	1L	21	*IHC:* ≥1 *ELISA:* ≥ 15 ng/mL HER2 antigen shed	Single-arm: Cisplatin and gemcitabine D1 + D8 then trastuzumab – single arm	1° ORR 2° 1-y survival	ORR: 38% 1-y survival: 62%
Krug et al, [24] 2005	Phase 2	1L	64	*IHC*: 2+/3+	Single arm: Docetaxel/ paclitaxel and trastuzumab - single arm	1° ORR 2° mOS	ORR: 23% docetaxel and trastuzumab and 32% paclitaxel and trastuzumab mOS: 16 mo and 14 mo
Peters et al, [29] 2019	Phase 2	NCT02289833 -2L+	49	*IHC*: 2+/3+	Single-arm: Trastuzumab-emtansine	1° ORR 2° DOR, CBR, PFS, OS	ORR: 20% IHC 3+ and 0% IHC 2+ PFS: 2.6 vs 2.7 mo (IHC 2+ vs 3+) mOS 12.2 vs 15.3 mo (IHC 2+ vs 3+)
Smit et al, [30] 2024	DESTINY-Lung01: Phase 2	NCT03505710 -2L+	49 (22 with amplifications)	*FISH*: *HER2*/ CEN17 ratio ≥2	Single arm: Trastuzumab deruxtecan	1° ORR 2° PFS, OS	ORR: 55% PFS: 8.2 mo OS: 17.8 mo
Meric-Bernstam et al, [28] 2024	DESTINY-PanTumor02: Phase 2	NCT04482309 -2L+	267 (amplifications not specified)	*IHC*: 2+ or 3+	Single arm: Trastuzumab deruxtecan	1° ORR 2° DOR, PFS, OS	ORR IHC 2+ or 3+: 37.1% IHC 3+ subgroup (N = 75): DOR: 11.3 mo mPFS: 6.9 mo mOS: 13.4 mo
Heymach et al, [31] 2024	Beamion-LUNG-1: Phase 1b	NCT04886804 – 2L+	66 (17 with amplifications)	*IHC:* 2+ or 3+ *FISH:* not published	Single arm: Zongertinib (BID vs QD)	1° ORR 2° DCR PFS	ORR with IHC overexpression: 39% DCR with IHC overexpression: 83%

	Lung04: Phase 3		ongoing	amplifications excluded, mutations identified by NGS	deruxtecan vs investigator's choice chemotherapy	2° OS, ORR, DOR	

***MET* Amplification Trials**

Author (Year)	Cohort (Phase)	Trial Identifier	Study Population (*MET* Amplification Subgroup)	*MET* Amplification Criteria	Intervention and Comparator	Endpoints	Findings
De Novo MET amplification trials							
Wolf et al, [37] 2024	GEOMETRY mono-1: Phase 2	NCT02414139 – 2L+	364 (210 *amplification)* Advanced NSCLC	*FISH:* CNG ≥5	Single arm: Capmatinib	1° ORR 2° DOR, DCR, PFS	ORR for CNG≥10: 29% previously treated and 40% treatment naive
Camidge et al, [44] 2021	PROFILE 1001: Phase 2	NCT00585195 – 1L	38	*FISH: MET*/CEP7 ratio ≥1.8	Single arm: Crizotinib	1° ORR 2° DOR, PFS	ORR: 28.9% (38.1% in *MET*:CEP7 ≥4) PFS: 6.7 mo (in *MET*:CEP7 ≥4)
Camidge et al, [48] 2024	LUMINOSITY: Phase 2	NCT03539536 – 2L+	172 (4 with *MET* amplification)	*FISH: MET*/CEP7 ratio ≥1.8	Single arm: Telisotuzumab vedotin	1° ORR 2° DOR, PFS	ORR: 28.6% mPFS: 5.7 mo mOS: 14.5 mo
Spira et al, (ongoing)	METalmark: Phase 1/2	NCT05488314 – 2L+	18 (2) advanced NSCLC line >1	Not specified	Amivantamab and capmatinib	1° Safety	Ongoing
Treatment Emergent *MET* Amplification Trials							
Wu et al, [54] 2020	INSIGHT: Phase 2	NCT01982955 – 2L+	55 (19 with *MET* amplifications)	*FISH:* CNG ≥5 and/or MET/CEP7 ≥2	Tepotinib + gefitinib vs Platinum doublet chemotherapy (after progression on gefitinib)	1° PFS 2° OS, Safety	MET amplification subgroup: mPFS: 16.6 vs 4.2 mo (HR = 0.13) mOS: 37.3 vs 13.1 mo (HR = 0.08) Favoring tepotinib + gefinitinb over chemo

(continued on next page)

(continued)

MET Amplification Trials

Author (Year)	Cohort (Phase)	Trial Identifier	Study Population (*MET* Amplification Subgroup)	*MET* Amplification Criteria	Intervention and Comparator	Endpoints	Findings
Hartmaier et al, [43] 2023	TATTON: Phase 1b	NCT02143466 – 2L+	120 (40 with centrally confirmed *MET* amplification)	*FISH:* CNG ≥5 and/or MET/CEP7 ≥2 *NGS:* ≥20% tumor cells, ≥5 CNG	Single arm: Savolitinib plus osimertinib	1° ORR 2° DCR	ORR for previously treated with osi: 31% ORR for treatment naïve: 70%
Cho et al, [45] 2023	CHRYSALIS: Phase 1	NCT02609776 – 2L+	45 (5 with *MET* amplifications)	*NGS:* CNG ≥ 3	Single arm: Amivatinimab	1° ORR 2° DOR, mPFS	ORR: 36% (60% for MET amplification subgroup) mPFS: 4.9 mo (6.7 in *EGFR* and *MET* resistance subgroup = 17) mDOR: 9.6 mo
Besse et al, [56] 2023	CHRYSALIS-2: Phase 1b	NCT04077463 – 2L+	77 (28 with *MET* overexpression)	*IHC:* 3+ on ≥25% of tumor cells	Single arm	1° ORR 2° PFS	ORR: 61% vs 12% favoring *MET*+ mPFS: NR vs 4.1 mo favoring *MET*+
Wu et al, [55] 2024	INSIGHT2: Phase 2	NCT03940703 – 2L+	128 (98 with centrally confirmed *MET* amplifications)	*FISH:* CNG ≥5 and/or MET/CEP7 ≥2 *cfDNA NGS:* ≥2.3	Tepotinib vs platinum + pemetrexed (after progression on first line osimertinib)	1° ORR 2° DOR, Safety	ORR = 50% Grade ≥3 TRAE's: 13%
Wu et al, [59] 2022	GEOMETRY-E: Phase 3	NCT04816214 – 2L+	Planned 225 patient enrollment	Not specified	Capmatinib + osimertinib vs platinum + pemetrexed	1° PFS 2° ORR, OiRR, DOR	Ongoing

Abbreviations: cfDNA, cell-free DNA; DOR, duration of response; EFS, event free survival; OiRR, overall intracranial response rate.

progressed on gefitinib and were found to have *MET* amplifications [54]. *MET* amplification was defined by a CNG ≥5 or MET/CEP7 ≥2 by FISH. The combination of gefitinib and tepotinib was well-tolerated. An exploratory subgroup analysis of 19 patients with confirmed *MET* amplifications demonstrated an mPFS of 16.6 versus 4.2 months and mOS of 37.3 versus 13.1 months favoring gefitinib and tepotinib over chemotherapy [54]. Unfortunately, the study was terminated early due to low recruitment. However, the larger 98-patient phase 2 INSIGHT2 trial evaluating the addition of tepotinib to osimertinib (after progression on EGFR TKI monotherapy) versus platinum-doublet chemotherapy, demonstrated a favorable 50% ORR with similar criteria for centrally confirmed *MET* amplifications by FISH (CNG ≥5, MET/CEP ratio ≥2) or NGS (CNG ≥2.3) [55]. INSIGHT2 trial participants generally tolerated the combination of tepotinib and osimertinib well, with only 13% experiencing grade greater than or equal to 3 adverse events. However, 4 patients (3%) died on treatment due to pneumonitis that was potentially related to treatment, noting a potential synergistic toxicity to monitor when combining EGFR and MET directed TKIs [55].

The MET-EGFR bispecific antibody, amivantamab, has also been successfully utilized in this context. The CHRYSALIS trial evaluated the efficacy of amivantamab in patients with advanced *EGFR* mutant NSCLC following progression on osimertinib [45]. Of 17 patients with *EGFR* or *MET* based mechanisms of resistance to osimertinib, amivantamab demonstrated a 47% ORR with a mPFS of 6.7 months [45]. These data led to the FDA approval of amivantamab in advanced *EGFR* mutant NSCLC following progression on a third-generation TKI. Notably of the 5 patients with *MET* amplifications, the ORR was 60% with one patient experiencing a complete response [45]. The phase 1b CHRYSALIS-2 study of osimertinib-relapsed, chemotherapy naïve patients treated with amivantamab identified 28 patients with *MET* overexpression by IHC (defined as ≥ 25% of tumor cells) [56]. This trial found that patients with *MET* overexpression treated with amivantamab had a significantly higher ORR (61% vs 12%) and longer mPFS (not reached vs 4.1 months) than patients without evidence of *MET* overexpression on IHC [56]. Interestingly, detection of MET-based resistance to osimertinib by NGS was not as good a predictor of response to amivantamab as detection of *MET* amplification [45,56]. Taken together, these findings suggest that amivantamab may be particularly effective in managing emergent *MET* amplifications for patients treated with *EGFR* directed TKIs.

In the real world setting, a single-institution retrospective case series of 12 patients with treatment emergent *MET* amplifications (CNG ≥3 on FISH), while on osimertinib managed with the addition of capmatinib experienced a 58% ORR and no grade greater than or equal to 3 toxicities. This cohort when pooled with 6 patients with *MET* overexpression by IHC had a mPFS of 18.1 months [57]. A larger multi-institutional retrospective cohort of patients with acquired *MET* resistance mutations to EGFR, ALK, and ROS1-directed TKIs found the mechanism of resistance in 90% (37 of 41) patients was a *MET* amplification [58]. Patients were then treated with MET-directed TKIs or chemotherapy and those treated with TKIs were found to have a significantly higher ORR (69.2% vs 20%) without a significant difference in progression-free survival (PFS) (5 vs 6 months) or overall survival (OS) (13 vs 11 months). There was no significant difference in adverse events or clinical outcomes between the MET inhibitors utilized (crizotinib, tepotinib, capmatinib) [6]. These retrospective studies demonstrate the clinical utility and tolerability of this TKI combination approach.

CLINICS CARE POINTS

- Gene copy number gain is a biologically heterogeneous process that drives cancer emergence, progression, and therapy resistance.
- Multiple techniques exist to directly or indirectly assess gene copy number gain such as IHC, FISH, and NGS. Each technique has advantages and limitations that are important to appreciate when ordering and interpreting patient test results.
- While the terms CNG and gene amplification are often used interchangeably, clinically relevant gene amplification does not have a universal definition and is based on clinical trial data demonstrating meaningful prognostic or therapeutic benefits.
- FISH remains the gold standard for identifying clinically relevant *ERBB2* and *MET* amplifications.
- IHC expression of HER2 is not a reliable predictor of responsiveness to HER2 directed therapies (other than trastuzumab deruxtecan) in NSCLC, but the identification of activating somatic mutations and *ERBB2* amplifications has been shown to predict response.
- Patients with progression on targeted therapies can benefit from repeat molecular profiling on tissue to evaluate for treatment emergent resistance alterations in targetable genes such as *ERBB2* and *MET*.

- Patients found to have *MET* amplifications while on treatment with *EGFR*-directed TKIs can effectively be managed with the addition of MET-directed TKIs or use of bispecific antibodies.
- Ongoing trials of combinations of TKIs, bispecific antibodies, and antibody drug conjugates are underway to improve clinical outcomes for patients with *MET* and *ERBB2* amplifications and these patients should be considered for clinical trials if eligible.

ACKNOWLEDGMENTS

The authors would like to thank Dr Jacqueline J Roth for her expertise and kind feedback on this article. Figures for this review were commissioned and produced by Tage Reinhart of Skimra Design Services.

DISCLOSURE

B.A. Bleiberg reports a consulting role with Janssen Pharmaceuticals. M.E. Marmarelis reports research funding from Eli Lilly (Inst), AstraZeneca, United Kingdom (Inst), Merck, United States (Inst), Genentech (Inst) consulting role with AstraZeneca, Novocure, Boehringer Ingelheim, Janssen, Takeda, Blueprint Pharmaceuticals, Bayer, Bristol Myers Squibb, Ikena, Regeneron, Daiichi Sankyo, Neuvogen; Honorarium from Thermo Fisher; Stock Merck, Johnson & Johnson. S.F. Priore has nothing to disclose.

REFERENCES

[1] Tanaka H, Watanabe T. Mechanisms underlying recurrent genomic amplification in human cancers. Trends Cancer 2020;6(6):462–77.
[2] Yi Z, Rong G, Guan Y, et al. Molecular landscape and efficacy of HER2-targeted therapy in patients with HER2-mutated metastatic breast cancer. npj Breast Cancer 2020;6(1):59.
[3] Martin V, Mazzucchelli L, Frattini M. An overview of the epidermal growth factor receptor fluorescence in situ hybridisation challenge in tumour pathology. J Clin Pathol 2009;62(4):314–24.
[4] Purshouse K, Pollard SM, Bickmore WA, et al. Imaging extrachromosomal DNA (ecDNA) in cancer. Histochem Cell Biol 2024;162(1):53–64.
[5] Talevich E, Shain AH, Botton T, et al. CNVkit: genome-wide copy number detection and visualization from targeted DNA sequencing. PLoS Comput Biol 2016;21(4):e1004873.
[6] Wolff AC, Hammond MEH, Allison KH, et al. HER2 testing in breast cancer: American society of clinical oncology/college of American pathologists clinical practice guideline focused update summary. J Oncol Pract 2018;14(7):437–41.
[7] Jennings LJ, Arcila ME, Corless C, et al. Guidelines for validation of next-generation sequencing–based oncology panels: a joint consensus recommendation of the association for molecular pathology and college of American pathologists. J Mol Diagn 2017;19(3):341–65.
[8] Mikhail FM, Biegel JA, Cooley LD, et al. Technical laboratory standards for interpretation and reporting of acquired copy-number abnormalities and copy-neutral loss of heterozygosity in neoplastic disorders: a joint consensus recommendation from the American College of Medical Genetics and Genomics (ACMG) and the Cancer Genomics Consortium (CGC). Genet Med 2019;21(9):1903–16.
[9] Chandramohan R, Reuther J, Gandhi I, et al. A validation framework for somatic copy number detection in targeted sequencing panels. J Mol Diagn : J Mod Dynam 2022;24(7):760–74.
[10] Lemes CC, Silva AGD, Ribeiro DA, et al. Challenges and solutions in FISH for formalin-fixed paraffin-embedded tissue: a scoping review. Microsc Res Tech 2025;88(1):270–8.
[11] Gown AM. Diagnostic immunohistochemistry: what can go wrong and how to prevent it. Archives of pathology & laboratory medicine 2016;140(9):893–8.
[12] Guo R, Berry LD, Aisner DL, et al. MET IHC is a poor screen for MET amplification or MET exon 14 mutations in lung adenocarcinomas: data from a tri-institutional cohort of the lung cancer mutation consortium. J Thorac Oncol 2019;14(9):1666–71.
[13] Hong L, Patel S, Drusbosky LM, et al. Molecular landscape of ERBB2 alterations in 3000 advanced NSCLC patients. npj Precis Oncol 2024;8(1):217.
[14] Odintsov I, Makarem M, Nishino M, et al. Prevalence and therapeutic targeting of high-level ERBB2 amplification in NSCLC. J Thorac Oncol 2024;19(5):732–48.
[15] Slamon DJ, Clark GM, Wong SG, et al. Human breast cancer: correlation of relapse and survival with amplification of the HER-2/neu oncogene. Science 1987;235-(4785):177–82.
[16] Lux MP, Nabieva N, Hartkopf AD, et al. Therapy landscape in patients with metastatic HER2-positive breast cancer: data from the PRAEGNANT real-world breast cancer registry. Cancers 2018;11(1):10.
[17] Bose R, Kavuri SM, Searleman AC, et al. Activating HER2 mutations in HER2 gene amplification negative breast cancer. Cancer Discov 2013;3(2):224–37.
[18] Slamon DJ, Leyland-Jones B, Shak S, et al. Use of chemotherapy plus a monoclonal antibody against HER2 for metastatic breast cancer that overexpresses HER2. N Engl J Med 2001;344(11):783–92.
[19] Robert N, Leyland-Jones B, Asmar L, et al. Randomized phase III study of trastuzumab, paclitaxel, and carboplatin compared with trastuzumab and paclitaxel in women with HER-2–overexpressing metastatic breast cancer. J Clin Oncol 2006;24(18):2786–92.

[20] Modi S, Jacot W, Yamashita T, et al. Trastuzumab deruxtecan in previously treated HER2-low advanced breast cancer. N Engl J Med 2022;387(1):9–20.

[21] Bardia A, Hu X, Dent R, et al. Trastuzumab deruxtecan after endocrine therapy in metastatic breast cancer. N Engl J Med 2024;391(22):2110–22.

[22] Li BT, Smit EF, Goto Y, et al. Trastuzumab deruxtecan in HER2-mutant non–small-cell lung cancer. N Engl J Med 2022;386(3):241–51.

[23] Lara PN, Laptalo L, Longmate J, et al. Trastuzumab plus docetaxel in HER2/neu–positive non–small-cell lung cancer: a California cancer consortium screening and phase II trial. Clin Lung Cancer 2004;5(4):231–6.

[24] Krug LM, Miller VA, Patel J, et al. Randomized phase II study of weekly docetaxel plus trastuzumab versus weekly paclitaxel plus trastuzumab in patients with previously untreated advanced nonsmall cell lung carcinoma. Cancer 2005;104(10):2149–55.

[25] Zinner RG, Glisson BS, Fossella FV, et al. Trastuzumab in combination with cisplatin and gemcitabine in patients with Her2-overexpressing, untreated, advanced non-small cell lung cancer: report of a phase II trial and findings regarding optimal identification of patients with Her2-overexpressing disease. Lung Cancer 2004; 44(1):99–110.

[26] Goto K, Goto Y, Kubo T, et al. Trastuzumab deruxtecan in patients with HER2-mutant metastatic non–small-cell lung cancer: primary results from the randomized, phase II DESTINY-Lung02 trial. J Clin Oncol 2023;41(31): 4852–63.

[27] Shih J-Y. ERBB2 amplification in NSCLC: how many faces? J Thorac Oncol 2024;19(5):668–70.

[28] Meric-Bernstam F, Makker V, Oaknin A, et al. Efficacy and safety of trastuzumab deruxtecan in patients with HER2-expressing solid tumors: primary results from the DESTINY-PanTumor02 phase II trial. J Clin Oncol 2024;42(1):47–58.

[29] Peters S, Stahel R, Bubendorf L, et al. Trastuzumab emtansine (T-DM1) in patients with previously treated HER2-overexpressing metastatic non–small cell lung cancer: efficacy, safety, and biomarkers. Clin Cancer Res 2019;25(1):64–72.

[30] Smit EF, Felip E, Uprety D, et al. Trastuzumab deruxtecan in patients with metastatic non-small-cell lung cancer (DESTINY-Lung01): primary results of the HER2-overexpressing cohorts from a single-arm, phase 2 trial. Lancet Oncol 2024;25(4):439–54.

[31] Heymach J, Opdam F, Barve MA, et al. Phase Ia/Ib trial of zongertinib (BI 1810631), a HER2-specific tyrosine kinase inhibitor (TKI), in patients (pts) with HER2 aberration-positive solid tumors: updated Phase Ia data from Beamion LUNG-1, including progression-free survival (PFS) data. J Clin Oncol 2024;42(16_suppl). https://doi.org/10.1200/JCO.2024.42.16_suppl.8514.

[32] Heymach JV, Opdam F, Barve M, et al. HER2-selective tyrosine kinase inhibitor, zongertinib (BI 1810631), in patients with advanced/metastatic solid tumors with HER2 alterations: a phase Ia Dose-escalation study. J Clin Oncol 2025;43(11):1337–47.

[33] Johnson ML, Soo RA, Wu Y-L, et al. Beamion LUNG-2: a phase III randomized controlled trial of zongertinib (BI 1810631) versus standard of care (SoC) in patients with locally advanced/metastatic non-squamous non-small cell lung cancer (NSCLC) harboring HER2 tyrosine kinase domain (TKD) mutations. J Clin Oncol 2024;42(16_suppl). https://doi.org/10.1200/JCO.2024.42.16_suppl.TPS8654.

[34] Passaro A, Brase JC, Xu J, et al. 1395TiP A randomized phase III trial evaluating oral BAY 2927088, compared with standard of care, as first-line treatment of locally advanced or metastatic NSCLC harboring HER2-activating mutations (SOHO-02). Ann Oncol 2024;35. https://doi.org/10.1016/j.annonc.2024.08.1450.

[35] Le X, Hong L, Hensel C, et al. Landscape and clonal dominance of co-occurring genomic alterations in non–small-cell lung cancer harboring MET exon 14 skipping. JCO Precision Oncology 2021;5(5). https://doi.org/10.1200/PO.21.00135:PO.21.00135.

[36] Qin K, Hong L, Zhang J, et al. MET amplification as a resistance driver to TKI therapies in lung cancer: clinical challenges and opportunities. Cancers 2023;15(3):612.

[37] Wolf J, Hochmair M, Han J-Y, et al. Capmatinib in MET exon 14-mutated non-small-cell lung cancer: final results from the open-label, phase 2 GEOMETRY mono-1 trial. Lancet Oncol 2024;25(10):1357–70.

[38] Go H, Jeon YK, Park HJ, et al. High MET gene copy number leads to shorter survival in patients with non-small cell lung cancer. J Thorac Oncol 2010;5(3):305–13.

[39] Heydt C, Becher A-K, Wagener-Ryczek S, et al. Comparison of in situ and extraction-based methods for the detection of MET amplifications in solid tumors. Comput Struct Biotechnol J 2019;17:1339–47.

[40] Smit EF, Dooms C, Raskin J, et al. Insight 2: a phase II study of tepotinib plus osimertinib in MET-amplified NSCLC and first-line osimertinib resistance. Future Oncol 2022;18(9):1039–54.

[41] Peng L, Li A, Liu S, et al. P85.02 NGS could not replace FISH regarding to MET amplification as an optimal biomarker. J Thorac Oncol 2021;16(3). https://doi.org/10.1016/j.jtho.2021.01.1224.

[42] Hartmaier RJ, Markovets AA, Ahn MJ, et al. Osimertinib + savolitinib to overcome acquired MET-mediated resistance in epidermal growth factor receptor–mutated, MET-amplified non–small cell lung cancer: TATTON. Cancer Discovery 2023;13(1):98–113.

[43] Xiang C, Lv X, Chen K, et al. Unraveling the significance of MET focal amplification in lung cancer: integrative NGS, FISH, and IHC investigation. Mod Pathol 2024; 37(4):100451.

[44] Camidge DR, Otterson GA, Clark JW, et al. Crizotinib in patients with MET-Amplified NSCLC. J Thorac Oncol 2021;16(6):1017–29.

[45] Cho BC, Kim D-W, Spira AI, et al. Amivantamab plus lazertinib in osimertinib-relapsed EGFR-mutant advanced

non-small cell lung cancer: a phase 1 trial. Nat Med 2023; 29(10):2577–85.

[46] Leighl N, Cho BC, Hiret S, et al. OA21.04 amivantamab in patients with advanced NSCLC and MET exon 14 skipping mutation: results from the CHRYSALIS study. J Thorac Oncol 2023;18(11). https://doi.org/10.1016/j.jtho.2023.09.105.

[47] Schmalz L, Bloomer C, Zhang W, et al. Durable response to amivantamab in treatment refractory NSCLC harboring EGFR and complex MET mutations: a case report. Lung Cancer 2023;186:107400.

[48] Camidge DR, Bar J, Horinouchi H, et al. Telisotuzumab vedotin monotherapy in patients with previously treated c-met protein–overexpressing advanced nonsquamous EGFR-wildtype non–small cell lung cancer in the phase II LUMINOSITY trial. J Clin Oncol 2024;42(25): 3000–11.

[49] Horinouchi H, Shibata Y, Looman J, et al. Phase 2 study of telisotuzumab vedotin (Teliso-V) monotherapy in patients with previously untreated MET-amplified locally advanced/metastatic non-squamous non-small cell lung cancer (NSQ NSCLC). J Clin Oncol 2023;41(16_suppl). https://doi.org/10.1200/JCO.2023.41.16_suppl.TPS9149.

[50] Spira AI, Cho BC, Kim TM, et al. Amivantamab plus capmatinib in advanced non-small cell lung cancer (NSCLC) harboring MET alterations: recommended phase 2 combination dose and preliminary dose-escalation results from the phase 1/2 METalmark study. J Clin Oncol 2024;42(16_suppl). https://doi.org/10.1200/JCO.2024.42.16_suppl.8619.

[51] Han Y, Yu Y, Miao D, et al. Targeting MET in NSCLC: an ever-expanding territory. JTO Clinical and Research Reports 2024;5(2):100630.

[52] Yu HA, Goldberg SB, Le X, et al. Biomarker-directed phase II platform study in patients with EGFR sensitizing mutation-positive advanced/metastatic non-small cell lung cancer whose disease has progressed on first-line osimertinib therapy (ORCHARD). Clin Lung Cancer 2021; 22(6):601–6.

[53] Ramalingam SS, Cheng Y, Zhou C, et al. Mechanisms of acquired resistance to first-line osimertinib: preliminary data from the phase III FLAURA study. Ann Oncol 2018;29-(suppl_8). https://doi.org/10.1093/annonc/mdy424.063.

[54] Wu Y-L, Cheng Y, Zhou J, et al. Tepotinib plus gefitinib in patients with EGFR-mutant non-small-cell lung cancer with MET overexpression or MET amplification and acquired resistance to previous EGFR inhibitor (INSIGHT study): an open-label, phase 1b/2, multicentre, randomised trial. Lancet Respir Med 2020;8-(11):1132–43.

[55] Wu Y-L, Guarneri V, Voon PJ, et al. Tepotinib plus osimertinib in patients with EGFR-mutated non-small-cell lung cancer with MET amplification following progression on first-line osimertinib (INSIGHT 2): a multicentre, open-label, phase 2 trial. Lancet Oncol 2024; 25(8):989–1002.

[56] Besse B, Baik CS, Marmarelis ME, et al. Predictive biomarkers for treatment with amivantamab plus lazertinib among EGFR-mutated NSCLC in the post-osimertinib setting: analysis of tissue IHC and ctDNA NGS. J Clin Oncol 2023;41(16_suppl). https://doi.org/10.1200/JCO.2023.41.16_suppl.9013.

[57] Elghawy O, Barsouk A, Reed-Guy L, et al. Brief report: osimertinib plus capmatinib for patients with MET-altered EGFR-mutant NSCLC following progression on front line therapy. Clin Lung Cancer 2025;26(2): 158–63.e2.

[58] Patil T, Staley A, Nie Y, et al. The efficacy and safety of treating acquired MET resistance through combinations of parent and MET tyrosine kinase inhibitors in patients with metastatic oncogene-driven NSCLC. JTO Clinical and Research Reports 2024;5(2):100637.

[59] Wu Y-L, Ahn M-J, Goto K, et al. Capmatinib plus osimertinib versus platinum-pemetrexed doublet chemotherapy as second-line therapy in patients with stage IIIb/IIIc or IV *EGFR*-mutant, T790M-negative NSCLC harboring *MET* amplification. JCO 2022;40:TPS9153-TPS9153. https://doi.org/10.1200/JCO.2022.40.16_suppl.TPS9153.

Advances in Molecular Pathology 8 (2025) 69–82

ADVANCES IN MOLECULAR PATHOLOGY

Perspectives on Homologous Recombination Repair Deficiency (HRD)

Updates on Testing to Treatments

Kathleen Gwilliam, PhD[1], Kendall E. Martin, PhD[1], Scott A. Turner, PhD*

Department of Pathology, Virginia Commonwealth University Health Center, 403 Nth 13th Street, Clinial Support Center, RM 247, Richmond, VA 23298, USA

KEYWORDS

• Homologous recombination deficiency • HRD • Homologous recombination repair • PARP inhibitors • PARPi • *BRCA1* • *BRCA2*

KEY POINTS

- Homologous recombination deficiency (HRD) occurs when cells are unable to repair double-stranded DNA breaks, resulting in loss of genomic stability. HRD is typically caused by pathogenic variants or epigenetic changes impacting genes in the homologous recombination repair (HRR) pathway, including *BRCA1, BRCA2, PALB2, RAD51*, and others.
- Several methods for detecting HRD in tumors include the sequencing of HRR pathway genes and biomarker testing to identify genomic scarring, including loss of heterozygosity, large-scale state transitions, and telomeric imbalances. This testing is commercially available and is recommended for treatment in several tumor types.
- Treatments for HRD-positive tumors include PARP inhibitors and platinum-based chemotherapy. HRD status is a key biomarker in predicting therapy response.

INTRODUCTION

The capability of a cell to correct mistakes made during DNA replication or to repair DNA damage from exogenous forces is essential for proper cell proliferation and survival. One of the key hallmarks of cancer is the ability of a cell to accumulate these genetic alterations, commonly referred to as genomic instability [1]. Genomic instability can result in the deregulation of the normal function of oncogenes and tumor suppressors and drive a cell toward either cell death or tumorigenesis. The cell has several innate pathways to repair DNA damage and protect the cell from the accumulation of these pathogenic variants. The molecular mechanisms for these pathways are dependent on the types of DNA damage incurred and are covered in other reviews [2–7]. The potential for genomic instability is highest when this damage results in double-stranded breaks in the DNA (DSBs). When this occurs, the cell depends on 2 pathways for repair; the error-prone process of non-homologous end-joining (NHEJ) or the higher fidelity process of homologous recombination repair (HRR). When a cell loses the ability to repair these DSBs with the more accurate homologous recombination, it will rely on non-homologous end-joining. In turn, there is a further accumulation of mutations, leading to genomic instability. The loss of HRR is a

[1] Co-first authors.

*Corresponding author. *E-mail address:* scott.turner@vcuhealth.org

https://doi.org/10.1016/j.yamp.2025.07.004 www.advancesinmolecularpathology.com
2589-4080/25/ © 2025 Elsevier Inc. All rights are reserved, including those for text and data mining, AI training, and similar technologies.

ABBREVIATIONS

ctDNA	cell-free tumor DNA
DSBs	double-stranded breaks
ER	Estrogen
FDA	Federal Drug Administration
FFPE	Formalin-Fixed Paraffin-Embedded
H&E	hematoxylin and eosin
HR	Homologous recombination
HRD	Homologous recombination deficiency
HRR	homologous recombination repair
ICL	interstrand crosslink
LOH	loss of heterozygosity
LSTs	Large-scale state transitions
mCRPC	metastatic castration-resistant prostate cancer
MMEJ	microhomology-mediated end-joining
NGS	next-generation sequencing
NHEJ	non-homologous end-joining
PARP	poly (ADP-ribose) polymerase
PR	Progesterone
SNP	single nucleotide polymorphism
TAI	telomere allelic imbalance
TMEJ	theta-mediated end joining
TNBCs	Triple negative breast cancers

common feature in several solid tumor types, including breast, ovarian, endometrial, pancreatic, and prostate cancers.

Over the past several decades, novel compounds have been identified, studied, and approved by the Federal Drug Administration (FDA) to treat patients whose tumors exhibit homologous recombination deficiency (HRD). The most common approach is to inhibit the functions of the protein poly (ADP-ribose) polymerase (PARP). PARP plays a role in DNA damage repair for single-stranded DNA breaks, and when inhibited these unrepaired breaks will often result in further DSBs [8]. While the independent loss of these 2 pathways may increase genomic instability, the combinatorial loss will result in cell death, a process known as synthetic lethality. The testing of various molecular biomarkers has been used to identify those tumors that are HRD-positive, a positive predictor of response to these therapies. This article will review the mechanisms of HRR, how HRD is identified in a tumor, the currently recommended and future treatments for HRD-positive tumors, and the limitations and challenges associated with the use of HRD in clinical care.

HOMOLOGOUS RECOMBINATION REPAIR PATHWAY

The HRR pathway involves numerous proteins that are activated and recruited when a double-stranded DNA break (DSB) occurs (Figs. 1A–F). The start of this signaling cascade occurs when ATM, along with the MRN complex, establishes the presence of a DSB and begins to phosphorylate downstream targets, including BRCA1, CHEK2, and p53. This phosphorylation initiates the process of activating cell cycle checkpoints, which is necessary to pause the cell cycle for DNA repair to occur [9–11]. CHEK2 also phosphorylates other proteins, including BRCA1, which interacts with BARD1 to sense the DSB and activate cell cycle checkpoints, arresting the cell cycle in the G2/M phase, whereby the sister chromatid serves as the repair template [12–14]. Following cell cycle arrest, BRCA1 and BRIP1, together, facilitate end resection by creating a 3′ single-stranded DNA overhang at the DSB, a step that is essential for the strand invasion process of homologous recombination (HR). PALB2 acts as a bridge between BRCA1 and BRCA2, binding to BRCA1 and recruiting BRCA2 to form the BRCA complex [15]. PALB2's role facilitates the ability of BRCA2 to interact with RAD51 to position it onto the single-stranded DNA at the DSB [16]. Specifically, BRCA2 ensures the formation and stabilization of the RAD51-ssDNA nucleoprotein filament that allows for homologous pairing and strand invasion to occur [17–20]. Pathogenic variants in the genes that encode these HRR pathway proteins may result in loss of protein function, which then impairs the cell's ability to repair DSBs via HR and leads to HRD.

HOMOLOGOUS RECOMBINATION DEFICIENCY

HRD is a contributing factor to the development of certain cancers, with some of the most prevalent including breast [21], ovarian [22,23], pancreatic [24], and prostate cancer [25–27]. These cancers can develop due to pathogenic variants in genes within the HRR pathway, with germline or somatic variants in *BRCA1* or *BRCA2* being the most common [28,29]. Additionally, variants in other genes involved in the HRR pathway, including *PALB2, BARD1, ATM, CHECK1, CHECK2, BRIP1,* and *RAD51*, can cause HRD [28]. Pathogenic variants in these HRR pathway genes, including *BRCA1* and *BRCA2*, can include missense and nonsense mutations, splice variants, deletions, and rearrangements. Currently, guidelines recommend the germline

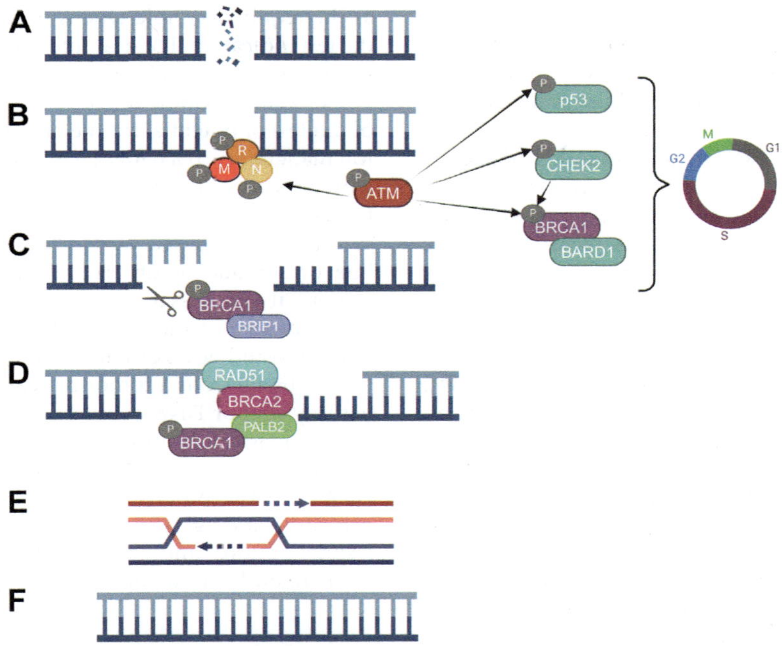

FIG. 1 Homologous recombination repair pathway. (**A**) A double-stranded DNA break (DSB) occurs. (**B**) The MRN complex and ATM detect the DSB, recruiting other proteins to activate cell cycle checkpoints for the HRR pathway to proceed. (**C**) At the DSB, BRCA1 and BRIP1 generate a 3′ ssDNA overhang. (**D**) BRCA2, as part of the BRCA complex (BRCA1, PALB2, and BRCA2), facilitates the loading of RAD51 onto the single-stranded DNA overhang, whereby a RAD51-DNA nucleoprotein filament is formed. (**E**) Homologous pairing and strand invasion occur, allowing for homologous recombination. (**F**) Repaired double-stranded DNA. (Created in BioRender. Gwilliam, K. (2025) https://BioRender.com/y1y3ksf).

testing of *BRCA1* and *BRCA2* in cases of breast, ovarian, pancreatic, and prostate cancer, as well as germline and somatic testing of additional HRR genes in ovarian and advanced prostate cancers. In addition to testing for pathogenic variants in HRR genes, HRD can be detected in a tumor by assessing genomic instability, testing that is currently recommended for ovarian cancer but not other cancer types. Determining the HRD status of a patient's tumor, either through genetic testing of HRR pathway genes or through the assessment of genomic instability, has become increasingly important as therapeutics have been developed to specifically target HRD-positive tumors, which may lead to a better prognosis.

TESTING TO IDENTIFY HOMOLOGOUS RECOMBINATION DEFICIENCY

Identification of Genomic Scarring

Failure to repair DNA damage via the HRR pathway will often lead to alternative pathways of DNA repair, most of which are more prone to errors. Errors during DNA repair may lead to genomic instability, which can include a genomic loss of heterozygosity, large-scale state transitions of the genome, and telomere allelic imbalance [30] Genomic loss of heterozygosity (LOH) is a loss of one of the 2 alleles, either due to DNA repair using the same allele as the template or a deletion of one of the alleles during repair. In HRD, LOH is often classified as a region greater than or equal to 15 Mb [31]. Large-scale state transitions (LSTs) encompass rearrangements within the chromosome such as deletions, translocations, and/or inversions, and telomere allelic imbalance (TAI) occurs when there is an unequal portion of the telomere of one allele in comparison to the other [32]. Testing for these different types of genomic instability or "scarring" through methods such as next-generation sequencing (NGS) can indicate if HRD is present. Specifically, this genomic scarring can be measured by an HRD score. LOH, LST, and TAI can each be tested simultaneously using NGS or chromosomal single nucleotide polymorphism (SNP) microarray platforms. Scores are independently assigned for LOH, LST, and TAI through bioinformatic analysis of the NGS or chromosomal SNP microarray results, which establishes the amount of LOH, LST, and TAI present in the regions of the genome tested. An HRD score is then calculated by combining the LOH, LST, and TAI scores [33]. HRD score is most commonly established using NGS platforms such as the MyChoice CDx Myriad HRD Companion Diagnostic Test. However, studies have shown that comparable HRD scores can be determined using chromosomal SNP microarrays, which are more cost-effective, although not standard in diagnostic HRD testing to determine therapeutic options [34]. Cutoffs for HRD scores and their implications for an effective response to a particular treatment varies based on cancer type. In ovarian cancer, the presence of HRD is confirmed by an HRD score greater than or equal to 42, with some studies showing a lower score of greater than or equal to 33 is effective [35,36]. However, while different platforms use similar calculations to generate the HRD score, there are calculation variations among these different tests that affect the score. Additionally, the clinical utility of these scores can vary by cancer type and subtype [37,38]. Some testing platforms, such as the FoundationOne CDx (Foundation Medicine), only test for the presence of LOH, but not LSTs or TAIs and determine HRD based on the presence of variants in HRR pathway genes, including *BRCA1* and *BRCA2*, and LOH. As HRD testing grows in utility, the standardization of these scores and their implications for treatment selection for each cancer type will be essential.

Testing for Germline and/or Somatic Variants in Homologous Recombination Deficiency

When choosing which test is appropriate to assess variants or genomic instability due to HRD it is important to select the test that is specific to variants common to that cancer type [39]. For example, if a patient with breast cancer only needs to be tested for germline variants in *BRCA1* and *BRCA2*, the most cost and time-effective test would be a gene-specific assay, such as the BRACAnalysis CDx (Myriad) test. This test identifies variants through a combination of Sanger sequencing and multiplex PCR of *BRCA1* and *BRCA2*. However, in the case of ovarian cancer, it would be beneficial to test for both *BRCA1* and *BRCA2* variants along with genomic instability, using an assay such as the MyChoice CDx Myriad HRD Companion Diagnostic Test. It is also essential to determine whether the goal is to identify germline or somatic variants, as the required sample type is different depending on the test indication. For example, when testing for germline variants, whole blood is preferred and there should be no contamination of the specimen with the tumor of interest or potential for the presence of a hematological malignancy. If a patient has a hematological cancer, a blood sample or buccal swab would not be suitable for testing as the variants present may confound the results and the detected variant could be either of germline or somatic origin. For somatic testing in solid tumors, it is necessary to ensure that the specimen is representative of the tumor of interest. The preferred sample would be a Formalin-Fixed Paraffin-Embedded (FFPE) tissue from a tumor resection or biopsy. Alternatively, tumor DNA could be obtained from the patient's plasma by isolating cell-free tumor DNA (ctDNA) which is present due to the tumor shedding DNA into the bloodstream through various mechanisms, including apoptosis. An overview of HRD testing options and the specimen requirements for each are outlined in Table 1.

Testing of Homologous Recombination Repair Gene Promoter Methylation

HRD is not only caused by changes to the DNA sequence of HRR genes but also changes in methylation patterns of the promoters of specific HRR genes. For instance, breast and ovarian cancers can be HRD-positive due to the abnormal methylation of the promoter region of *BRCA1* or *RAD51C*. Although clinical studies have shown that the heterozygous methylation of *BRCA1* or *RAD51C* does not lead to a disruption of the HRR pathway, individuals with the homozygous methylation of *BRCA1* or *RAD51C* have shown positive response to HRD-targeted treatment in ovarian cancer [40,41]. Therefore, quantitative clinical assays to test for *BRCA1* or *RAD51C* methylation that show at least 70% methylation of the promoter region may be useful in developing an HRD treatment plan. Clinically validated qualitative assays that use blood and/or tumor FFPE samples include a *BRCA1* methylation-specific digital drop PCR (MS-ddPCR) [40], bisulfite conversion followed by pyrosequencing at CpG sites of *BRCA1* [42], and an NGS-based *BRCA1* and *RAD51C* promoter methylation assay [43].

Testing for RAD51 Foci Formation

Another method to determine the presence of HRD is through a RAD51 foci assay. Fixed tissue or fixed sorted cells undergo immunohistochemistry, with antibodies specific to RAD51 and Geminin, a marker of cell

TABLE 1
Homologous Recombination Deficiency (HRD) Tests by the Assay Target Type

HRD Test Type	Test Name	Germline or Somatic Testing	Indicated Cancers[a]	Specimen Types
BRCA variant test (*BRCA1, BRCA2*)	Ion Torrent™ Oncomine™ *BRCA* Research Assay GX	Germline or Somatic	Breast, Ovarian, Pancreatic, Prostate	WB, FFPE
	Myriad BRACAnalysis CDx®	Germline	Breast, Ovarian, Pancreatic, Prostate	WB
	Quest Diagnostics™ BRCA Panel (BRCA1, BRCA2)	Germline	Breast, Ovarian, Pancreatic, Prostate	WB, SA, BS, CF
	Invitae® BRCA1 and BRCA2 Panel	Germline	Breast, Ovarian, Pancreatic, Prostate	WB SA, BS, gDNA
	Ambry Genetics® BRCA1/2 3-mutation panel	Germline	Breast, Ovarian, Pancreatic, Prostate	WB, SA, BS, CF, gDNA
	Ambry Genetics® BRCA1/2 seq and del/dup	Germline	Breast, Ovarian, Pancreatic, Prostate	WB, SA, BS, CF, gDNA
HRR gene variant test (gene content varies)	Ion Torrent™ Oncomine™ HRR Pathway Predesigned Panel	Somatic	Not Indicated	FFPE
	QIAGEN® QIAseq HRR Panel	Somatic	Not Indicated	FFPE, P, FT
	FoundationOne®CDx	Somatic	Prostate, Ovarian	FFPE
	FoundationOne®Liquid CDx	Somatic	Prostate	WB
	Ion Torrent™ Oncomine™ BRCA Expanded Panel	Somatic	Not Indicated	FFPE
BRCA variant test HRR variant test Genomic instability test[b]	Ion Torrent™ Oncomine™ Comprehensive Assay Plus	Somatic	Not Indicated	FFPE
BRCA variant test and Genomic instability test[b]	FoundationOne®CDx	Somatic	Pancreatic, Ovarian	FFPE
	MyChoice®CDx Myriad HRD Companion Diagnostic Test	Germline and Somatic	Ovarian	FFPE

Abbreviations: BS, buccal swab; CF, cultured skin fibroblast; FFPE, formalin fixed paraffin embedded tissue; FT, fresh or frozen tissue; P, plasma; SA, saliva; WB, whole blood.

[a] Cancers indicated by the laboratory or assay manufacturer.

[b] Genomic instability testing biomarkers and scoring systems vary by assay.

proliferation (S/G2 phase of the cell cycle) [44]. If the HRR pathway is functional, RAD51 foci form. Therefore, in HRD-positive cancers, there would be a decrease or the absence of RAD51 foci. Additionally, the RAD51 foci assay is a cost and time-effective method to determine the HRD status of a tumor without having to identify the specific cause of HRD. This assay also detects the current HRD status of the tumor, unlike genomic scarring assays that would return HRD-positive results even if the function of the HRR pathway had been restored, which can occur during treatment when a pathogenic variant reverts to a wild-type state. Future studies to better quantify the amount of RAD51 foci in specific cancer types and how it affects therapeutic efficacy will allow for better treatment selection and prognosis.

Alternative Methods in Development

Other testing methodologies are being developed to accompany the use of molecular HRD testing. One study has shown the ability to predict HRD in breast and ovarian cancers using hematoxylin and eosin

(H&E)-stained histopathological slides from primary breast and ovarian cancers and a deep learning artificial intelligence program, DeepHRD [45]. DeepHRD was able to correctly determine the HRD status of fresh frozen and FFPE breast and ovarian cancer H&E stained slides and could also differentiate between cancers that had a complete, partial, or absent treatment response [45]. Further studies will be needed to test the clinical utility of platforms such as DeepHRD, but these tests could provide a beneficial primary step to an HRD diagnosis.

The determination of HRD tumor status is now recommended for therapeutic selection across several cancer types. However, as described, current testing limitations need to be addressed to fully realize the potential of HRD as a biomarker. Currently, there is a lack of biomarker and scoring standardization. Without further standardization, the assessment of clinical utility in various tumors will be challenging to establish.

THERAPEUTICS FOR HOMOLOGOUS RECOMBINATION DEFICIENCY-POSITIVE CANCERS

Homologous Recombination Deficiency Targeted Therapeutics and Synthetic Lethality

Establishing the HRD status of a patient's tumor has become increasingly important as targeted therapies have been developed for HRD-positive tumors. As HRD-positive tumors contain pathogenic variants in HRR pathway genes, these tumor cells are unable to repair DNA damage via HR. Therefore, HRD-targeting treatments aim to exploit an impaired repair pathway by inducing DNA damage, which is then unable to be repaired by HR in HRD-positive cells, ultimately leading to cell death [25,46]. Currently, DNA damage can be caused by chemotherapy that directly alters DNA structure or through the generation of DSBs by targeted therapy via synthetic lethality [25]. Synthetic lethality is a genetic interaction between 2 genes for which the loss of a single gene has no impact on cell survival, but the loss of both genes results in cell death [47]. As HRD-positive cells have at least one pathogenic variant that impacts DSB repair, therapies have been developed to target an additional gene within the DNA damage response pathway, further impacting these cells' ability to repair DSBs [47,48]. At present, there are currently 2 classes of drugs that have been approved by the FDA to treat HRD-positive tumors: interstrand crosslink (ICL) inducing platinum-based chemotherapies and synthetic lethal poly (ADP-ribose) polymerase inhibitors (PARPis). Additional synthetic lethal treatments, polymerase theta inhibitors, are currently being investigated in early-stage trials.

Platinum-Based Therapies

Platinum-based chemotherapies have been in use since 1971 and function by generating interstrand crosslinks (ICLs), which are covalent bonds that form between the 2 opposite strands of a DNA double helix. ICLs prevent DNA strand separation, thereby limiting transcription and DNA replication, which are vital for cell survival [49,50]. One mechanism by which ICLs are repaired is through the HRR pathway [50,51]. Therefore, HRD-positive cells treated with ICL-inducing platinum-based therapies undergo cell death, as they are unable to repair ICLs via HR [25,51]. Thus, while platinum-based chemotherapies have been used to treat various cancer types since 1971, in recent years they have been particularly effective in HRD-positive tumor types. Specifically, cisplatin, carboplatin, and oxaliplatin are often used as first-line therapy for patients with HRD-positive tumors [32,52–55].

Poly (ADP-Ribose) Polymerase Inhibitors

Similar to ICL-inducing platinum-based therapies, poly (ADP-ribose) polymerase inhibitors (PARPis) take advantage of the impaired HRR pathway to target HRD-positive tumor cells [56]. PARP proteins are involved in the DNA damage response pathway by localizing to ssDNA breaks and recruiting the cellular machinery necessary to repair the break [56,57]. When PARP is inhibited, the ssDNA breaks are unable to be repaired, leading to the formation of DSBs. HRD-positive cells are unable to repair these DSBs via the HRR pathway, resulting in cell death. Thus, PARPis are synthetic lethal whereby the combination of the inhibition of PARP along with a pathogenic variant in an HRR gene causes cell death [25,56,57]. A summary of PARPis currently used to treat HRD-positive cancer can be found in Table 2.

Polymerase Theta Inhibitors

A new HRD-positive cancer therapy currently in the early stages of clinical trials targets a different part of the DNA damage response pathway: polymerase theta (POLθ). POLθ, encoded by the gene *POLQ*, has been shown to function in DSB repair through the microhomology-mediated end-joining (MMEJ) pathway, also called

TABLE 2
PARP Inhibitors Used in HRD-Positive Tumors

Cancer	Therapy	Genetic Testing	Trial Name	Phase	Clinical Trial ID
Breast	Talazoparib	Germline *BRCA1/2*	EMBRACA	III	NCT01945775
	Olaparib	Germline *BRCA1/2*	OlmpiAD	III	NCT02000622
	Olaparib	Germline *BRCA1/2*	OlympiA	III	NCT02032823
	Olaparib	Somatic *BRCA1/2*	TBCRC048	II	NCT03344965
Ovarian	Olaparib	Germline or Somatic *BRCA1/2*	SOLO-1	III	NCT01844986
	Niraparib	BRCA status WT or unknown, HRD	PRIMA	III	NCT02655016
	Olibarib + Bevacizumab	BRCA status WT or unknown; HRD	PAOLA-1	III	NCT02477644
	Rucaparib	Germline or Somatic *BRCA1/2*	ARIEL3	III	NCT01968213
Prostate	Olaparib	Germline or Somatic HRR mutation (*BRCA1, BRCA2, ATM, BARD1, BRIP1, CDK12, CHEK1, CHEK2, FANCL, PALB2, RAD51B, RAD51C, RAD51D, or RAD54L*)	PROfound	III	NCT02987543
	Rucaparib	Germline or Somatic *BRCA1/2*	TRITON2	II	NCT02952534
	Niraparib + Abiraterone	Germline or Somatic *BRCA1/2*	MAGNITUDE	III	NCT03748641
	Olaparib + Abiraterone	Germline or Somatic *BRCA1/2*	PROpel	III	NCT03732820
	Talazoparib + Enzalutamide	Germline or Somatic HRR mutation (*BRCA1, BRCA2, ATM, ATR, CDK12, CHEK2, FANCA, MLH1, MRE11A, NBN, PALB2,* or *RAD51C*)	TALAPRO-2	III	NCT03395197
Pancreatic	Olaparib	Germline *BRCA1/2*	POLO	III	NCT02184195
	Rucaparib	Germline or Somatic *BRCA1/2* or *PALB2*		II	NCT03140670

Abbreviation: WT, wild-type.

polymerase theta-mediated end joining (TMEJ) [58,59]. This error-prone repair pathway is not commonly used in healthy cells. However, POLθ is upregulated in cells that are HR deficient, likely to compensate for the loss of the HRR pathway [59,60]. Therefore, new therapies aim to inhibit POLθ to further impair HRD-positive cells' ability to repair DSBs [60,61]. As HRD-positive tumors have also been shown to develop resistance to PARPis and platinum-based therapies, POLθ inhibitors also hold promise in treating patients who have developed resistance to other treatment types [62,63]. Currently, there are multiple POLθ inhibitors in Phase I clinical trials to test their effectiveness both as single agents and in combination with a PARPi as a treatment for patients with HRD-positive tumors [61,64](Table 3). Although the clinical utility of POLθ inhibitors is still in the early stages of investigation, they hold promise for the future of HRD-positive tumor treatment.

BRCA1 and/or *BRCA2* Variant Reversion After Treatment

It is possible in cases undergoing treatment for the original HRD causing variants to revert to a wild-type sequence [65]. Even though genomic scarring has likely occurred at this point, this reversion of the variant will lead to a now HR-proficient tumor that will be resistant to PARPi treatment or any other treatment that targets HRD. Therefore, it is important to closely monitor treatment response and to perform follow-up molecular testing to check the status of the baseline variant or perform a RAD51 foci assay that will check for overall HRD.

Overall, treatments for HRD-positive tumors exploit the cells' inability to repair DNA damage via HRR, thus leading to targeted cell death. Presently, there are FDA-approved therapies for the most common HRD-associated cancers: breast, ovarian, prostate, and pancreatic cancers.

TABLE 3
Current POLθ Clinical Trials for HRD-Positive Tumors

Clinical Trial ID	Therapy	Phase	Combination	Genetic Testing
NCT05898399	ART6043	I/II	Monotherapy; Olaparib; Niraparib	Loss of function of known DNA damage response (DDR) genes
NCT04991480	ART4215	I	Monotherapy; Talazoparib; Niraparib	*BRCA1/2* mutation for some parts
NCT06077877	GSK4524101	I/II	Monotherapy; Niraparib	No genetic testing required; must have advanced or metastatic solid tumor that has exhausted all standard of care treatment options
NCT05687110	Novobiocin	I	Monotherapy	*BRCA1/2, PALB2, RAD51C, RAD51D, ATM, BARD1, BLM, BRIP1, CDK12, FANCA, FANCC, FANCD2, FANCE, FANCF, FANCM, MRE11A, NBN (NBS1), RAD50,* and *RAD51B*
NCT06545942	MOMA-313	I	Monotherapy; Olaparib; Niraparib	HR-deficient alterations

TREATMENT GUIDELINES FOR HOMOLOGOUS RECOMBINATION REPAIR DEFICIENCY-POSITIVE CANCERS

With advancements in testing, it has become possible to identify HRD in an increasing number of tumors. It has been shown that nearly 51% of high-grade serous ovarian carcinomas have alterations in HRR genes [66] and a similarly high percentage of triple-negative breast cancers (50%–60%) have been shown to be HRD-positive [67,68]. Although the rates are slightly lower, HRD is also present in both pancreatic (19%–30%) and prostate (19%) cancers [24,69,70]. Therefore, HRD testing has been incorporated into the national treatment guidelines for these cancer types.

Breast Cancer

Triple negative breast cancers (TNBCs), that is, tumors that are negative for the estrogen (ER), progesterone (PR), and human epidermal growth factor 2 (HER2) receptors, account for around 15% of all breast cancers [71]. Both platinum-based therapies and PARPis have been evaluated in the treatment of HRD-positive TNBCs [55,72–76](Table 2). However, current guidelines have only been established for patients harboring germline *BRCA1* and/or *BRCA2* variants. For TNBCs, platinum-based therapies (carboplatin and cisplatin) and PARPis (olaparib and talazoparib) are both considered first-line treatments in patients with germline pathogenic *BRCA1/2* variants and a PD-L1 combined positive score <10 [55,72–76], with PARPis as a second line treatment for any germline pathogenic *BRCA1/2* variant. PARPis have also been shown to be effective in hormone receptor-positive, HER2-negative breast cancers in patients with germline pathogenic *BRCA1/2* variants [74]. Although platinum therapies have been shown to have an effect in patients with germline pathogenic *BRCA1/2* variants, they are less effective in patients with somatic *BRCA1/2* variants [72]. In a phase II clinical trial, the PARPi olaparib was effective in patients with somatic pathogenic *BRCA1/2* variants or germline variants in *PALB2*; however, this study showed a limited response in patients with germline variants in the other HRR genes, *ATM* and *CHEK2*, suggesting that different HRR gene variants react differently to PARP inhibition [77]. Further studies are needed to investigate the effectiveness of PARPis in patients with breast cancer with germline or somatic variants in other HRR genes.

Ovarian Cancer

While the treatment guidelines for breast cancer are primarily centered around germline pathogenic *BRCA1/2* variants, the guidelines for ovarian cancer include broader HRD testing. Molecular testing is recommended to detect pathogenic *BRCA1/2* variants (both somatic and germline) and HRD status in the absence of a *BRCA1/2* mutation in both diagnostic and recurrent cases [78]. First line treatment for ovarian cancer includes platinum-based therapies, which have been shown to be effective in the case of HRD-positive tumor types [79–81]. Additionally, 3 PARPis have been approved by the FDA for use in ovarian cancer: olaparib, niraparib, and rucaparib [82–84] (see Table 2). Olaparib has been approved for use in patients with pathogenic *BRCA1/2* variants who have shown sensitivity to platinum-based therapies [84]. Additionally, olaparib can be used in combination with bevacizumab in patients who are HRD-positive, regardless of *BRCA1/2* mutation status [82]. Niraparib may be used in patients who have already received first-line platinum-based therapies and have either a pathogenic *BRCA1/2* variant or are HRD-positive [83]. Lastly, rucaparib is recommended for patients with pathogenic *BRCA1/2* variants who have already been treated with 2 or more lines of chemotherapy and is preferred for patients with platinum-resistant disease [85–87].

Prostate Cancer

Prostate cancer is the second most common cancer in men worldwide [88]. Platinum-based therapies have been shown to primarily be effective against metastatic castration-resistant prostate cancer (mCRPC) [89–92]. As such, current guidelines only list platinum-based therapies as a first-line treatment for CRPCs with use in conjunction with other therapies. It has been shown that patients with HRD-positive tumors, which account for roughly 25% of CRPCs, are likely to gain the greatest benefit from platinum-based therapies [89,93–95]. Additionally, PARPis have been shown to be an effective treatment in CRPCs that are HRD-positive. There are currently four PARPis that have been FDA approved for prostate cancer: olaparib, rucaparib, niraparib, and talazoparib [96–99] (see Table 2). Olaparib and rucaparib are among the preferred regimens for patients who have previously received novel hormone therapy and have a germline pathogenic *BRCA1/2* variant [98]. Under certain circumstances, olaparib can also be used in patients with pathogenic variants in HRR genes other than *BRCA1/2* [99]. It has also been shown that PARPis can be used in conjunction with hormone therapies in patients with HRD who have not previously received treatment for mCRPC [96,97]. Niraparib plus abiraterone may be used in patients with germline pathogenic *BRCA1/2* variants [96] and talazoparib plus enzalutamide can be used for patients with pathogenic variants in any HRR gene [97]. Interestingly, it has been suggested that PARP-1 can promote androgen receptor activity and that androgen receptor inhibitors can mimic HRR pathway gene variants by down-regulating DNA repair genes [100–103]. This suggests that the combination of a PARPi and an androgen receptor inhibitor may also provide benefit to patients with HR-proficient tumors, as the androgen receptor inhibition could behave similarly to a pathogenic HRR pathway gene variant. In phase II clinical trial, olaparib plus abiraterone produced a clinical benefit in patients with mCRPC regardless of HRD status [104]. However, further studies are needed to determine if PARPis combined with hormone therapy is a viable treatment in patients without HRD.

Pancreatic Cancer

Despite accounting for only 5% of cancer diagnoses, pancreatic cancer is the third most common cause of cancer-related death in the United States [105]. Combination chemotherapy that includes a platinum-based compound (either oxaliplatin or cisplatin) is a first-line therapy for pancreatic cancer. This combination chemotherapy has a higher success rate in patients with pathogenic *BRCA1/2* variants or other indicators of HRD positivity [24,106–109]. Currently, there is only one PARPi that has been FDA-approved for pancreatic cancer: olaparib [110] (see Table 2). Per the treatment guidelines, olaparib can be used as a maintenance therapy for patients with germline pathogenic *BRCA1/2* variants that have shown a response to platinum-based therapies. In addition, rucaparib has shown promise for patients who have responded to platinum-based therapy and have a germline or somatic pathogenic *BRCA1/2* variant or those with a pathogenic variant in *PALB2* [111]. So, while rucaparib has been deemed potentially useful in certain circumstances in individuals with pancreatic cancer per the treatment guidelines, it has not yet been FDA approved for this use.

In summary, both platinum-based chemotherapies and PARPis are FDA-approved for use in HRD-positive breast, ovarian, prostate, and pancreatic cancers. While *BRCA1* and *BRCA2* are currently the most commonly tested genes to determine HRD status in breast, ovarian, prostate, and pancreatic cancers, current and future studies will continue to elucidate the effects of pathogenic variants in other HRR pathway genes in response to HRD-targeted treatment.

CHALLENGES AND SUMMARY

HRD status is quickly becoming a more widely used biomarker for making treatment decisions across a growing number of tumor types. However, there are still several challenges in determining HRD status and its use as a biomarker for treatment that need to be considered. The general limitations of using FFPE samples for somatic testing, including sample insufficiency and tumor heterogeneity may limit HRD-testing availability in some cases. Further work needs to focus on establishing the use of scant (fine needle aspirates, and so forth) or non-invasive samples (ctDNA from plasma) for HRD testing. The biological complexity of HRR means there are several different mechanisms for which HRD can arise, making testing design challenging. Inconsistency in current methodologies can often lead to different results depending on which markers of HRD were measured. Furthermore, the lack of standardization in HRD calculations and clear cutoff thresholds for determining HRD status will continue to limit the establishment of further clinical utility. In consideration of these challenges and limitations, efforts should be taken to combine testing methodologies (variant testing and genomic instability) to improve the sensitivity and specificity of these tests. Additionally, if assay calculation and reported cutoffs continue to be assay-dependent then further efforts need to be taken to standardize the utility of these values. Finally, the complexity of this testing will continue to require clear communication between the health care team (molecular pathologist, oncologist, genetic counselors) and the laboratory to ensure proper interpretation of these results and their implications in treatment and care.

CLINICS CARE POINTS

- Homologous recombination deficiency (HRD) status should be determined using comprehensive testing approaches (genomic instability measurements and homologous recombination repair pathway gene testing) for accurate classification.
- HRD status can be used as a biomarker for patient response to FDA-approved therapies (PARP inhibitors and platinum-based chemotherapy) for patients with ovarian, breast, prostate, and pancreatic cancers.

DISCLOSURE

The authors have nothing to disclose.

REFERENCES

[1] Hanahan D. Hallmarks of cancer: new dimensions. Cancer Discov 2022;12(1):31–46.
[2] Rahimian E, Amini A, Alikarami F, et al. DNA repair pathways as guardians of the genome: therapeutic potential and possible prognostic role in hematologic neoplasms. DNA Repair 2020;96:102951.
[3] Hakem R. DNA damage repair; the good, the bad, and the ugly. EMBO J 2008;27(4):589–605.
[4] Lieber MR. The mechanism of human nonhomologous DNA end joining. J Biol Chem 2008;283(1):1–5.
[5] San Filippo J, Sung P, Klein H. Mechanism of eukaryotic homologous recombination. Annu Rev Biochem 2008;77:229–57.
[6] David SS, O'Shea VL, Kundu S. Base-excision repair of oxidative DNA damage. Nature 2007;447(7147):941–50.
[7] Jiricny J. The multifaceted mismatch-repair system. Nat Rev Mol Cell Biol 2006;7(5):335–46.
[8] Chen A. PARP inhibitors: its role in treatment of cancer. Chin J Cancer 2011;30(7):463–71.
[9] Qiu S, Huang J. MRN complex is an essential effector of DNA damage repair. J Zhejiang Univ - Sci B 2021;22(1):31–7.
[10] Roy R, Chun J, Powell SN. BRCA1 and BRCA2: different roles in a common pathway of genome protection. Nat Rev Cancer 2011;12(1):68–78.
[11] Abraham RT. Cell cycle checkpoint signaling through the ATM and ATR kinases. Genes Dev 2001;15(17):2177–96.
[12] Zhao W, Steinfeld JB, Liang F, et al. BRCA1-BARD1 promotes RAD51-mediated homologous DNA pairing. Nature 2017;550(7676):360–5.
[13] Zhang J, Willers H, Feng Z, et al. Chk2 phosphorylation of BRCA1 regulates DNA double-strand break repair. Mol Cell Biol 2004;24(2):708–18.
[14] Lee JS, Collins KM, Brown AL, et al. hCds1-mediated phosphorylation of BRCA1 regulates the DNA damage response. Nature 2000;404(6774):201–4.
[15] Hartford SA, Chittela R, Ding X, et al. Interaction with PALB2 is essential for maintenance of genomic integrity by BRCA2. PLoS Genet 2016;12(8):e1006236.
[16] Prakash R, Zhang Y, Feng W, et al. Homologous recombination and human health: the roles of BRCA1, BRCA2, and associated proteins. Cold Spring Harb Perspect Biol 2015;7(4):a016600.
[17] Appleby R, Joudeh L, Cobbett K, et al. Structural basis for stabilisation of the RAD51 nucleoprotein filament by BRCA2. Nat Commun 2023;14(1):7003.
[18] Jensen RB, Carreira A, Kowalczykowski SC. Purified human BRCA2 stimulates RAD51-mediated recombination. Nature 2010;467(7316):678–83.
[19] Thorslund T, McIlwraith MJ, Compton SA, et al. The breast cancer tumor suppressor BRCA2 promotes the specific targeting of RAD51 to single-stranded DNA. Nat Struct Mol Biol 2010;17(10):1263–5.
[20] Liu J, Doty T, Gibson B, et al. Human BRCA2 protein promotes RAD51 filament formation on RPA-covered single-stranded DNA. Nat Struct Mol Biol 2010;17(10):1260–2.
[21] Yndestad S, Engebrethsen C, Herencia-Ropero A, et al. Homologous recombination deficiency across subtypes of primary breast cancer. JCO Precis Oncol 2023;7:e2300338.

[22] Mangogna A, Munari G, Pepe F, et al. Homologous recombination deficiency in ovarian cancer: from the biological rationale to current diagnostic approaches. J Pers Med 2023;13(2). https://doi.org/10.3390/jpm13020284.

[23] Miller RE, Leary A, Scott CL, et al. ESMO recommendations on predictive biomarker testing for homologous recombination deficiency and PARP inhibitor benefit in ovarian cancer. Ann Oncol 2020;31(12):1606–22.

[24] Park W, Chen J, Chou JF, et al. Genomic methods identify homologous recombination deficiency in pancreas adenocarcinoma and optimize treatment selection. Clin Cancer Res 2020;26(13):3239–47.

[25] Stewart MD, Merino Vega D, Arend RC, et al. Homologous recombination deficiency: concepts, definitions, and assays. Oncologist 2022;27(3):167–74.

[26] Mekonnen N, Yang H, Shin YK. Homologous recombination deficiency in ovarian, breast, colorectal, pancreatic, non-small cell lung and prostate cancers, and the mechanisms of resistance to PARP inhibitors. Front Oncol 2022;12:880643.

[27] Scott RJ, Mehta A, Macedo GS, et al. Genetic testing for homologous recombination repair (HRR) in metastatic castration-resistant prostate cancer (mCRPC): challenges and solutions. Oncotarget 2021;12(16):1600–14.

[28] Heeke AL, Pishvaian MJ, Lynce F, et al. Prevalence of homologous recombination-related gene mutations across multiple cancer types. JCO Precis Oncol 2018; 2018. https://doi.org/10.1200/PO.17.00286.

[29] Hodgson D, Lai Z, Dearden S, et al. Analysis of mutation status and homologous recombination deficiency in tumors of patients with germline BRCA1 or BRCA2 mutations and metastatic breast cancer: OlympiAD. Ann Oncol 2021;32(12):1582–9.

[30] Herzog TJ, Vergote I, Gomella LG, et al. Testing for homologous recombination repair or homologous recombination deficiency for poly (ADP-ribose) polymerase inhibitors: a current perspective. Eur J Cancer 2023;179:136–46.

[31] Abkevich V, Timms KM, Hennessy BT, et al. Patterns of genomic loss of heterozygosity predict homologous recombination repair defects in epithelial ovarian cancer. Br J Cancer 2012;107(10):1776–82.

[32] Birkbak NJ, Wang ZC, Kim JY, et al. Telomeric allelic imbalance indicates defective DNA repair and sensitivity to DNA-damaging agents. Cancer Discov 2012; 2(4):366–75.

[33] Knijnenburg TA, Wang L, Zimmermann MT, et al. Genomic and molecular landscape of DNA damage repair deficiency across the cancer genome atlas. Cell Rep 2018;23(1):239–54.e6.

[34] Tsantikidi A, Papazisis K, Floros T, et al. RediScore: prospective validation of a pipeline for homologous recombination deficiency analysis. Oncol Lett 2023; 26(5):480.

[35] How JA, Jazaeri AA, Fellman B, et al. Modification of homologous recombination deficiency score threshold and association with long-term survival in epithelial ovarian cancer. Cancers (Basel) 2021;13(5). https://doi.org/10.3390/cancers13050946.

[36] Denkert C, Romey M, Swedlund B, et al. Homologous recombination deficiency as an ovarian cancer biomarker in a real-world cohort: validation of decentralized genomic profiling. J Mol Diagn 2022;24(12):1254–63.

[37] Lotan TL, Kaur HB, Salles DC, et al. Homologous recombination deficiency (HRD) score in germline BRCA2- versus ATM-altered prostate cancer. Mod Pathol 2021; 34(6):1185–93.

[38] Lenz L, Neff C, Solimeno C, et al. Identifying homologous recombination deficiency in breast cancer: genomic instability score distributions differ among breast cancer subtypes. Breast Cancer Res Treat 2023; 202(1):191–201.

[39] Hirsch S, Gieldon L, Sutter C, et al. Germline testing for homologous recombination repair genes-opportunities and challenges. Genes Chromosomes Cancer 2021; 60(5):332–43.

[40] Nesic K, Kondrashova O, Hurley RM, et al. Acquired RAD51C promoter methylation loss causes PARP inhibitor resistance in high-grade serous ovarian carcinoma. Cancer Res 2021;81(18):4709–22.

[41] Kondrashova O, Topp M, Nesic K, et al. Methylation of all BRCA1 copies predicts response to the PARP inhibitor rucaparib in ovarian carcinoma. Nat Commun 2018;9(1):3970.

[42] Sahnane N, Rivera D, Libera L, et al. Pyrosequencing assay for BRCA1 methylation analysis: results from a cross-validation study. J Mol Diagn 2023;25(4): 217–26.

[43] Fink JL, Jaradi B, Stone N, et al. Validation and performance of quantitative BRCA1 and RAD51C promoter hypermethylation testing in breast and ovarian cancers. J Mol Diagn 2025;27(2):139–53.

[44] Castroviejo-Bermejo M, Cruz C, Llop-Guevara A, et al. A RAD51 assay feasible in routine tumor samples calls PARP inhibitor response beyond BRCA mutation. EMBO Mol Med 2018;10(12). https://doi.org/10.15252/emmm.201809172.

[45] Bergstrom EN, Abbasi A, Díaz-Gay M, et al. Deep learning artificial intelligence predicts homologous recombination deficiency and platinum response from histologic slides. J Clin Oncol 2024;42(30): 3550–60.

[46] Kolesnichenko M, Scheidereit C. Synthetic lethality by PARP inhibitors: new mechanism uncovered based on unresolved transcription-replication conflicts. Signal Transduct Target Ther 2024;9(1):179.

[47] Topatana W, Juengpanich S, Li S, et al. Advances in synthetic lethality for cancer therapy: cellular mechanism and clinical translation. J Hematol Oncol 2020; 13(1):118.

[48] Murai J, Pommier Y. BRCAness, homologous recombination deficiencies, and synthetic lethality. Cancer Res 2023;83(8):1173–4.

[49] Basourakos SP, Li L, Aparicio AM, et al. Combination platinum-based and DNA damage response-targeting cancer therapy: evolution and future directions. Curr Med Chem 2017;24(15):1586–606.

[50] Deans AJ, West SC. DNA interstrand crosslink repair and cancer. Nat Rev Cancer 2011;11(7):467–80.

[51] Hashimoto S, Anai H, Hanada K. Mechanisms of interstrand DNA crosslink repair and human disorders. Genes Environ 2016;38:9.

[52] Kondo T, Kanai M, Kou T, et al. Association between homologous recombination repair gene mutations and response to oxaliplatin in pancreatic cancer. Oncotarget 2018;9(28):19817–25.

[53] Byrski T, Dent R, Blecharz P, et al. Results of a phase II open-label, non-randomized trial of cisplatin chemotherapy in patients with BRCA1-positive metastatic breast cancer. Breast Cancer Res 2012;14(4):R110.

[54] Yang D, Khan S, Sun Y, et al. Association of BRCA1 and BRCA2 mutations with survival, chemotherapy sensitivity, and gene mutator phenotype in patients with ovarian cancer. JAMA 2011;306(14):1557–65.

[55] Silver DP, Richardson AL, Eklund AC, et al. Efficacy of neoadjuvant Cisplatin in triple-negative breast cancer. J Clin Oncol 2010;28(7):1145–53.

[56] Lord CJ, Ashworth A. PARP inhibitors: synthetic lethality in the clinic. Science 2017;355(6330):1152–8.

[57] Satoh MS, Lindahl T. Role of poly(ADP-ribose) formation in DNA repair. Nature 1992;356(6367):356–8.

[58] Ceccaldi R, Liu JC, Amunugama R, et al. Homologous-recombination-deficient tumours are dependent on Polθ-mediated repair. Nature 2015;518(7538):258–62.

[59] Brambati A, Barry RM, Sfeir A. DNA polymerase theta (Polθ) - an error-prone polymerase necessary for genome stability. Curr Opin Genet Dev 2020;60:119–26.

[60] Schrempf A, Slyskova J, Loizou JI. Targeting the DNA repair enzyme polymerase θ in cancer therapy. Trends Cancer 2021;7(2):98–111.

[61] Bazan Russo TD, Mujacic C, Di Giovanni E, et al. Polθ: emerging synthetic lethal partner in homologous recombination-deficient tumors. Cancer Gene Ther 2024;31(11):1619–31.

[62] Zatreanu D, Robinson HMR, Alkhatib O, et al. Polθ inhibitors elicit BRCA-gene synthetic lethality and target PARP inhibitor resistance. Nat Commun 2021;12(1):3636.

[63] Zhou J, Gelot C, Pantelidou C, et al. A first-in-class polymerase theta inhibitor selectively targets homologous-recombination-deficient tumors. Nat Cancer 2021;2(6):598–610.

[64] Smith CM, Gupta GP. Polymerase θ inhibition steps on the cGAS pedal. J Clin Investig 2023;133(11). https://doi.org/10.1172/JCI170660.

[65] Mayor P, Gay LM, Lele S, et al. BRCA1 reversion mutation acquired after treatment identified by liquid biopsy. Gynecol Oncol Rep 2017;21:57–60.

[66] Cancer Genome Atlas Research Network. Integrated genomic analyses of ovarian carcinoma. Nature 2011;474(7353):609–15.

[67] Wang Z, Lu Y, Han M, et al. Association between homologous recombination deficiency status and carboplatin treatment response in early triple-negative breast cancer. Breast Cancer Res Treat 2024;208(2):429–40.

[68] Imanishi S, Naoi Y, Shimazu K, et al. Clinicopathological analysis of homologous recombination-deficient breast cancers with special reference to response to neoadjuvant paclitaxel followed by FEC. Breast Cancer Res Treat 2019;174(3):627–37.

[69] Casolino R, Paiella S, Azzolina D, et al. Homologous recombination deficiency in pancreatic cancer: a systematic review and prevalence meta-analysis. J Clin Oncol 2021;39(23):2617–31.

[70] Cancer Genome Atlas Research Network. The molecular taxonomy of primary prostate cancer. Cell 2015;163(4):1011–25.

[71] Belli C, Duso BA, Ferraro E, et al. Homologous recombination deficiency in triple negative breast cancer. Breast 2019;45:15–21.

[72] Tutt A, Tovey H, Cheang MCU, et al. Carboplatin in BRCA1/2-mutated and triple-negative breast cancer BRCAness subgroups: the TNT Trial. Nat Med 2018;24(5):628–37.

[73] Isakoff SJ, Mayer EL, He L, et al. TBCRC009: a multicenter phase II clinical trial of platinum monotherapy with biomarker assessment in metastatic triple-negative breast cancer. J Clin Oncol 2015;33(17):1902–9.

[74] Tutt ANJ, Garber JE, Kaufman B, et al. Adjuvant olaparib for patients with BRCA1- or BRCA2-mutated breast cancer. N Engl J Med 2021;384(25):2394–405.

[75] Robson M, Im SA, Senkus E, et al. Olaparib for metastatic breast cancer in patients with a germline BRCA mutation. N Engl J Med 2017;377(6):523–33.

[76] Litton JK, Rugo HS, Ettl J, et al. Talazoparib in patients with advanced breast cancer and a germline BRCA mutation. N Engl J Med 2018;379(8):753–63.

[77] Tung NM, Robson ME, Ventz S, et al. Tbcrc 048: phase II study of olaparib for metastatic breast cancer and mutations in homologous recombination-related genes. J Clin Oncol 2020;38(36):4274–82.

[78] Heitz F, Ataseven B, Staniczok C, et al. Implementing HRD testing in routine clinical practice on patients with primary high-grade advanced ovarian cancer. Cancers (Basel) 2023;15(3). https://doi.org/10.3390/cancers15030818.

[79] Vencken PMLH, Kriege M, Hoogwerf D, et al. Chemosensitivity and outcome of BRCA1- and BRCA2-associated ovarian cancer patients after first-line chemotherapy compared with sporadic ovarian cancer patients. Ann Oncol 2011;22(6):1346–52.

[80] Tan DSP, Rothermundt C, Thomas K, et al. "BRCAness" syndrome in ovarian cancer: a case-control study describing the clinical features and outcome of patients with epithelial ovarian cancer associated with BRCA1 and BRCA2 mutations. J Clin Oncol 2008;26(34):5530–6.

[81] Pennington KP, Walsh T, Harrell MI, et al. Germline and somatic mutations in homologous recombination genes predict platinum response and survival in ovarian, fallopian tube, and peritoneal carcinomas. Clin Cancer Res 2014;20(3):764–75.

[82] Ray-Coquard I, Leary A, Pignata S, et al. Olaparib plus bevacizumab first-line maintenance in ovarian cancer: final overall survival results from the PAOLA-1/ENGOT-ov25 trial. Ann Oncol 2023; 34(8):681–92.

[83] González-Martín A, Pothuri B, Vergote I, et al. Niraparib in patients with newly diagnosed advanced ovarian cancer. N Engl J Med 2019;381(25):2391–402.

[84] Moore K, Colombo N, Scambia G, et al. Maintenance olaparib in patients with newly diagnosed advanced ovarian cancer. N Engl J Med 2018;379-(26):2495–505.

[85] Balasubramaniam S, Beaver JA, Horton S, et al. FDA approval summary: rucaparib for the treatment of patients with deleterious BRCA mutation-associated advanced ovarian cancer. Clin Cancer Res 2017;23-(23):7165–70.

[86] Kristeleit R, Shapiro GI, Burris HA, et al. A phase I-II study of the oral PARP inhibitor rucaparib in patients with germline BRCA1/2-mutated ovarian carcinoma or other solid tumors. Clin Cancer Res 2017;23(15): 4095–106.

[87] Coleman RL, Oza AM, Lorusso D, et al. Rucaparib maintenance treatment for recurrent ovarian carcinoma after response to platinum therapy (ARIEL3): a randomised, double-blind, placebo-controlled, phase 3 trial. Lancet 2017;390(10106):1949–61.

[88] Sung H, Ferlay J, Siegel RL, et al. Global cancer statistics 2020: GLOBOCAN estimates of incidence and mortality worldwide for 36 cancers in 185 countries. CA Cancer J Clin 2021;71(3):209–49.

[89] Schmid S, Omlin A, Higano C, et al. Activity of platinum-based chemotherapy in patients with advanced prostate cancer with and without DNA repair gene aberrations. JAMA Netw Open 2020;3(10):e2021692.

[90] Hager S, Ackermann CJ, Joerger M, et al. Anti-tumour activity of platinum compounds in advanced prostate cancer-a systematic literature review. Ann Oncol 2016;27(6):975–84.

[91] Aparicio AM, Harzstark AL, Corn PG, et al. Platinum-based chemotherapy for variant castrate-resistant prostate cancer. Clin Cancer Res 2013;19(13):3621–30.

[92] Leal F, García-Perdomo HA. Effectiveness of platinum-based chemotherapy in patients with metastatic prostate cancer: systematic review and meta-analysis. Clin Genitourin Cancer 2019;17(3):e627–44.

[93] Pomerantz MM, Spisák S, Jia L, et al. The association between germline BRCA2 variants and sensitivity to platinum-based chemotherapy among men with metastatic prostate cancer. Cancer 2017;123(18): 3532–9.

[94] Cheng HH, Pritchard CC, Montgomery B, et al. Prostate cancer screening in a new era of genetics. Clin Genitourin Cancer 2017;15(6):625–8.

[95] Mota JM, Barnett E, Nauseef JT, et al. Platinum-based chemotherapy in metastatic prostate cancer with DNA repair gene alterations. JCO Precis Oncol 2020; 4:355–66.

[96] Chi KN, Rathkopf D, Smith MR, et al. Niraparib and abiraterone acetate for metastatic castration-resistant prostate cancer. J Clin Oncol 2023;41(18):3339–51.

[97] Agarwal N, Azad AA, Carles J, et al. Talazoparib plus enzalutamide in men with first-line metastatic castration-resistant prostate cancer (TALAPRO-2): a randomised, placebo-controlled, phase 3 trial. Lancet 2023;402(10398):291–303.

[98] Abida W, Patnaik A, Campbell D, et al. Rucaparib in men with metastatic castration-resistant prostate cancer harboring a BRCA1 or BRCA2 gene alteration. J Clin Oncol 2020;38(32):3763–72.

[99] de Bono J, Mateo J, Fizazi K, et al. Olaparib for metastatic castration-resistant prostate cancer. N Engl J Med 2020;382(22):2091–102.

[100] Schiewer MJ, Goodwin JF, Han S, et al. Dual roles of PARP-1 promote cancer growth and progression. Cancer Discov 2012;2(12):1134–49.

[101] Polkinghorn WR, Parker JS, Lee MX, et al. Androgen receptor signaling regulates DNA repair in prostate cancers. Cancer Discov 2013;3(11):1245–53.

[102] Li L, Karanika S, Yang G, et al. Androgen receptor inhibitor-induced "BRCAness" and PARP inhibition are synthetically lethal for castration-resistant prostate cancer. Sci Signal 2017;10(480). https://doi.org/10.1126/scisignal.aam7479.

[103] Asim M, Tarish F, Zecchini HI, et al. Synthetic lethality between androgen receptor signalling and the PARP pathway in prostate cancer. Nat Commun 2017;8(1):374.

[104] Clarke N, Wiechno P, Alekseev B, et al. Olaparib combined with abiraterone in patients with metastatic castration-resistant prostate cancer: a randomised, double-blind, placebo-controlled, phase 2 trial. Lancet Oncol 2018;19(7):975–86.

[105] Rahib L, Smith BD, Aizenberg R, et al. Projecting cancer incidence and deaths to 2030: the unexpected burden of thyroid, liver, and pancreas cancers in the United States. Cancer Res 2014;74(11):2913–21.

[106] Sehdev A, Gbolahan O, Hancock BA, et al. Germline and somatic DNA damage repair gene mutations and overall survival in metastatic pancreatic adenocarcinoma patients treated with FOLFIRINOX. Clin Cancer Res 2018;24(24):6204–11.

[107] Yu S, Agarwal P, Mamtani R, et al. Retrospective survival analysis of patients with resected pancreatic ductal adenocarcinoma and a germline BRCA or PALB2 mutation. JCO Precis Oncol 2019;3:1–11.

[108] Wattenberg MM, Asch D, Yu S, et al. Platinum response characteristics of patients with pancreatic ductal

adenocarcinoma and a germline BRCA1, BRCA2 or PALB2 mutation. Br J Cancer 2020;122(3):333–9.
[109] O'Reilly EM, Lee JW, Zalupski M, et al. Randomized, multicenter, phase II trial of gemcitabine and cisplatin with or without veliparib in patients with pancreas adenocarcinoma and a germline BRCA/PALB2 mutation. J Clin Oncol 2020;38(13):1378–88.
[110] Golan T, Hammel P, Reni M, et al. Maintenance olaparib for germline BRCA-mutated metastatic pancreatic cancer. N Engl J Med 2019;381(4):317–27.
[111] Reiss KA, Mick R, O'Hara MH, et al. Phase II study of maintenance rucaparib in patients with platinum-sensitive advanced pancreatic cancer and a pathogenic germline or somatic variant in BRCA1, BRCA2, or PALB2. J Clin Oncol 2021;39(22):2497–505.

Advances in Molecular Pathology 8 (2025) 83–95
ADVANCES IN MOLECULAR PATHOLOGY

A Review of Molecular Techniques and Biomarkers for the Diagnosis of Tumors of the Central Nervous System

Derek Wong, PhD*
Department of Pathology and Laboratory Medicine, Division of Genomic Diagnostics, The Children's Hospital of Philadelphia, University of Pennsylvania Perelman School of Medicine, Philadelphia, PA, USA

KEYWORDS
• Central nervous system tumors • World health organization • Molecular diagnostics • Molecular techniques
• Next-generation sequencing • Molecular pathology • Methylation profiling • Fusion profiling

KEY POINTS

- Molecular information is incorporated into the World Health Organization classification system and is essential diagnostic criteria for specific entities.
- Comprehensive DNA and RNA profiling provides the highest diagnostic yield.
- Molecular profiling should be performed in tandem with histology to provide an integrated diagnosis.

INTRODUCTION

Tumors of the central nervous system (CNS) encompass a diverse group of neoplasms that arise within the brain and spinal cord. Given the complexity and the varied nature of CNS tumors, accurate diagnosis is crucial for guiding treatment decisions, predicting patient outcomes, and improving overall survival rates. Over the past decades, diagnostic approaches for brain tumors have undergone a significant transformation— from the reliance on histologic examination to the integration of diagnostic molecular biomarkers into the World Health Organization (WHO) classification of CNS tumors [1].

Starting in the 1920s, neurosurgeon Harvey Cushing and pathologist Percival Bailey laid the foundation of neuropathology and introduced the concept of tumor grading and classification [2]. Though Cushing and Bailey's histologic approach was rudimentary, classifying tumors into broad categories based largely on macroscopic features (cellular characteristics, anatomic location, and growth patterns), it set the foundation for understanding brain tumors. The development of immunohistochemistry (IHC) in the mid-twentieth century significantly advanced the diagnosis of brain tumors allowing pathologists to more accurately identify tumor based on both tissue/cell morphology and IHC characteristics. In 1979, the introduction of the WHO classification system for CNS tumors marked a major milestone, which provided a standardized and systematic approach to categorize CNS tumors based on histologic findings and introduced the concept of tumor grading, distinguishing between benign and malignant tumors [3].

Over the past 2 decades, molecular diagnostics have revolutionized our understanding of brain tumors. Histology-based classification systems, while still valuable, were not sufficient in distinguishing tumors with similar morphologic features or tumors with nontypical morphologic features. Advances in molecular biology, including the discovery of genetic mutations, chromosomal abnormalities, and epigenetic changes, have provided valuable tools for more

*Corresponding author. *E-mail address:* Wongd3@chop.edu

https://doi.org/10.1016/j.yamp.2025.05.007
www.advancesinmolecularpathology.com
2589-4080/25/ © 2025 Elsevier Inc. All rights are reserved, including those for text and data mining, AI training, and similar technologies.

ABBREVIATIONS	
CNS	central nervous system
CPC	choroid plexus carcinoma
CPP	choroid plexus papilloma
ctDNA	circulating tumor DNA
DA	diffuse astrocytoma
ddPCR	digital droplet polymerase chain reaction
DHG	diffuse hemispheric glioma
DMG	diffuse midline glioma
FISH	fluorescence in situ hybridization
IDH	isocitrate dehydrogenase
IHC	immunohistochemistry
LRS	long-read sequencing
MB-G3	medulloblastoma, Group 3
MB-G4	medulloblastoma, Group 4
MB-SHH	medulloblastoma, SHH-activated
MB-WNT	medulloblastoma, WNT-activated
NGS	next-generation sequencing
PA	pilocytic astrocytoma
PCR	polymerase chain reaction
PF	posterior fossa
PF-EPN-A	posterior fossa ependymoma, type A
PF-EPN-B	posterior fossa ependymoma, type B
pHGG	pediatric high-grade glioma
pLGG	pediatric low-grade gliomas
PXA	pleomorphic xanthoastrocytoma
qPCR	quantitative polymerase chain reaction
RNA-seq	RNA sequencing
SP	spinal
SP-EPN	spinal ependymoma
SP-MPE	myxopapillary ependymoma
SP-MYCN	spinal ependymoma, MYCN amplified
SRS	short-read sequencing
ST	supratentorial
ST-EPN-RELA	supratentorial ependymoma, ZFTA fusion-positive
ST-EPN-YAP1	supratentorial ependymoma, YAP1 fusion-positive
WHO	World Health Organization

accurate tumor classification and prognosis which enable pathologists to classify tumors at a much more granular level. In 2016, the WHO classification of CNS tumors incorporated, for the first time, molecular biomarkers into the diagnostic criteria for diffuse adult gliomas, creating distinct molecular entities independent of histology [4]. The WHO continues to refine and integrate molecular biomarkers into diagnostic criteria as our understanding of the molecular pathogenesis of CNS tumors increases. In 2021, DNA methylation profiles were introduced adding global genomic profiling to CNS tumor classification [5]. Today, multi-omic diagnostics are routinely performed on CNS tumors and are an integral part of diagnostic pathology.

CURRENT TECHNIQUES

Immunohistochemistry and fluorescence in situ hybridization

IHC and fluorescence in situ hybridization (FISH) are histology-based (in situ) molecular techniques. IHC detects expression of a specific target antigen within a tissue sample using antibodies tagged with a colorimetric label. IHC is the "bread and butter" in diagnostic pathology but is heavily reliant on the specificity and availability of antibodies and limited to known antigens (Fig. 1). In contrast, FISH uses fluorescently labeled DNA probes to detect the presence, location, and quantity of specific target DNA sequences and can be used for detecting chromosomal rearrangements and copy number changes (deletions, duplications, and amplifications) (Fig. 2). FISH can also be used to assess for fusions using break apart or come-together probes [6].

Polymerase chain reaction and Sanger sequencing

Polymerase chain reaction (PCR) is a fundamental molecular technique that allows for the analysis of specific DNA sequences following target amplification (Fig. 3A). Primers can be designed for a specific region of interest and then analyzed using Sanger sequencing which is based on the introduction of labeled dideoxynucleotides which stop replication when incorporated into a growing DNA strand (see Fig. 3C–D). Sanger sequencing is often used to investigate specific point mutations. Other common PCR-based diagnostic assays include real-time quantitative PCR (qPCR) and digital droplet PCR (ddPCR) which provide quantitation by assessing a fluorescent signal following each PCR cycle (see Fig. 3B). Both qPCR and ddPCR are highly sensitive and can be used to assess gene expression, amplification, copy number, or specific variants.

Methylation analysis

In addition to sequence analysis, molecular diagnostics also includes epigenetic markers such as DNA

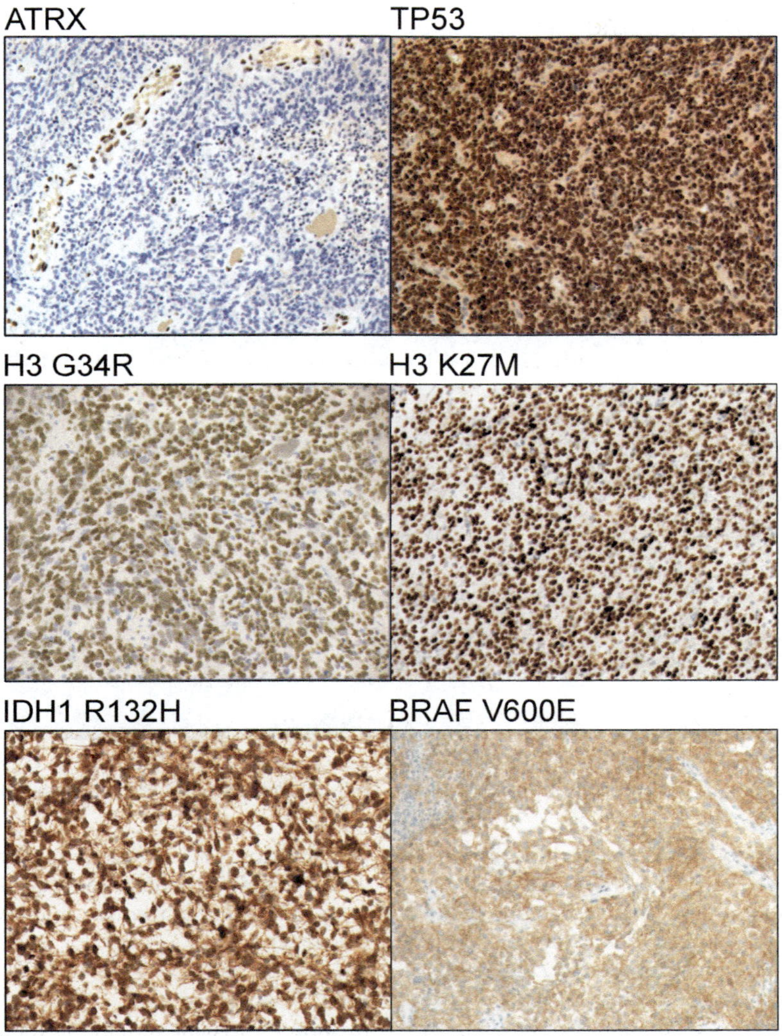

FIG. 1 IHC images showing loss of ATRX (*ATRX* mutation), TP53 overexpression (*TP53* mutation), and presence of mutant proteins H3 G34R, H3 K27M, IDH1 R132H, and BRAF V600E. Target antigens are stained in brown while blue staining (hematoxylin) are cell nuclei.

methylation. The most common epigenetic-based diagnostic test in CNS tumors is assessing the promoter methylation of *MGMT* (O-6-*methylguanine-DNA methyltransferase*) in glioblastoma (GBM) [7]. This is performed using methylation-specific PCR where half of the sample is treated with sodium bisulfite which converts unmethylated cytosine into uracil through deamination. Primers that are designed to target the methylated and unmethylated sequences are then used for PCR amplification. The amount of PCR amplification that occurs in the bisulfite-treated sample, compared with the untreated sample, can be used to determine the methylation level in MGMT promoter.

Array-based technologies

Moving from targeted analyses, array-based technologies were one of the first technologies that provided a genome-wide view for copy number alterations using fluorescently labeled DNA samples hybridized onto chips (10^3–10^6 targets). The 2 main array-based

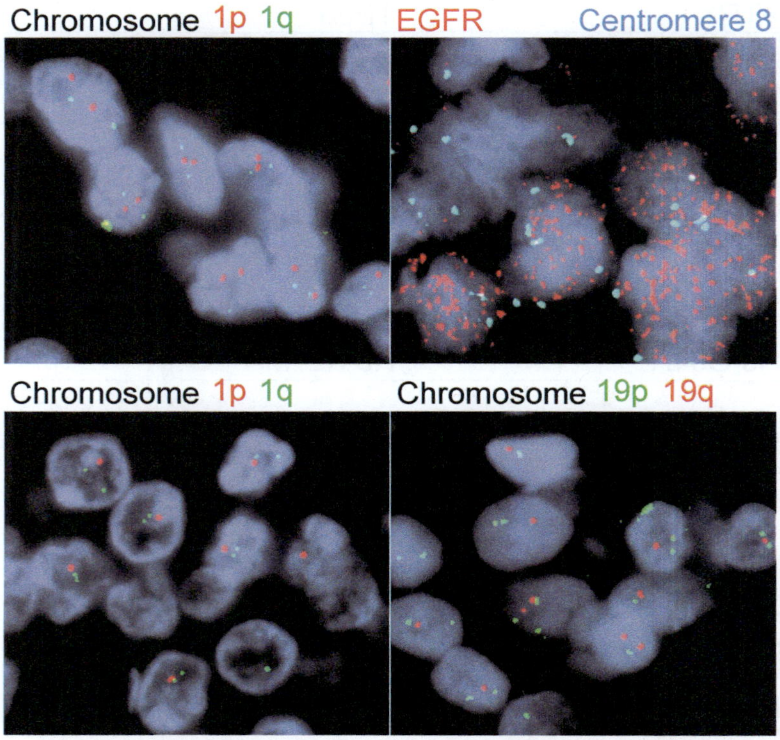

FIG. 2 FISH images showing balanced copy number (2 copies each, upper left), 1p loss (1 red, 2 green, lower left), 19q loss (1 red, 2 green, lower right), and *EGFR* amplification (red amplification, upper right).

technologies, comparative genomic hybridization and single nucleotide polymorphism (SNP)-based arrays, are able to detect copy neutral loss of heterozygosity, which is a common mechanism that results in biallelic inactivation of tumor suppressor genes (*TP53*, *PTEN*, and *RB1*). SNP arrays are limited to the regions captured by the probe design and do not supply sequence information or exact breakpoints.

Next-generation sequencing

The most comprehensive and inclusive method of molecular profiling is next-generation sequencing (NGS), which allows for rapid and high-throughput analysis of DNA sequences. Unlike Sanger, which sequences one DNA fragment at a time, NGS sequences millions of DNA fragments simultaneously and has become the gold standard in molecular diagnostics. NGS is most often performed by targeting a select number of genes or regions of interest through hybrid capture or PCR amplification to generate a library which is analyzed on a flow cell. Large somatic panels [8] have become integral to routine clinical workups (see Fig. 3E). Copy number alterations can also be analyzed with the addition of a genome-wide backbone, similar to in SNP arrays or through shallow sequencing of the whole genome (0.1–1x) [9].

RNA fusion

In addition to gene mutations and copy number alterations, cancers can also be driven by the production of an oncogenic fusion gene. Detection of these fusion events can be challenging at the DNA level because genomic instability and structural rearrangements, a hallmark of cancer, are common events that do not often produce a functional fusion transcript. Many fusions also occur within large introns which would not be feasible to capture in a DNA panel which targets coding exons. To combat these challenges, diagnostic laboratories routinely utilize NGS analysis of RNA to profile for expressed fusion genes. The most common method of detection uses a panel such as the Illumina TruSight or Archer FusionPlex that enriches for genes of interest using hybrid capture or anchored multiplex PCR technologies [10]. The use of RNA also provides

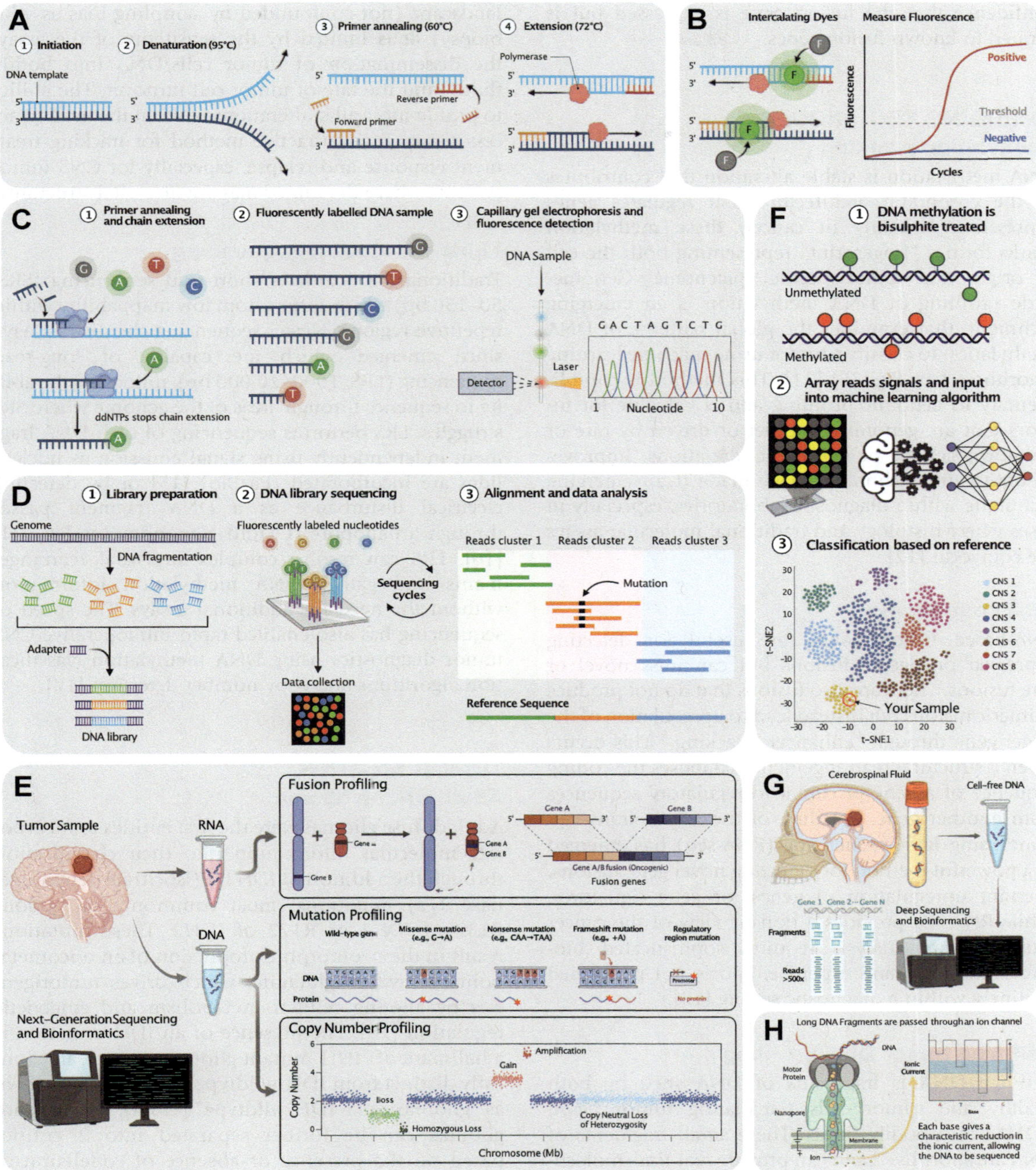

FIG. 3 Molecular diagnostic techniques. Illustration showing the steps of PCR **(A)**, qPCR **(B)**, Sanger sequencing **(C)**, next generation sequencing **(D)**, and DNA methylation array **(F)**. **(E)** shows the components of DNA/RNA analysis of tumors using next-generation sequencing and the alteration types that can be identified. **(G)** shows cell-free DNA sequencing using deep sequencing and **(H)** shows the process of sequencing long reads using nanopore sequencing technology.

confidence that the fusion gene is expressed but is limited to known fusion genes.

EMERGING TECHNIQUES

Methylation profiling

DNA methylation is stable alteration that contributes to the chromatin architecture that regulates genes expression. Similarly in cancer, these methylation marks form a "fingerprint" representing both the cell of origin and tumor-specific epigenome. Genome-wide profiling of DNA methylation is an emerging technique that examines the global patterns of DNA methylation to classify a tumor using machine learning algorithms (see Fig. 3F) [11]. This method is complimentary to genomic profiling and is valuable for tumors that are genomically quiet or driven by rare or unknown genetic or epigenetic alterations. Improvements to this technology have made it an emerging technique within diagnostic laboratories, especially in cases where histology and traditional molecular assays are equivocal [12].

RNA sequencing

RNA-based fusion panels are useful for detecting expressed oncogenic fusions but can miss novel or rare fusions. There are also fusions that do not produce chimeric fusions but instead lead to upregulation of the target gene through "enhancer hijacking." This occurs when a structural rearrangement juxtaposes the coding sequence of a gene proximal to regulatory sequences from another gene. Profiling of the whole transcriptome using RNA sequencing (RNA-seq) has emerged as a powerful method for detecting novel gene fusions, aberrant upregulation of genes, or gene signatures. While RNA-seq provides a holistic view of the cancer transcriptome, analysis requires sophisticated bioinformatic tools and expertise, and is not performed routinely within a diagnostic setting [13].

Cell-free tumor DNA profiling

Cell-free DNA is fragments of DNA shed by both healthy and tumor cells (circulating tumor DNA; ctDNA) into bodily fluids. These small fragments of DNA are short-lived and can provide real-time molecular information about the originating cell such as mutations and DNA methylation [14]. Improvements to the sensitivity of NGS technologies have enabled deep profiling of ctDNA to detect somatic variants as low as 0.1% (see Fig. 3G). While ctDNA analysis can provide a more holistic view of a tumor's genomic landscape (not confounded by sampling bias as with biopsy), it is limited by the sensitivity of the assay, the dissemination of tumor cells/DNA into bodily fluids, and the rate of tumor cell turnover. The ability to profile molecular alterations without the need to access tissue is an attractive method for tracking treatment response and relapse, especially for CNS tumor patients where the tumor may involve vital structures.

Third-generation sequencing

Traditional NGS utilizes short-read sequencing (SRS; 50–150 bp) which suffers from low mappability within repetitive regions. Newer sequencing chemistries have since emerged which are capable of long-read sequencing (LRS; 1000–20,000 bp), unlocking the ability to sequence through areas of the genome where SRS struggles. LRS performs sequencing of each DNA fragment independently using signal emission as nucleotides are incorporated (PacBio) [15] or by detecting electrical disturbance as a DNA fragment passes through a nanopore (Oxford Nanopore; see Fig. 3H) [16]. LRS can resolve complex structural rearrangements and gather DNA methylation information without the need for additional assays. The speed of sequencing has also enabled rapid intraoperative CNS tumor diagnostics using DNA methylation classification algorithms and copy number detection [17].

TUMOR ENTITIES

Adult diffuse glioma

Adult diffuse gliomas were the first entities to incorporate molecular information into their classification through the addition of *IDH1/2* (isocitrate dehydrogenase 1/2) mutations, most commonly on codons R132 of *IDH1* or R172 of *IDH2*. These mutations result in the neomorphic production of an oncometabolite, 2-hydroxyglutarate, which drives tumorigenesis by altering cellular metabolism and epigenetic regulation [18]. The presence of an IDH mutation is a hallmark of "IDH-mutant gliomas," which are clinically distinct from IDH-wildtype gliomas, also known as "glioblastoma, IDH-wildtype" (GBM). IDH-mutant gliomas can be further separated into 2 entities based on the presence or absence of codeletion of chromosomes 1p and 19q [19]. Gliomas that harbor 1p/19q codeletion are classified as "oligodendroglioma, IDH-mutant, and 1p19/q co-deleted" and often also harbor mutations in *CIC*, *FUBP1*, and *TERT* promoter mutations [20]. IDH-mutant gliomas that lack 1p/19q codeletion are classified as "astrocytoma, IDH-mutant" and often harbor mutations in *TP53* and *ATRX* [21]. In both subtypes, loss of *CDKN2A/B* indicates a more aggressive tumor and higher WHO CNS grade [22].

Glioblastoma, IDH-wildtype (GBM) encompasses a heterogenous group of aggressive high-grade gliomas [23]. Common molecular alterations for this entity include concurrent gain of chromosome 7 and loss of chromosome 10 (+7/−10 signature), *TERT* promoter mutations, and *EGFR* activating alterations or amplification. Mutations in the promoter region of the *TERT* gene (telomerase reverse transcriptase), C228T and C250T, lead to the reactivation of telomerase enabling tumor cells to maintain their telomere length and sustain their proliferative potential [24]. Activation of the MAPK or PIK3-AKT-mTOR pathways is frequently seen in GBM with the most common alteration being *EGFR* (epidermal growth factor receptor) amplification, rearrangement (in-frame deletion of exons 2–7; EGFRvIII), and activating mutations (A289, G598, and R108). Dysregulation of the DNA damage repair pathway through inactivation of *TP53* or amplification of *MDM2/4* is also commonly seen in GBM. Oncogenic fusions, while rarer, are observed in GBM with the most frequent involving *MET* (promiscuous), *FGFR3* (*FGFR3::TACC3*), and *NTRK1/2/3* (promiscuous) [25]. Lastly, the methylation status of the *MGMT* (O6-methylguanine-DNA methyltransferase) promoter is another critical molecular marker useful for treatment planning. *MGMT* is a DNA repair enzyme, and its promoter methylation leads to the silencing of this gene, making the tumor more sensitive to alkylating agents like temozolomide (TMZ) [26] (Fig. 4A).

Meningioma

Meningiomas are the most common primary CNS tumor and typically arise from the meninges in patients >65 years of age. While historically classified based on histologic appearance and graded according to their degree of malignancy (Grades 1–3), the molecular diagnostics of meningiomas has advanced significantly. Meningiomas can be classified into 2 large subgroups based on *NF2* status. Biallelic inactivation of *NF2* on chromosome 22q can be achieved through a combination of mutations, deletions, or loss of heterozygosity within the *NF2* locus [27]. Higher grade meningiomas are characterized by increased genomic instability and often exhibit more complex changes such as losses of chromosomes 1p, 2, 3p, 4, 6, 7p, 8, 10q, 14q, 18, homozygous loss of *CDKN2A/B*, and *TERT* promoter mutations [28].

Non-*NF2* meningiomas are a more heterogeneous group of tumors, the most common being recurrent mutations in *AKT1* (p.E17K), *TRAF7*, *SMO* (p.L412F and p. W535L), *KLF4* (p.K409Q), and *PIK3CA* (p.E545K and p. H1047R) [29,30]. Alterations in *AKT1*, *SMO*, and *PIK3CA* are strongly correlated to meningothelial, and *KLF4* and *TRAF7* alterations are correlated to the secretory subtypes of meningioma. Unlike *NF2*-driven meningioma, these tumors exhibit balanced genomes, and grading relies on histopathological correlates.

Rarer non-*NF2* alterations include *POLR2A*, *PBRM1*, *BAP1*, *SMARCE1*, and *YAP1*. *POLR2A* hotspot mutations (p.Q403K and p.L438_His439del) are frequently identified in Grade 1, benign meningiomas [31]. Papillary and rhabdoid meningiomas, which show overlapping histologic features, also share overlapping alterations in *PBRM1* and *BAP1*, suggesting shared pathogenesis [32,33]. Nuclear loss of SMARCE1 is present in nearly all clear cell meningiomas which often harbor somatic variants in *SMARCE1* [34]. Lastly, alterations involving *YAP1* can be identified in pediatric onset meningioma [35] (see Fig. 4B).

Pediatric low-grade glioma

Pediatric low-grade gliomas (pLGG) are the most common type of CNS tumor in children, comprising a diverse group of tumors that generally have a favorable prognosis. Nearly all pLGG are driven by activation of the MAPK pathway through alterations in *BRAF*, *FGFR1/2/3*, *NTRK1/2/3*, and *NF1* [36,37]. Although molecular diagnostics is informative for determining targetable mutations, diagnosis of these entities still rely heavily on histopathology due to the broad overlap of driver mutations across several histologic subtypes.

The most common alterations in pLGG lead to the activation of *BRAF* with the 2 most common alterations being *BRAF* p.V600E and *KIAA1549::BRAF* fusions [38]. *BRAF* fusions, such as the *KIAA1549::BRAF* fusion, are most commonly observed in "pilocytic astrocytoma" (PA), though alternate fusion partners with *BRAF*, while rare, can also be identified [39]. If loss of chromosome 1p is also identified, these tumors are often classified as "diffuse leptomeningeal glioneuronal tumor" which have a poorer prognosis [40]. In contrast, the activating *BRAF* p.V600E variant is more common in "pleomorphic xanthoastrocytoma" (PXA), "diffuse astrocytoma—MAPK altered" (DA), and "ganglioglioma" [41]. DA can also be driven by alterations in *FGFR1/2/3* with the diagnosis relying on histopathology and ruling out other entities. Alterations in *FGFR1* such as the hotspot mutations p.

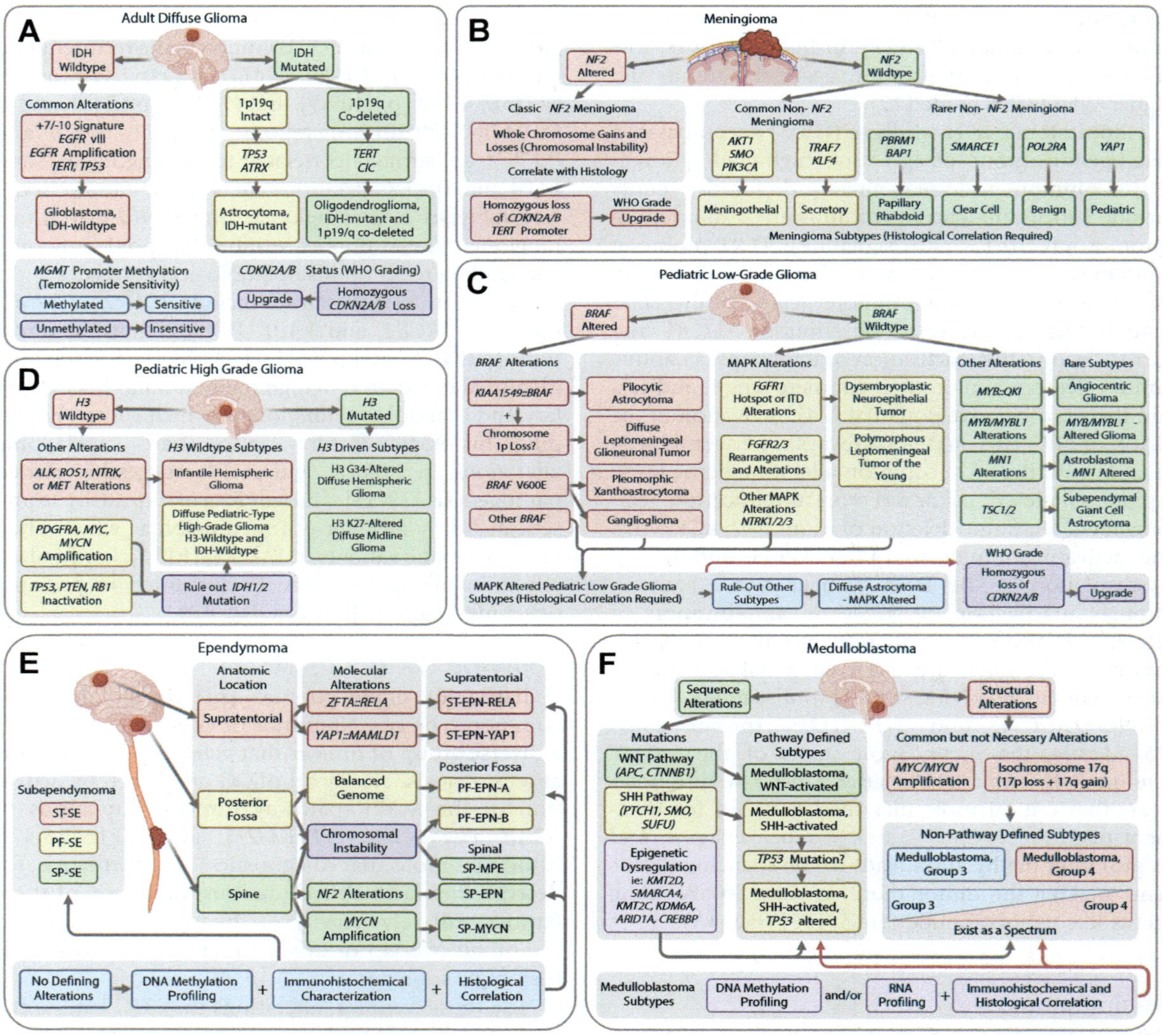

FIG. 4 Diagnostic algorithms for brain tumors. Diagnostic algorithm schematics for adult diffuse glioma **(A)**, meningioma **(B)**, pediatric low-grade glioma **(C)**, pHGG **(D)**, ependymoma **(E)**, and medulloblastoma **(F)**. All molecular diagnostic algorithms should also take into account histologic and immunophenotyping correlation to synthesize an integrated diagnosis.

N546K and p.K656E and internal tandem duplications within the *FGFR1* kinase domain are most prevalent in "dysembryoplastic neuroepithelial tumor", while alterations such as fusion events involving *FGFR2* or *FGFR3* are more commonly associated with "polymorphous leptomeningeal tumor of the young" [42]. Fusions involving the *NTRK1/2/3* genes can be observed across several subtypes of pLGG with *NTRK2* being the most common. Most importantly, within this group of pLGG, many of these activating alterations can be inhibited by small molecular inhibitors targeting *BRAF*, *TRK1/2/3* (*NTRK1/2/3*), and *FGFR1/2/3* [43].

Some rarer pLGG subtypes have defining genomic alterations. Rearrangements involving *MYB/MYBL1* are defining for "*MYB/MYBL1*-altered diffuse astrocytoma" [44] with *MYB::QKI* fusions being commonly associated with angiocentric glioma [45]. Another subtype, driven by rearrangements in *MN1*, "Astroblastoma, *MN1*-altered," is a more recent addition to the WHO that relies on molecular information, as these tumors show histologic overlap with several other entities [46]. Lastly, "subependymal giant cell astrocytoma" is highly associated with alterations in *TSC1/2* and the genetic disorder tuberous sclerosis [47].

Few subtypes of pLGG can be classified solely on molecular information and often require correlation with histology. However, grading of several entities, such as PA, PXA, and DA can be heavily influenced by the loss of cell cycle regulators *CDKN2A/B*. Alterations in *CDKN2A/B* are associated with a more aggressive clinical course, higher-grade histology, and may suggest a need for more aggressive treatment and closer monitoring [36] (see Fig. 4C).

Pediatric high-grade glioma

Pediatric high-grade glioma (pHGG) encompasses a diverse and aggressive group of tumors that are often resistant to conventional therapies: surgery, radiation, and chemotherapy. Defining molecular alterations in these tumors involves mutations affecting histone *H3*, 1 of the 4 subunits that make up a histone tetramer. Histones are protein complexes that organize DNA structure (chromatin) and aid in gene regulation. Alterations in *H3* most often affect codons K27 or G34 which can be classified into 2 distinct subtypes [48]. Codon 27 mutations (most commonly p.K27M) dysregulate chromatin structure and gene expression through inhibition of the polycomb repressive complex 2; and are defining for "H3K27-altered diffuse midline glioma" (DMG) [49]. Alternatively, codon 34 mutations (most commonly p.G34R), result in global DNA hypomethylation due to inhibition of the methyltransferases SETD2 and DNMT1, and are defining for "H3G34-altered diffuse hemispheric glioma" (DHG) [50]. Both alterations result in the expression of "oncohistones" which drive pathogenesis but also have distinct oncogenic pathways and mechanisms leading to differences in the anatomic location (midline vs hemispheric) and molecular landscape of DHG and DMG [51].

pHGG that lack alterations in *H3* are heterogenous. One subset, termed "infantile hemispheric glioma" are driven by alterations, often fusions, in receptor tyrosine kinases such as *ALK*, *ROS1*, *NTRK*, and *MET* and arises in infants (>1 years) [52]. The remainder of these CNS tumors is termed "diffuse pediatric-type high-grade glioma H3-wildtype and IDH-wildtype," and alterations in *IDH1/2* and *H3* must be first ruled out. Many of these tumors are driven by amplification of *MYC*, *MYCN*, or *PDGFRA*, or activating alterations in *EGFR*. Inactivating mutations in tumor suppressor genes such as *PTEN*, *RB1*, and *TP53* are also frequently observed [53]. Importantly, loss of function of *TP53* which regulates the cell cycle, DNA repair, and apoptosis, is often associated with a more aggressive phenotype and poorer prognosis (see Fig. 4D).

Ependymoma

Molecular and clinicopathologic analysis of ependymoma have resulted in a classification system based both on the location of the tumor and molecular markers. Anatomically, ependymoma are stratified into supratentorial (ST), posterior fossa (PF), and spinal (SP) which can be further classified based on molecular alterations [54].

ST ependymoma can be divided into 2 molecular groups that are both driven by fusions. *ZFTA::RELA* (previously known as *C11orf95::RELA*) which activates the NF-kB pathway [55] are defining for "supratentorial ependymoma, ZFTA fusion-positive; ST-EPN-RELA," and *YAP1::MAMLD1*, which activates the Hippo pathway [56], are defining for "supratentorial ependymoma, YAP1 fusion-positive; ST-EPN-YAP1." While these 2 fusions are the most common, fusions of *RELA* and *YAP1* with alternative partners have also been observed.

PF ependymomas can be classified into 2 subtypes [57]. "posterior fossa ependymoma, type A; PF-EPN-A" is the most common subgroup in children and is characterized by a lack of recurrent copy number alterations. Due to this lack of genomic markers, it can be challenging to confidently classify PF-EPN-A using solely DNA analysis, thus, diagnosis is often paired with DNA methylation and immunohistochemical phenotyping. In contrast, "posterior fossa ependymoma, type B; PF-EPN-B" occurs more frequently in adults with a more favorable prognosis and is characterized by chromosomal instability with frequent loss of chromosomes 6, 10, 17, and 22, and gain of chromosomes 1q, 5, 8, and 18.

"Spinal ependymoma; SP-EPN" are most often low-grade tumors with favorable prognosis. The most common alteration observed in SP-EPN is loss of chromosome 22 and mutations in *NF2*. One subtype is driven by chromosomal instability, gains and loss of whole chromosomes, which are classified as "myxopapillary ependymoma; SP-MPE." And lastly, an aggressive subtype of spinal ependymoma is driven by amplification of *MYCN*, "spinal ependymoma, MYCN amplified; SP-MYCN" [58].

Low-grade ependymal tumors called subependymoma can also occur in all 3 anatomic compartments and do not have any defining molecular features (ST-SE, PF-SE, and SP-SE). Studies have shown that those that arise in the spine are more likely to have loss of chromosome 6q. However, diagnosis relies on histomorphology. While some ependymoma subtypes have defining molecular alterations, DNA methylation profiling integrated with histomorphology is more reliable in precisely classifying these tumors (see Fig. 4E).

Medulloblastoma

Medulloblastoma is the most common malignant pediatric CNS tumor and arises primarily in the cerebellum. Advances in understanding the molecular and genomic landscape of medulloblastoma over the past 2 decades have resulted in the ability to stratify tumors based on molecular markers and have enhanced our ability to predict prognosis and tailor treatment. Medulloblastomas can be classified into 4 subtypes: "medulloblastoma, WNT-activated; MB-WNT," "medulloblastoma, SHH-activated; MB-SHH," "medulloblastoma, Group 3, MB-G3," and "medulloblastoma, Group 4; MB-G4" [59]. The WNT and SHH subtypes are characterized by alterations that activate the WNT (*CTNNB1* and *APC*) and SHH (*PTCH1*, *SMO*, and *SUFU*) signaling pathways, respectively. The common CNV of WNT-activated MB is loss of chromosome 6. Other commonly mutated genes in the SHH subtype are *TP53* and *TERT* promoter mutations. Group 3 and Group 4 tumors are less well-defined genomically compared with WNT and SHH subtypes and often exist as a heterogenous spectrum between G3 and G4 [60]. Both subtypes are associated with poorer outcomes, especially those that harbor amplification of *MYC/MYCN*; with *MYC* amplification restricted to Group 3 tumors. Group 3 and 4 medulloblastomas also frequently harbor loss of chromosome 17p and gain of 17q caused by an isochromosome 17q. Due to the overlapping genomic features of Group 3 and 4 medulloblastomas, it is difficult to distinguish them based solely on DNA-based analysis. RNA transcriptome and DNA methylation analysis can distinguish these 2 subtypes. Aside from subtype-specific alterations, mutations in epigenetic modifier proteins such as *KMT2D*, *SMARCA4*, *KMT2C*, *KDM6A*, *ARID1A*, and *CREBBP* are common across all 4 subtypes (see Fig. 4F).

Other tumors

In addition to the broad tumor groups listed earlier, CNS tumors include a wide array of rarer subtypes that are associated with specific molecular markers (a few highlighted). Craniopharyngiomas, locally aggressive tumors that arise from the craniopharyngeal duct can be divided into 2 subtypes. Adamantinomatous craniopharyngiomas arise primarily in children and are characterized by *CTNNB1* exon 3 mutations, and papillary craniopharyngiomas are more common in adults and are characterized by *BRAF* V600E mutations [61]. Choroid plexus tumors can be divided into 2 subtypes, "choroid plexus papilloma; CPP" and "choroid plexus carcinoma; CPC." CPP are benign neoplasms that exhibit hyperdiploidy while CPC harbor biallelic mutations of *TP53* in addition to hyperdiploidy [62]. Atypical teratoid/rhabdoid tumor is a highly aggressive embryonal CNS tumor that affect young children and is universally characterized by biallelic loss of *SMARCB1* [63], or less commonly, *SMARCA4* [64]. Pineoblastomas are embryonal tumors that arise in the pineal parenchyma and can be grouped into an mRNA processing-altered subtype, which harbors alterations in *DICER1*, *DROSHA*, and *DGCR8*; and an *RB1*-altered subtype [65]. Lastly, embryonal tumor with multilayered rosettes typically harbor focal amplification of a microRNA cluster on chromosome 19q13.42 (C19MC) or C19MC::*TTYH1* fusion event [66].

SUMMARY

The diagnostic process for CNS tumors involves a multifaceted approach that integrates clinical, histopathological, and molecular data, resulting in an accurate integrated diagnosis crucial for determining patient prognosis and therapeutic options. The evolution of brain tumor diagnostics has been marked by a shift from histology-based approaches to a more comprehensive, molecular paradigm driven by advancements in technology, from IHC to NGS and now DNA methylation profiling. This shift has led to the advent of personalized medicine where therapeutic decisions can be made dependent on the molecular landscape of an individual tumor. The accuracy and importance of molecular profiling are also tightly intertwined with ongoing research to further understand tumor biology and identify novel biomarkers. As diagnostic technologies continue to advance, the integration of genomics, histology, imaging, clinical correlates, and artificial intelligence will likely further refine our ability to detect, classify, and treat brain tumors with greater precision.

CLINICS CARE POINTS

- In some tumor subtypes, molecular testing can establish a classification based on WHO guidelines.
- However, not all molecular biomarkers are specific to one tumor subtype and many require correlation with histopathology and clinical presentation.

ACKNOWLEDGMENT

Dr Wong would like to thank Drs Stephen Yip, MD, PhD (BC Cancer Agency/Vancouver General Hospital) and Mariarita Santi, MD, PhD (Children's Hospital of Philadelphia) for providing images for the immunohistochemisty and FISH sections of this article. Additionally, he would like to thank members of the Division of Genomic Diagnostics at the Children's Hospital of Philadelphia for their input.

DISCLOSURE

The author has nothing to disclose.

REFERENCES

[1] Central nervous system tumours. Lyon: International agency for research on cancer; 2021.
[2] Ferguson S, Lesniak MS. Percival Bailey and the classification of brain tumors. Neurosurg Focus 2005;18:e7.
[3] Zülch KJ. Principles of the new World Health Organization (WHO) classification of brain tumors. Neuroradiology 1980;19:59–66.
[4] Louis DN, Perry A, Reifenberger G, et al. The 2016 World Health organization classification of tumors of the central nervous system: a summary. Acta Neuropathol 2016;131:803–20.
[5] Louis DN, Perry A, Wesseling P, et al. The 2021 WHO classification of tumors of the central nervous system: a summary. Neuro Oncol 2021;23:1231–51.
[6] Wong D, Yip S, Sorensen PH. Methods for identifying patients with tropomyosin receptor kinase (TRK) fusion cancer. Pathol Oncol Res 2020;26:1385–99.
[7] Brandner S, McAleenan A, Kelly C, et al. MGMT promoter methylation testing to predict overall survival in people with glioblastoma treated with temozolomide: a comprehensive meta-analysis based on a Cochrane Systematic Review. Neuro Oncol 2021;23:1457–69.
[8] Surrey LF, MacFarland SP, Chang F, et al. Clinical utility of custom-designed NGS panel testing in pediatric tumors. Genome Med 2019;11:32.
[9] Adalsteinsson VA, Ha G, Freeman SS, et al. Scalable whole-exome sequencing of cell-free DNA reveals high concordance with metastatic tumors. Nat Commun 2017;8:1324.
[10] Heydt C, Wlwer CB, Velazquez Camacho O, et al. Detection of gene fusions using targeted next-generation sequencing: a comparative evaluation. BMC Med Genomics 2021;14:62.
[11] Capper D, Jones DTW, Sill M, et al. DNA methylation-based classification of central nervous system tumours. Nature 2018;555:469–74.
[12] Capper D, Stichel D, Sahm F, et al. Practical implementation of DNA methylation and copy-number-based CNS tumor diagnostics: the Heidelberg experience. Acta Neuropathol 2018. https://doi.org/10.1007/s00401-018-1879-y.
[13] Byron SA, Van Keuren-Jensen KR, Engelthaler DM, et al. Translating RNA sequencing into clinical diagnostics: opportunities and challenges. Nat Rev Genet 2016;17:257–71.
[14] Cescon DW, Bratman SV, Chan SM, et al. Circulating tumor DNA and liquid biopsy in oncology. Nat Cancer 2020;1:276–90.
[15] Eid J, Fehr A, Gray J, et al. Real-time DNA sequencing from single polymerase molecules. Science 2009;323:133–8.
[16] Wang Y, Zhao Y, Bollas A, et al. Nanopore sequencing technology, bioinformatics and applications. Nat Biotechnol 2021;39:1348–65.
[17] Vermeulen C, Pagès-Gallego M, Kester L, et al. Ultra-fast deep-learned CNS tumour classification during surgery. Nature 2023;622:842–9.
[18] Turcan S, Rohle D, Goenka A, et al. IDH1 mutation is sufficient to establish the glioma hypermethylator phenotype. Nature 2012;483:479–83.
[19] Eckel-Passow JE, Lachance DH, Molinaro AM, et al. Glioma groups based on 1p/19q, IDH, and TERT promoter mutations in tumors. N Engl J Med 2015;372:2499–508.
[20] Yip S, Butterfield YS, Morozova O, et al. Concurrent CIC mutations, IDH mutations, and 1p/19q loss distinguish oligodendrogliomas from other cancers. J Pathol 2012;226:7–16.
[21] Brat DJ, Verhaak RGW, Aldape KD, et al, Cancer Genome Atlas Research Network. Comprehensive, integrative genomic analysis of diffuse lower-grade gliomas. N Engl J Med 2015;372:2481–98.
[22] Aoki K, Nakamura H, Suzuki H, et al. Prognostic relevance of genetic alterations in diffuse lower-grade gliomas. Neuro Oncol 2018;20:66–77.
[23] Brennan CW, Verhaak RGW, McKenna A, et al. The somatic genomic landscape of glioblastoma. Cell 2013;155:462–77.
[24] Bell RJA, Rube HT, Kreig A, et al. The transcription factor GABP selectively binds and activates the mutant TERT promoter in cancer. Science 2015;348:1036–9.
[25] You G, Fan X, Hu H, et al. Fusion genes altered in adult malignant gliomas. Front Neurol 2021;12:715206.
[26] Hegi ME, Diserens AC, Gorlia T, et al. MGMT gene silencing and benefit from temozolomide in glioblastoma. N Engl J Med 2005;352:997–1003.
[27] Ruttledge MH, Sarrazin J, Rangaratnam S, et al. Evidence for the complete inactivation of the NF2 gene in the majority of sporadic meningiomas. Nat Genet 1994;6:180–4.
[28] Bi WL, Greenwald NF, Abedalthagafi M, et al. Genomic landscape of high-grade meningiomas. NPJ Genomic Med 2017;2:15.
[29] Abedalthagafi M, Bi WL, Aizer AA, et al. Oncogenic PI3K mutations are as common as AKT1 and SMO mutations in meningioma. Neuro Oncol 2016;18:649–55.

[30] Clark VE, Erson-Omay EZ, Serin A, et al. Genomic analysis of non-NF2 meningiomas reveals mutations in TRAF7, KLF4, AKT1, and SMO. Science 2013;339:1077–80.
[31] Clark VE, Harmancı AS, Bai H, et al. Recurrent somatic mutations in POLR2A define a distinct subset of meningiomas. Nat Genet 2016;48:1253–9.
[32] Williams EA, Wakimoto H, Shankar GM, et al. Frequent inactivating mutations of the PBAF complex gene PBRM1 in meningioma with papillary features. Acta Neuropathol 2020;140:89–93.
[33] Shankar GM, Santagata S. BAP1 mutations in high-grade meningioma: implications for patient care. Neuro Oncol 2017;19:1447–56.
[34] Sievers P, Sill M, Blume C, et al. Clear cell meningiomas are defined by a highly distinct DNA methylation profile and mutations in SMARCE1. Acta Neuropathol 2021; 141:281–90.
[35] Sievers P, Chiang J, Schrimpf D, et al. YAP1-fusions in pediatric NF2-wildtype meningioma. Acta Neuropathol 2020;139:215–8.
[36] Ryall S, Zapotocky M, Fukuoka K, et al. Integrated molecular and clinical analysis of 1,000 pediatric low-grade gliomas. Cancer Cell 2020;37:569–83.e5.
[37] Zhang J, Wu G, Miller CP, et al. Whole-genome sequencing identifies genetic alterations in pediatric low-grade gliomas. Nat Genet 2013;45:602–12.
[38] Dougherty MJ, Santi M, Brose MS, et al. Activating mutations in BRAF characterize a spectrum of pediatric low-grade gliomas. Neuro Oncol 2010;12:621–30.
[39] Jones DTW, Kocialkowski S, Liu L, et al. Tandem duplication producing a novel oncogenic BRAF fusion gene defines the majority of pilocytic astrocytomas. Cancer Res 2008;68:8673–7.
[40] Deng MY, Sill M, Chiang J, et al. Molecularly defined diffuse leptomeningeal glioneuronal tumor (DLGNT) comprises two subgroups with distinct clinical and genetic features. Acta Neuropathol 2018;136:239–53.
[41] Schindler G, Capper D, Meyer J, et al. Analysis of BRAF V600E mutation in 1,320 nervous system tumors reveals high mutation frequencies in pleomorphic xanthoastrocytoma, ganglioglioma and extra-cerebellar pilocytic astrocytoma. Acta Neuropathol 2011;121:397–405.
[42] Surrey LF, Jain P, Zhang B, et al. Genomic analysis of dysembryoplastic neuroepithelial tumor spectrum reveals a diversity of molecular alterations dysregulating the MAPK and PI3K/mTOR pathways. J Neuropathol Exp Neurol 2019;78:1100–11.
[43] Plant-Fox AS, Tabori U. Future perspective of targeted treatments in pediatric low-grade glioma (pLGG): the evolution of standard-of-care and challenges of a new era. Childs Nerv Syst 2024;40:3291–9.
[44] Moreira DC, Qaddoumi I, Spiller S, et al. Comprehensive analysis of MYB/MYBL1-altered pediatric-type diffuse low-grade glioma. Neuro Oncol 2024;26:1327–34.
[45] Bandopadhayay P, Ramkissoon LA, Jain P, et al. MYB-QKI rearrangements in angiocentric glioma drive tumorigenicity through a tripartite mechanism. Nat Genet 2016;48:273–82.
[46] Lehman NL, Usubalieva A, Lin T, et al. Genomic analysis demonstrates that histologically-defined astroblastomas are molecularly heterogeneous and that tumors with MN1 rearrangement exhibit the most favorable prognosis. Acta Neuropathol Commun 2019;7:42.
[47] Bongaarts A, Giannikou K, Reinten RJ, et al. Subependymal giant cell astrocytomas in Tuberous Sclerosis Complex have consistent TSC1/TSC2 biallelic inactivation, and no BRAF mutations. Oncotarget 2017;8:95516–29.
[48] Schwartzentruber J, Korshunov A, Liu XY, et al. Driver mutations in histone H3.3 and chromatin remodelling genes in paediatric glioblastoma. Nature 2012;482: 226–31.
[49] Lewis PW, Müller MM, Koletsky MS, et al. Inhibition of PRC2 activity by a gain-of-function H3 mutation found in pediatric glioblastoma. Science 2013;340:857–61.
[50] Jain SU, Khazaei S, Marchione DM, et al. Histone H3.3 G34 mutations promote aberrant PRC2 activity and drive tumor progression. Proc Natl Acad Sci U S A 2020;117:27354–64.
[51] Sturm D, Witt H, Hovestadt V, et al. Hotspot mutations in H3F3A and IDH1 define distinct epigenetic and biological subgroups of glioblastoma. Cancer Cell 2012;22: 425–37.
[52] Guerreiro Stucklin AS, Ryall S, Fukuoka K, et al. Alterations in ALK/ROS1/NTRK/MET drive a group of infantile hemispheric gliomas. Nat Commun 2019;10:4343.
[53] Wu G, Diaz AK, Paugh BS, et al. The genomic landscape of diffuse intrinsic pontine glioma and pediatric non-brainstem high-grade glioma. Nat Genet 2014;46: 444–50.
[54] Pajtler KW, Witt H, Sill M, et al. Molecular classification of ependymal tumors across all CNS compartments, histopathological grades, and age groups. Cancer Cell 2015;27:728–43.
[55] Parker M, Mohankumar KM, Punchihewa C, et al. C11orf95–RELA fusions drive oncogenic NF-κB signalling in ependymoma. Nature 2014;506:451–5.
[56] Pajtler KW, Wei Y, Okonechnikov K, et al. YAP1 subgroup supratentorial ependymoma requires TEAD and nuclear factor I-mediated transcriptional programmes for tumorigenesis. Nat Commun 2019;10:3914.
[57] Witt H, Mack SC, Ryzhova M, et al. Delineation of two clinically and molecularly distinct subgroups of posterior fossa ependymoma. Cancer Cell 2011;20:143–57.
[58] Ghasemi DR, Sill M, Okonechnikov K, et al. MYCN amplification drives an aggressive form of spinal ependymoma. Acta Neuropathol 2019;138:1075–89.
[59] Northcott PA, Buchhalter I, Morrissy AS, et al. The whole-genome landscape of medulloblastoma subtypes. Nature 2017;547:311–7.
[60] Cavalli FMG, Remke M, Rampasek L, et al. Intertumoral heterogeneity within medulloblastoma subgroups. Cancer Cell 2017;31:737–54.e6.

[61] An W, Li S, An Y, et al. Molecular subtypes of adamantinomatous craniopharyngiomas. Neuro Oncol 2025; noaf030. https://doi.org/10.1093/neuonc/noaf030.

[62] Thomas C, Soschinski P, Zwaig M, et al. The genetic landscape of choroid plexus tumors in children and adults. Neuro Oncol 2021;23:650–60.

[63] Versteege I, Svenet N, Lange J, et al. Truncating mutations of hSNF5/INI1 in aggressive paediatric cancer. Nature 1998;394:203–6.

[64] Holdhof D, Johann PD, Spohn M, et al. Atypical teratoid/rhabdoid tumors (ATRTs) with SMARCA4 mutation are molecularly distinct from SMARCB1-deficient cases. Acta Neuropathol 2021;141:291–301.

[65] Li BK, Vasiljevic A, Dufour C, et al. Pineoblastoma segregates into molecular sub-groups with distinct clinico-pathologic features: a Rare Brain Tumor Consortium registry study. Acta Neuropathol 2020;139:223–41.

[66] Lambo S, Gröbner SN, Rausch T, et al. The molecular landscape of ETMR at diagnosis and relapse. Nature 2019;576:274–80.

SECTION: PHARMACOGENOMICS

Advances in Molecular Pathology 8 (2025) 97–112
ADVANCES IN MOLECULAR PATHOLOGY

Economic Analysis of Pharmacogenomics

Challenges and Progress

Simran D.S. Maggo, PhD[a,*], Jenny C. Nguyen, PharmD[b], Cynthia L. Gong, PharmD, PhD[c]

[a]Bernard J. Dunn School of Pharmacy, Shenandoah University, Building 1775 N Sector Ct, Winchester, VA 22601, USA; [b]Personalized Care Program, Children's Hospital Los Angeles, 4650 W Sunset Boulevard, Los Angeles, CA 90027, USA; [c]Curta Inc., Seattle, WA, USA

KEYWORDS
• Pharmacogenomics • Pharmacogenetics • Economic modeling • Cost-effectiveness

KEY POINTS

- Pharmacogenomic (PGx) testing improves medication efficacy and safety, but its widespread adoption depends on demonstrating cost-effectiveness and addressing economic and health care system challenges.
- Economic evaluations, including cost-effectiveness and budget impact analyses, show PGx's potential value in oncology, cardiology, psychiatry, and other therapeutic areas.
- Economic barriers to pharmacogenomic testing coverage include variability in reimbursement policies, uncertain return on investment for payers, and limited evidence from budget impact models demonstrating long-term cost savings.

INTRODUCTION

The field of pharmacogenomics (PGx) has advanced remarkably in the past decade, generating significant interest from institutions desiring to implement personalized medicine approaches as part of routine clinical care. PGx testing identifies specific polymorphisms related to drug metabolism which can optimize dosing for medications, resulting in significantly reduced adverse events and improved patient health outcomes. While the clinical benefits of PGx testing have been increasingly recognized, its economic viability remains a pivotal factor for its widespread adoption [1]. Demonstrating cost-effectiveness, which weighs the costs of testing and implementation against health outcomes and cost savings, is essential for its integration into routine care.

Since 2010, significant advances in PGx technologies, coupled with a growing emphasis on value-based health care, have spurred numerous studies exploring the economic impact of PGx testing. These evaluations span a variety of therapeutic areas, such as oncology, cardiology, and psychiatry. Despite the clinical benefits, however, challenges such as high initial implementation costs (eg, electronic medical record integration, workforce-education), varying payer reimbursement policies, lack of clinical expertise and/or education to interpret PGx test results, and inequities in access continue to pose barriers to its broader adoption [1–3].

In this article, we conduct a targeted literature review to provide examples of economic evaluations of PGx testing covering a wide range of therapeutic areas, followed by a discussion of methodological considerations for cost-effectiveness studies, implementation challenges, and policy implications.

*Corresponding author. *E-mail address:* simran.maggo@su.edu

https://doi.org/10.1016/j.yamp.2025.05.006
www.advancesinmolecularpathology.com
2589-4080/25/ © 2025 Elsevier Inc. All rights are reserved, including those for text and data mining, AI training, and similar technologies.

ABBREVIATIONS

CPIC	Clinical Pharmacogenetics Implementation Consortium
ICER	incremental cost-effectiveness ratio
PGx	pharmacogenomics
PMPM	per-member-per-month
PMPY	per-member-per-year
QALY	quality-adjusted life year
TAU	treatment as usual
WTP	willingness-to-pay

METHODS

This targeted literature review maps existing literature on economic analyses of PGx between January 1, 2014, and December 31, 2024, following standard methodological procedures for conducting systematic reviews [4–6]. Details for the search and screening strategy are provided in the following sections.

Search Strategy

A targeted literature search was conducted using PubMed and Embase to identify articles evaluating the economic impact of PGx. The following search query was used for both databases, with number of results for PubMed shown in Table 1.

Abstract and Title Screening

The articles from PubMed and Embase were imported into the Rayyan (Cambridge, MA - 02,142, US) web-based tool for systematic review management [7]. Duplicates were automatically identified and manually verified. Two independent reviewers conducted an initial screening of the titles, abstracts, and, where necessary, methods sections to identify the economic implications of PGx either through direct studies or via modeling approaches. Exclusion criteria included articles that did not report specifically on PGx, did not include an economic analysis (eg, cost-effectiveness, budget impact, or cost analysis), or was simply a review or background paper of PGx testing more generally. Following the initial screening, the 2 reviewers cross-validated each other's selections to ensure consistency of screening. Discrepancies were resolved through review by a third, independent reviewer.

Data Extraction

Data extracted for articles retained for full-text review included geographic setting, perspective (eg, payer or societal), type of PGx test being evaluated and relevant gene(s) and/or allele(s) tested, clinical implication (assessment of drug efficacy or adverse events), analysis type (eg, cost-effectiveness or cost analysis), model framework (eg, Markov vs decision tree), time horizon of the analysis, total cost estimated for PGx versus no testing or standard of care/treatment as usual, total quality-adjusted life years (QALYs), if applicable, and the incremental cost-effectiveness ratio (ICER) or total cost-savings calculated to determine whether PGx testing was generally considered cost-effective or cost saving. Data were also collected on the threshold used to determine cost-effectiveness and the primary data source for conducting the analysis.

Data Analysis

Data were qualitatively reviewed to identify common trends among analyses to date and gaps in the current literature that may help address future policy regarding routine implementation of, and reimbursement for, PGx testing. Recommendations related to methodology for future research to support increased access to PGx testing were also developed based on data extracted.

REVIEW OF LITERATURE

The literature search yielded 912 articles from Embase and 493 articles from PubMed. Upon deduplication, a total of n = 429 articles remained. After abstract

TABLE 1
Search Terms and Results (PubMed)

Search	Terms	Citations
#1	(“Pharmacogenomics”[Title/Abstract] OR “Pharmacogenetics”[Title/Abstract])	15,788
#2	(“cost-effectiveness”[Title/Abstract] OR “economic evaluation”[Title/Abstract] OR “health economics”[Title/Abstract])	99,551
#3	#1 AND #2	533
#4	#3 AND (“2014/01/01”[Date - Publication]: “2024/12/31”[Date - Publication]) AND NOT (“Animals”[MeSH] NOT “Humans”[MeSH]). Filters: Language, English	497

and title screening, 72 articles remained, of which a further 14 were excluded as they were commentaries or existing reviews, resulting in 58 articles being retained for full-text screening. Most articles (n = 43) were cost-effectiveness studies, with the majority specifically being cost-utility studies, that is, the outcome was cost per QALY. Only 2 studies provided cost outcomes in terms of clinical event (cost per severe hypoglycemia event per 100,000 patients) [8] and adverse event (cost per adverse event averted) [9]. The remaining articles were cost-analyses (n = 14), primarily claims database analyses (n = 9) or analyses using a combination of literature, clinical trials, and electronic health records to supply input parameters (n = 5). A summary of the review is presented in Table 2.

Pharmacogenomic Testing

As presented in Fig. 1, focus areas for the cost-effectiveness and clinical utility of PGx testing were psychiatry (eg, antidepressants, antipsychotics), cardiovascular drugs (eg, warfarin, clopidogrel, antihypertensives, ivabradine), oncology, hypersensitivity reactions, and immunosuppressants. The primary genes assessed included *CYP2C19, CYP2D6, CYP2C9, VKORC1, DPYD, TPMT, SLCO1B1*, and various *HLA* genes and variants. Some studies did not focus on a single medical specialty and were classified under general medicine (n = 5) [10–14] or multiple specialties (n = 2) [15,16]. Together, these accounted for 7 studies (12.1% of the total reviewed research), all of which found pharmacogenomic testing to be cost-effective. Notably, general medicine and several psychiatry-focused studies frequently employed multi-gene panels (eg, GeneSight, IDgenetix) rather than single-gene assessments, suggesting a preference for broader pharmacogenetic evaluations to inform prescribing.

Across the included studies, we observed the following:

- Psychiatry (n = 17) [17–33]: PGx testing primarily assessed the role of *CYP2D6* and *CYP2C19* in guiding antidepressant therapy (eg, citalopram, sertraline, amitriptyline) and antipsychotic medication (eg, aripiprazole, risperidone). Of these, n = 15 studies (88.2%) found PGx testing to be cost-effective. Several different multi-gene panels were mentioned for this specialty including Genesight (Mason, Ohio, US) [34] (n = 5) [18,20,23,27,32], YouScript's (Seattle, Washington, US), Genelex [35] (n = 1) [10], and Idgenetix (Friendswood, Texas, US) [36] (n = 2) [21,33]. These studies largely assessed the economics of using a PGx panel test to guide initial, or subsequent antidepressant therapy after initial failure or inefficacy. Furthermore, this subgroup also included 2 studies focused on evaluating *HLA*-testing prior to the prescription of clozapine to prevent agranulocytosis [24,29]. One study found PGx testing for venlafaxine was not cost-effective, but it was only 12-weeks long, thus limiting the duration during which benefits could be realized [25]. Additionally, Clinical Pharmacogenetics Implementation Consortium (CPIC) guidelines currently provide recommendations for venlafaxine and CYP2D6 poor metabolizers only, with no guidance for other phenotypes due to insufficient evidence. Consequently, the low prevalence of poor metabolizers may not justify the cost of PGx testing when only considering this medication. Additionally, the model was derived from a single venlafaxine study, potentially introducing bias, and its extrapolation to other antidepressants may have compromised the accuracy of cost-effectiveness estimates, as gene-drug interactions are not universally transferable.
- Cardiology (n = 17): Included warfarin (n = 8) [37–43], clopidogrel (n = 3) [44–46], antihypertensives (n = 2) [47,48], statins (n = 2) [49,50], and ivabradine (n = 1) [51]; one study evaluated clopidogrel, statins, and warfarin [52]. Warfarin dosing was frequently evaluated, particularly the role of *CYP2C9* and *VKORC1* in preventing bleeding events. Overall, 14 (82.4%) found PGx testing to be cost-effective in this specialty. Despite numerous studies evaluating the cost-effectiveness of PGx testing for warfarin, results remain mixed. This variability is likely associated with factors such as the declining clinical use of warfarin in favor of direct oral anticoagulants, differences in genotyping costs and turnaround times, and variability in patient risk profiles. Additionally, genotype-guided dosing does not fully account for non-genetic influences on warfarin response, and real-world adoption has been limited by inconsistent guideline implementation. As a result, the economic value of warfarin PGx testing is highly context-dependent.
- Oncology (n = 6) [53–58]: Testing focused on genes such as *DPYD, UGT1A1, TPMT*, and *NUDT15* influencing chemotherapy response and resultant ADRs, with all (100%) finding PGx testing cost-effective. Specifically under this clinical area, tamoxifen (n = 2) [55,57] was evaluated with respect to the impact of *CYP2D6* variants on tamoxifen metabolism, with both studies reporting cost-effectiveness. Both studies originating out of China focused on the

TABLE 2
Summary of Economic Evaluations for PGx Testing

Authors & Year	Country	Clinical Specialty	Gene(s)	Medication(s)	Clinical Outcome	Perspective	Economic Model Type	Methodological Details	Total Cost	Total QALYs	ICER	WTP Threshold	Cost-Effective or Cost-Saving	Data	Time Horizon
Moretti et al, [9] 2017	Canada	Analgesia	*CYP2D6*	Codeine	ADRs	Payer and Societal	Cost-effectiveness	Decision tree	Screening societal: $537 Screening payer: $498 No screen societal: $184 No screen payer: $146	Screening societal: 0.1339 adverse events Screening payer: 0.1309 adverse events No screen societal: 0.1687 adverse events No screen payer: 0.1656 adverse events	Societal: $10,443/ adverse event averted Payer: $10,174/ adverse event averted	NA	Yes	Literature	Lifetime
Chong et al, [37] 2014	Thailand	Cardiovascular	*CYP2C9, VKORC1*	Warfarin	Efficacy and ADRs	Payer	Cost-effectiveness	Hybrid decision tree-Markov model	PGx: 34,837,741 THB Usual care: 31,878,125 THB	39,421 (PGx) 39,419 (usual care)	14,777,042 THB/QALY ($49,234/QALY)	160,000 THB/ QALY ($5333/ QALY)	No	Literature	Lifetime
Mitropoulou et al, [38] 2015	Croatia	Cardiovascular	*CYP2C9, VKORC1*	Warfarin	Efficacy and ADRs	Payer	Cost-effectiveness	Decision tree	PGx: €538.70 Control: €219.70	0.954 (PGx) 0.944 (control)	€31,225/QALY	€50,000/QALY	Yes	Prospective single-center study (hospital)	1 y
Jiang et al, [45] 2016	United States	Cardiovascular	*CYP2C19*	Clopidogrel	Efficacy	Payer	Cost-effectiveness	Decision tree discrete event simulation	Universal clopidogrel testing, base case: $6047 GT-guided escalation: $6493 Universal ticareglor testing: $8832	Universal clopidogrel: 0.948 GT-guided escalation: 0.959 Universal ticagrelor: 0.969	GT-guided escalation: $42,365/QALY Universal ticagrelor: $227,044/QALY	$100,000/QALY	Yes	Real-world effectiveness data	1 y
Verhoef et al, [39] 2016	UK and Sweden	Cardiovascular	*CYP2C9, VKORC1*	Warfarin	Efficacy and ADRs	Payer	Cost-effectiveness	Markov	UK, standard care: £8614 UK, PGx: £8640 Sweden, standard care: 88,072 SEK Sweden, PGx: 88,453 SEK	UK, standard care: 7.9141 UK, PGx: 7.9180 Sweden, standard care: 7.5321 Sweden, PGx: 7.5336	£6702/QALY 253,848 SEK/QALY	£20,000/QALY 500,000 SEK/QALY	Yes	Clinical trial	Lifetime
Martes-Martinez et al, [68] 2017	Puerto Rico	Cardiovascular	*CYP2C9, VKORC1*	Warfarin	Efficacy and ADRs	Payer (Veterans Affairs)	Cost-effectiveness	Markov	PGx: $35,751 Standard care: $35,480	7.1261 (PGx) 7.1240 (standard)	$127,501/QALY	$50,000/QALY	No	Electronic health records	Lifetime
Mitchell et al, [49] 2018	Canada	Cardiovascular	Hypothetical test	Statins	ADRs	Payer	Cost-effectiveness	Discrete event simulation	PGx: CAD$61,139 No screening: CAD$57,437	PGx: 8.51 No screening: 7.64	CAD$4273/QALY	CAD$50,000/ QALY	Yes	Literature	Lifetime
Kelley et al, [47] 2018	United States	Cardiovascular	*ADRB1, ADRB2, SCNN1A, ADD1, SLC12A3, WNK1, ACE, AGT, AGTR1, CYP2D6, REN*	Antihypertensives	Efficacy and ADRs	Payer (per authors, however inclusion of indirect costs implies societal)	Cost analysis	Simulation	PGx, untreated: $13,309 per patient SOC, untreated: $15,813 per patient PGx, treated: $2502 per patient SOC, treated: $3778 per patient	NA	PGx cost savings: $4228 over 3 y PGx cost savings: $1409 per patient	NA	Yes	Literature	3 y
Fragoulakis V, et al, [46] 2019	Spain	Cardiovascular	*CYP2C19*	Clopidogrel	Efficacy	Payer	Cost-effectiveness	Decision tree	PGx: €2971 No PGx: €3205	PGx: 0.9446 No PGx: 0.9379	Dominant	NR	Yes	Electronic health records	12 mo, 24 mo, lifetime

Dong et al, [52] 2020	United States	Cardiovascular	*CYP2C19, SLCO1B1, CYP2C9, VKORC1*	Clopidogrel, statins, warfarin	Efficacy and ADRs	Payer	Cost-effectiveness	Hybrid decision tree-Markov model	Multigene PGx, 12 mo: $2151 Single-gene PGx, 12 mo: $2193 TAU, 12 mo: $1969 Multigene PGx, 24 mo: $3598 Single-gene PGx, 24 mo: $3640 TAU, 24 mo: $3412 Multigene PGx, lifetime: $5434 Single-gene PGx, lifetime: $5484 TAU, lifetime: $5250	Multigene PGx, 12 mo: 0.853 Single-gene PGx, 12 mo: 0.853 TAU, 12 mo: 0.850 Multigene PGx, 24 mo: 1.663 Single-gene PGx, 24 months: 1.663 TAU, 24 mo: 1.658 Multigene PGx, lifetime: 13.215 Single-gene PGx, lifetime: 13.213 TAU, lifetime: 13.166	12 mo: $59,876/QALY 24 mo: $33,512/QALY Lifetime: $3780/QALY Single-gene testing dominated by multigene	$50,000/QALY	Yes	Literature	12 mo, 24 mo, lifetime
Eljilany et al, [40] 2023	Qatar	Cardiovascular	*CYP2C9*	Warfarin	ADRs	Health system	Cost-benefit	Decision tree	Standard: $2388 PGx: $1659	NA	PGx cost savings per patient: $727	NA	Yes	Randomized controlled trial	1 y
Koufaki et al, [44] 2023	Spain	Cardiovascular	*CYP2C19*	Clopidogrel	Efficacy and ADRs	Payer	Cost-effectiveness	NR	PGx: €882.50 Control: €1755.40	PGx: 0.84 Control: 0.76	Dominant	€50,000/QALY	Yes	Randomized controlled trial	18 mo
Hafeez et al, [43] 2024	Canada	Cardiovascular	*CYP2C9, VKORC1, CYP4F2*	Warfarin	Efficacy and ADRs	Payer	Cost-effectiveness	Hybrid decision tree-Markov model	Standard warfarin: $219,093 CAD PGx warfarin: $219,672 CAD PGx rivaroxaban: $236,599 CAD PGx apixaban: $241,374 CAD	Standard warfarin: 10.59 PGx warfarin: 10.63 PGx rivaroxaban: 10.82 PGx apixaban: 10.96	PGx warfarin: $17,584 CAD/QALY PGx rivaroxaban: $77,777 CAD/QALY PGx apixaban: $60,397 CAD/QALY	$50,000 CAD/ QALY	Yes - PGx warfarin only	Literature	Lifetime
Anand et al, [41] 2024	India	Cardiovascular	*CYP2C9, VKORC1*	Warfarin	Efficacy and ADRs	Patient	Cost-effectiveness	Markov	PGx: ₹100,417 No PGx: ₹93,505	PGx: 4.08 No PGx: 3.83	₹27,341/QALY	₹71,630/QALY	Yes	Randomized controlled trial	Lifetime
Baranova et al, [48] 2017	Netherlands	Cardiovascular	Pharmacogenomics panel (unspecified)	Angiotensin-converting enzyme (ACE) inhibitors	ADRs	Payer	Cost-effectiveness	Decision tree	NR	NR	NR	€20,000–80,000/ QALY	Yes, assuming very high sensitivity, decent specificity, and low price	NR	NR
Iliza et al, [51] 2016	Canada	Cardiovascular	Pharmacogenomics panel (unspecified)	Ivabradine	Efficacy	Payer	Cost-effectiveness	Markov	NR	NR	$57,275/QALY	$70,000/QALY	Yes	NR	Lifetime
Mitchell et al, [50] 2017	Canada	Cardiovascular	*SLCO1B1*	Statins	ADRs	Payer	Cost-effectiveness	Markov	PGx: $41,439 CAD No PGx: $41,501 CAD	PGx: 7.18 No PGx: 6.95	PGx dominant, assuming test cost of <$356 CAD	$1000 CAD/ QALY	Yes (dominant)	Literature	20 y
Verhoef et al, [42] 2015	Netherlands	Cardiovascular	*CYP2C9, VKORC1*	Warfarin	ADRs	Payer	Cost-effectiveness	Hybrid decision tree-Markov model	PGx phenprocoumon: £9677 Clinical phenprocoumon: £9644 PGx acenocoumarol: £9649 Clinical acenocoumarol: £9616	PGx phenprocoumon: 9.5210 Clinical phenprocoumon: 9.5198 PGx acenocoumarol: 9.5201 Clinical acenocoumarol: 9.5187	Phenprocoumon: £28,349/QALY Acenocoumarol: £24,427/QALY	€20,000/QALY	No	Randomized controlled trial; literature	Lifetime
Fokoun et al, [8] 2021	France	Endocrinology	*CYP2C9*	Glimepiride	ADRs	Payer	Cost-effectiveness	Decision tree	No Pgx: €6,915,299 PGx: €58,463,498	No PGx: 3800 (number of severe hypoglycemia events) PGx: 3678 (number of severe hypoglycemia events)	€421,834/severe hypoglycemia event per 100,000 patients	NA	Unclear	Literature	1 y
Sluiter, et al, [25] 2019	Netherlands	Gastroenterology	*TPMT*	Thiopurines	ADRs	Societal	Cost-effectiveness	Prospective cohort study	PGx: €2181 No PGx: €2232	PGx: 0.302 No PGx: 0.301	Dominant	€20,000/QALY	Yes	Randomized controlled trial	20 wk

(continued on next page)

TABLE 2
(continued)

Authors & Year	Country	Clinical Specialty	Gene(s)	Medication(s)	Clinical Outcome	Perspective	Economic Model Type	Methodological Details	Total Cost	Total QALYs	ICER	WTP Threshold	Cost-Effective or Cost-Saving	Data	Time Horizon
Brixner, et al, [10] 2016	United States	General Medicine	*CYP2D6, CYP2C19, CYP2C9, CYP3A4, CYP3A5, VKORC1*	Any medications with pharmacogenomic associations - polypharmacy	Efficacy and ADRs	Payer	Cost analysis	Prospective case-control propensity score matched	NR	NA	$25,903 median cost-savings with PGx testing $44,723 mean cost-savings with PGx testing	NA	Yes	Claims	4 mo
Sugarman et al, [10] 2016	United States	General Medicine	*CYP1A2, CYP2C9, CYP2C19, CYP2D6, CYP3A4, CYP3A5, HTR2A, HTR2C, SLC6A4, SLC6A2, COMT, OPRM1, SLCO1B1, VKORC1, MTHFR*	Any medications with pharmacogenomic associations - polypharmacy	Efficacy and ADRs	Health system	Cost analysis	Retrospective analysis comparing those with and without medication changes	NR	NA	$3000 per patient' per stay $145,664 cost-savings	NA	Yes	Electronic health records	
Chan et al, [12] 2019	Singapore	General Medicine	Pharmacogenomics panel (unspecified)	Any medications with pharmacogenomic associations	Efficacy and ADRs	Health system	Cost analysis	Propensity score matched case control study	Total cost of ADRs: $570,404 Total cost of ADRs with PGx association: $214,902	NA	Total potential cost savings: $96,258	NA	Yes	Electronic health records	
Bain et al, [13] 2020	United States	General Medicine	Pharmacogenomics panel (unspecified)	Any medications with pharmacogenomic associations	Efficacy and ADRs	Payer	Cost analysis	Retrospective case analysis	Costs calculated as costs avoided assuming recommendation accepted	NA	Total savings if all recommendations included: $233,945 ($1985 per patient) Total savings if percentage of recommendations included: $162,031 ($1373 per patient)	NA	Yes	Clinical trial	90 d
Fragala et al, [14] 2024	United States	General Medicine	Pharmacogenomics panel (unspecified)	Any medications with pharmacogenomic associations	Efficacy and ADRs	Payer	Cost analysis	Propensity score matched case control study	PGx: $1516 PMPM No PGx: $1559 PMPM	NA	PGx cost savings PMPM: $128	NA	Yes	Claims	13 mo
Rens et al, [70] 2020	Brazil, South Africa, and India	Infectious diseases	*NAT2*	Isoniazid	Efficacy	Payer	Cost-effectiveness	Decision tree	PGx, Brazil: $964 No PGx, Brazil: $952 PGx, South Africa: $385 No PGx, South Africa: $352 PGx, India: $84 No PGx, India: $71	PGx, Brazil: 19.75 No PGx, Brazil: 19.72 PGx, South Africa: 16.93 No PGx, South Africa: 16.91 PGx, India: 18.61 No PGx, India: 18.59	PGx, Brazil: $476/QALY PGx, South Africa: $1780/QALY PGx, India: $546/QALY	Brazil: $8921 South Africa: $6340 India: $2016	Yes	Literature	Lifetime
Chen et al, [60] 2016	Hong Kong	Neurology	*HLA-B*15:02*	Carbamazepine	ADRs	Payer	Cost-effectiveness	Decision tree	No screening: $164 Current situation: $205 Ideal situation: $171 Extended screening: $320	No screening: 0.8273 Current: 0.8278 Ideal: 0.8279 Extended: 0.8281	Current situation: $85,697/QALY Ideal situation: $11,090/QALY Extended screening: $197,158/QALY	$90,000/QALY	No	Clinical Data Repository of the Hospital Authority	1 y
Plumpton et al, [62] 2015	UK	Neurology	*HLA-A*31:01*	Carbamazepine	ADRs	Payer	Cost-effectiveness	Hybrid decision tree-Markov model	PGx: £10,808 No PGx: £10,508	PGx: 15.77 SOC: 15.75	£12,808/QALY	£20,000/QALY	Yes	Randomized controlled trial	Lifetime
Plumpton et al, [15] 2019	UK	Neurology, Rheumatology, Infectious diseases	*HLA-A*31:01, HLA-B*15:02, HLA-B*57:01, HLA-B*58:01, HLA-B (158T), and HLA-DQB1 (126Q)*	Carbamazepine, phenytoin, allopurinol, abacavir, clozapine	ADRs	Payer	Cost-effectiveness	Decision tree	Varying	Varying	Dominant (multigene test only) Varying for single-gene test, depending on cost of genetic test	£30,000/QALY	Yes	Literature	Lifetime

Zhou et al, [16] 2021	Global	Neurology, Rheumatology, Infectious diseases	*HLA-B*57:01, HLA-B*15:02, HLA-A*31:01, HLA-B*58:01*	Carbamazepine, abacavir, allopurinol	ADRs	NR	Cost-effectiveness	Costs are calculated as treatment costs plus cost of adverse drug reaction, plus cost of genetic test if applicable	Varying depending on country	Varying depending on country	Varying depending on country	$10,000 - $100,000/ QALY, depending on country	Yes	Literature	NR
Butzke et al, [53] 2016	Germany	Oncology	*UGT1A1*	Irinotecan	ADRs	Payer	Cost-effectiveness	Hybrid decision tree-Markov model	PGx + dose reduction: €23,414 no PGx: €23,995 PGx + growth factors: €34,187	PGx + dose reduction: 1.1292 No PGx: 1.1290 PGx + growth factors: 1.1292	PGx + dose reduction: dominant vs no PGx PGx + growth factors: €65,000,000/QALY	€50,000/QALY	Yes*	Literature	Lifetime
Dionne et al, [54] 2018	Canada	Oncology	Hypothetical test	Anthracyclines	ADRs	Payer	Cost-effectiveness	Decision tree	No screening: CAD$8667 Pgx: CAD$8172	No screening: 2.67 potential years of life lost per patient PGx: 2.24 potential years of life lost per patient	NR	NR	Yes	Literature	Lifetime
Wei et al, [55] 2020	China	Oncology	*CYP2D6*	Tamoxifen	Efficacy	Payer	Cost-effectiveness	Markov	No PGx: $57,499 PGx: $75,466	No PGx: 7.351 PGx: 10.933	$5016/QALY	$26,508/QALY	Yes	Literature	20 y
Fragoulakis et al, [56] 2023	Italy	Oncology	*DPYD, UGT1A1*	Fluoropyrimidines and irinotecan	ADRs	Payer	Cost-effectiveness	NR	PGx: €380 Control: €560	PGx: 0.80 Control: 0.81	€13,418/QALY	€50,000/QALY	Yes	Randomized controlled trial	18 mo
Wei et al, [55] 2020.	China	Oncology	*CYP2D6*	Tamoxifen	Efficacy and ADRs	Societal	Cost-effectiveness	Hybrid decision tree-Markov model	Tamoxifen, no PGx: $63,879 Toremifene, no PGx: $90,157 PGx: $95,021	Tamoxifen, no PGx: 8.16 Toremifene, no PGx: 12.90 PGx: 13.86	$5056/QALY (vs. toremifene, no PGx)	$26,508/QALY	Yes	Literature	30 y
Fuerte et al, [58] 2024	United States	Oncology	*TPMT, NUDT15*	Mercaptopurine	ADRs	Health system	Budget impact	Markov	Not reported	NA	Cost savings per patient: $26,028	NA	Yes	Literature	16 wk
Fagerness et al, [17] 2014	United States	Psychiatry	*CYP2C19, CYP2D6, SLC6A4, CACNA1C, DRD2, COMT, MTHFR*	Antidepressants & Antipsychotics	Efficacy and ADRs	Payer	Cost analysis	Prospective case-control propensity score matched	NR	NA	Total cost savings: $298 per patient mean difference Total cost savings baseline: $562 mean baseline difference	NA	Yes	IMS Claims	Lifetime
Winner et al, [18] 2015	United States	Psychiatry	Genesight Test	Antidepressants & Antipsychotics	Efficacy and ADRs	Payer	Cost analysis	Prospective case-control propensity score matched	NR	NA	Annual drug spend savings: $1035 per member per year Total annual medication cost savings: $2774 when adhering to report recommendations	NA	Yes	Claims	1 y
Hornberger et al, [19] 2015	United States	Psychiatry	*CYP2D6, CYP2C19, CYP2C9, CYP1A2, SLC6A4, HTR2A.*	Antidepressants & Antipsychotics	Efficacy and ADRs	Societal	Cost-effectiveness	Hybrid decision tree-Markov model	PGx: $272,251 TAU: $275,515	PGx: 13.624 TAU: 13.308	Dominant (0.316 QALYs gained, $3764 saved)	$50,000/QALY	Yes	Literature	Lifetime
Brown et al, [20] 2017	United States	Psychiatry	Genesight Test	Antidepressants & Antipsychotics	Efficacy and ADRs	Payer	Cost analysis	Retrospective analysis comparing those with and without PGx-congruent recommendations by HCPs	PCPs: $3998 vs incongruent decisions OB/ GYN: $2296 vs incongruent decisions Psych: $1308 vs incongruent decisions	NA	NA	NA	Yes	Claims	1 y
Groessl et al, [21] 2018	United States	Psychiatry	*CYP1A2, CYP2C9, CYP2C19, CYP2D6, CYP3A4, CYP3A5, SLC6A4, COMT, HTR2A, MTHFR*	Antidepressants & Antipsychotics	Efficacy and ADRs	Societal	Cost-effectiveness	Markov	PGx: $44,697 SOC: $47,295	PGx: 2.07 SOC: 1.97	Dominant (0.1 QALYs gained, $2598 saved)	$50,000/QALY	Yes	Literature	3 y

(*continued on next page*)

TABLE 2
(continued)

Authors & Year	Country	Clinical Specialty	Gene(s)	Medication(s)	Clinical Outcome	Perspective	Economic Model Type	Methodological Details	Total Cost	Total QALYs	ICER	WTP Threshold	Cost-Effective or Cost-Saving	Data	Time Horizon
Perlis et al, [22] 2018	United States	Psychiatry	Genecept assay (*CYP2D6, CYP2C19, CYP3A4* and some pharmacodynamic variants)	Antidepressants & Antipsychotics	Efficacy and ADRs	Payer	Cost analysis	Retrospective case-control propensity score matched	PGx: $1895 TAU: $3123	NA	Mean difference: $1229 cost-savings with PGx	NA	Yes	Claims	6 mo
Benitez et al, [23] 2018	United States	Psychiatry	Genesight Test (*CYP2D6, CYP2C19, CYP2C9, CYP2B6, CYP3A4, CYP1A2, SLC6A4,* and *HTR2A*)	Antidepressants & Antipsychotics	Efficacy and ADRs	Payer	Cost analysis	Retrospective case-control	TAU: $23,132 PGx: $17,627	NA	PGx cost-savings total: $5505 PGx cost-savings PMPM over 24 mo: $0.07 (assumes 20% of prescribers use PGx)	NA	Yes	Claims	12 mo
Girardin et al, [24] 2019	United States	Psychiatry	*HLA-DQB1 (126Q), HLA-B (158T)*	Clozapine	ADRs	Payer	Cost-effectiveness	Decision tree	Current: $13,694 PGx: $13,091 Clozapine substitution: $13,738	Current: 669.9 quality-adjusted life days PGx: 669.8 quality-adjusted life days Clozapine: 660.2 quality-adjusted life days	Dominant	$50,000/QALY	Yes	Literature	Lifetime
Sluiter et al, [25] 2019	Netherlands	Psychiatry	*CYP2D6*	Venlafaxine	Efficacy and ADRs	Societal	Cost-effectiveness	Markov	PGx: €970 No PGx: €881	PGx: 0.146 No PGx: 0.145	€77,406/QALY	€80,000/QALY	No	Literature	12 wk
Tanner et al, [26] 2020	Canada	Psychiatry	Pharmacogenomics panel (unspecified)	Antidepressants & Antipsychotics	Efficacy and ADRs	Payer	Cost-effectiveness	Hybrid decision tree-Markov model	NR	NR	Dominant	$50,000/QALY	Yes	Literature	Lifetime
Jablonski et al, [27] 2020	United States	Psychiatry	Genesight Test	Antidepressants & Antipsychotics	Efficacy and ADRs	Payer	Cost analysis	Prospective case-control	NR	NA	Congruent prescribing cost-savings, >65 y: $3497 PMPY Congruent prescribing cost-savings, <65 y: $2467 PMPY	NA	Yes	Claims	1 y
Fabbri et al, [28] 2021	UK	Psychiatry	83 genes	Antidepressants & Antipsychotics	Efficacy and ADRs	Payer	Cost-effectiveness	Markov	NR	NR	PGx: £3937/QALY No PGx: £2341/QALY	NR	No	Literature	3 y
Ninomiya et al, [29] 2021	Japan & UK	Psychiatry	*HLA-B*59:01, HLA-B 158T, HLA-DQB1 126Q*	Clozapine	ADRs	Payer	Cost-effectiveness	Markov	No PGx Japan: £16,487 No PGx UK: £4211 PGx Japan: £16,552 PGx UK: £4281	No PGx Japan: 6.22608 No PGx UK: 5.82665 PGx Japan: 6.22917 PGx UK: 5.82990	Japan: £20,995/QALY UK: £21,373/QALY	Japan: £37,650/QALY UK: £30,000/QALY	Yes	Literature	10 y
Ghanbarian et al, [30] 2023	Canada	Psychiatry	*CYP2D6, CYP2C19*	Antidepressants	Efficacy and ADRs	Payer	Cost-effectiveness	Decision tree	PGx: $8.96 B CAD SOC: $9.92 B CAD	PGx: 2,234,977 SOC: 2,160,954	Dominant	$50,000 CAD/QALY	Yes	Literature	20 y
Lopez-Saavedra et al, [31] 2024	Spain	Psychiatry	*CYP2D6, CYP2C19*	Antidepressants	Efficacy and ADRs	Societal	Cost-effectiveness	Markov microsimulation	No PGx: €3173 PGx: €1687	No PGx: 2.64 PGx: 2.84	Dominant	€21,000/QALY	Yes	Literature	3 y
Roe et al, [32] 2018	United States	Psychiatry	Genesight Test	Antidepressants & Antipsychotics	Efficacy and ADRs	Payer	Cost analysis	Retrospective case control	NR	NA	PGx cost-savings PMPY: $6747 (GAD) PGx cost-savings PMPY: $3738 *(MDD)*	NA	Yes	Claims	1 y
Najafzadeh et al, [33] 2017	United States	Psychiatry	*CYP1A2, CYP2C9, CYP2C19, CYP2D6, CYP3A4, CYP3A5, SLC6A4, COMT, HTR2A, MTHFR*	Antidepressants & Antipsychotics	Efficacy and ADRs	Societal	Cost-effectiveness	Discrete event simulation	PGx: $14,214 TAU: $14,659	PGx: 2.09 TAU: 1.94	Dominant	$50,000/QALY	Yes	Literature	3 y

Wu et al, [67] 2015	United States	Respiratory	Hypothetical test	Inhaled Corticosteroids	Efficacy	Societal	Cost-effectiveness	Markov	$51,900 control $50,200 PGx	7.1 control 7.1 PGx	NR	NR	Yes	Literature	10 y
Li et al, [69] 2023	China	Respiratory	*ADRB2*	Long-acting -Beta2 receptor agonists	Efficacy	Payer	Cost-effectiveness	Markov	PGx: ¥11,477 No PGx: ¥11,812	PGx: 7.504 No Pgx: 7.503	Dominant	¥257,094/QALY	Yes	Literature	10 y
Ke et al, [61] 2017	Taiwan	Rheumatology	*HLA-B*58:01*	Allopurinol	ADRs	Payer	Cost-effectiveness	Decision tree	No screening, benzbromarone: NT$39,419 No screening, allopurinol: NT$39,476 Screening: NT$42,040 No screening, febuxostat: NT$43,548	No screening, benzbromarone: 0.943448 No screening, allopurinol: 0.940703 Screening: 0.9454617 No screening, febuxostat: 0.943448	No screening, allopurinol: dominated Screening: NT$234,611 No screening, febuxostat: dominated	NT$800,000/ QALY	Yes	Claims	Lifetime
Sluiter et al, [66] 2018	Netherlands	Substance Abuse	*OPRM1*	Naltrexone	Efficacy	Societal	Cost-effectiveness	Markov	PGx: €3611 No screening: €3544	PGx: 0.714 No screening: 0.709	€13,350/QALY	€80,000/QALY	Yes	Literature	1 y
Fragoulakis et al, [64] 2024	Austria	Transplant	*CYP3A5*	Tacrolimus	Efficacy	Payer	Cost-effectiveness	NR	PGx: €21,685 No PGx: €25,587	PGx: 0.900 No PGx: 0.851	Dominant	€50,000/QALY	Yes	Randomized controlled trial	Lifetime
Wang et al, [63] 2025	United States	Transplant	*CYP3A5*	Tacrolimus	Efficacy	Health system	Cost analysis	Decision tree	SOC: $154,033 per patient PGx: $136,808 per patient	NA	PGx cost-savings per patient: $17,225	NA	Yes	Literature, electronic health records	Drug initiation to discharge

Abbreviations: NA, not applicable, NR, not reported.

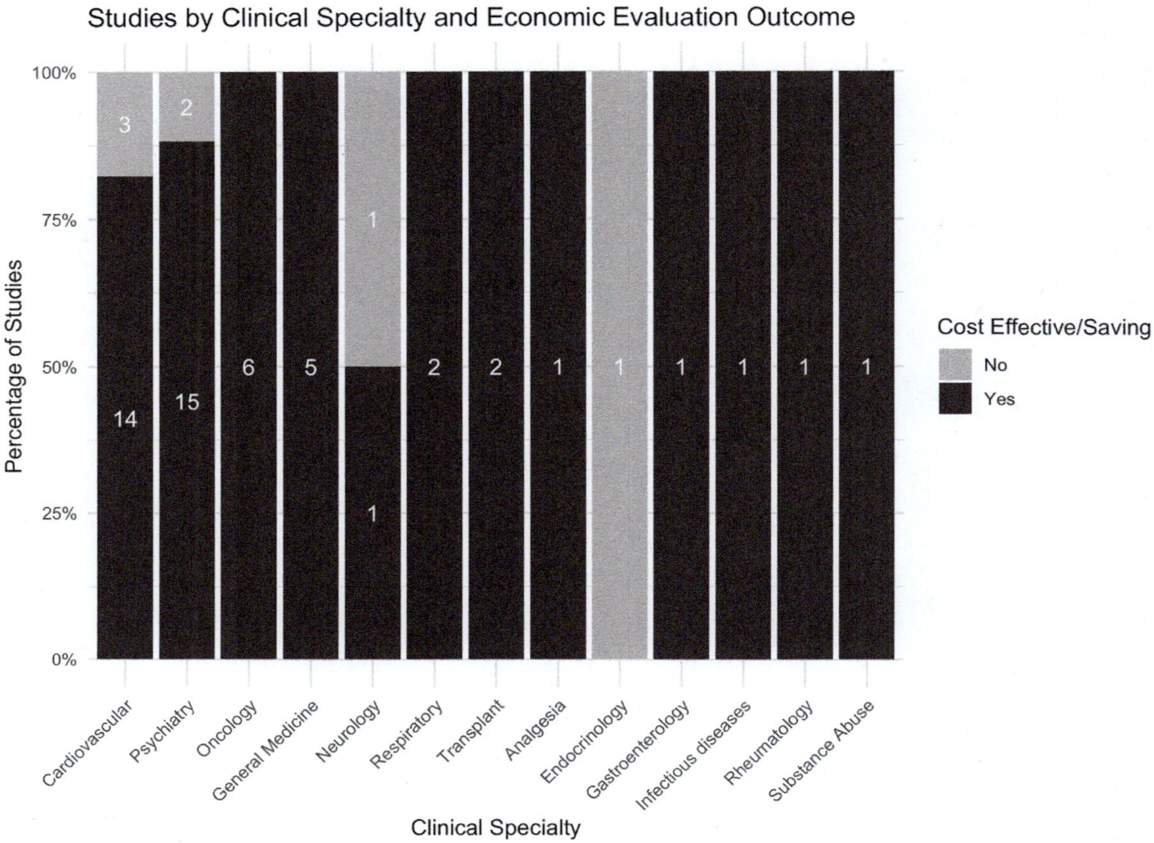

FIG. 1 Provides a graphical overview of each specialty and whether it was assessed as cost-effective/saving.

*CYP2D6*10* variant, which has a high population frequency in individuals of East-Asian descent [59].

- HLA-related hypersensitivity (n = 7) [15,16, 24,29,59–62]: PGx testing investigated hypersensitivity reactions to the drugs carbamazepine, phenytoin, allopurinol, abacavir, and clozapine mediated by *HLA* variants. Overall, 6 (86%) found PGx testing to be cost-effective.
- Tacrolimus (n = 2) [63,64]: PGx testing focused on *CYP3A5* genetic variants influencing tacrolimus metabolism and dosing, with both studies reporting cost-effectiveness.

Economic Approach

Most analyses were conducted from the payer perspective (n = 42), followed by societal (n = 9) [19,21,25,31,33,57,65–67], health system (n = 4) [11,12,40,63], patient (n = 1) [41], and not specified (n = 1) [16]. Nearly all papers (n = 50) found PGx testing to be either cost-effective or cost-saving relative to no testing or treatment as usual (TAU). Only 6 papers found PGx testing not cost-effective based on the country's specific willingness-to-pay (WTP) threshold; these included Thailand [37], Hong Kong [60], Puerto Rico [68], Netherlands [25,42], and the United Kingdom [28]. One analysis conducted from the French payer perspective was unclear, given that the outcome was the cost per severe hypoglycemia event per 100,000 patients [8]. Of the 6 papers that found PGx not to be cost-effective, half were analyses of PGx-guided warfarin dosing (n = 3) [37,42,68], while the others were in major depressive disorder [25,28] and epilepsy [60].

In terms of geography, most economic evaluations were conducted in non–United States settings (n = 38), including primarily Canada (n = 8) [9,26,

30,43,49–51,54], the United Kingdom (n = 5, 2 of which included other countries) [15,28,29,39,62], Netherlands (n = 5) [25,42,48,65,66]. China (n = 3) [55,57,69], and Spain (n = 3) [31,44,46]. Other countries included Austria (n = 1) [56], Brazil, South Africa, and India (n = 1) [70], Croatia (n = 1) [38], France (n = 1) [8], Germany (n = 1) [53], Hong Kong (n = 1) [60], Italy (n = 1) [56], India (n = 1) [41], Japan (n = 1, also included UK) [29], Puerto Rico (n = 1) [68], Qatar (n = 1) [40], Singapore (n = 1) [12], Sweden (n = 1, also included UK), Taiwan (n = 1) [61], and Thailand (n = 1) [37]. One paper was a global analysis across several different countries [16]. Of those analyses conducted in the United States (n = 20), all found PGx testing to be cost-effective or cost-saving, and in 2 papers, dominant (higher QALY gain and lower costs) compared to no testing [19,21]. These papers were primarily in psychiatry (n = 10) [17–24,32,33], followed by geriatrics (n = 3) [10,13,27], polypharmacy/medication management (n = 2) [11,14], acute coronary syndrome (n = 2) [45,52], hypertension (n = 1) [47], asthma (n = 1) [67], and pediatric transplant (n = 1) [63].

DISCUSSION

Methodological Considerations

Nearly all of the cost-effectiveness studies reviewed followed established economic modeling principles laid out in prior publications [71,72], providing useful insight into the relative cost and effectiveness of implementing PGx testing versus standard care or TAU. Despite indicating promising results for PGx, cost-effectiveness analyses are rarely a primary driving factor for policy decision-making in the United States, given the historic lack of consideration given to cost when considering the value of a given intervention, though this has recently changed [73]. Additional methods demonstrating cost-savings, such as retrospective and/or prospective claims database analyses like those identified in this review, can provide further evidence for proponents of PGx testing to advocate for more widespread adoption given the substantial potential downstream cost savings.

Notably, only 1 budget impact model from a health system perspective was identified in our review [63], despite budget impact models being a key tool for payers when making policy decisions. While many of the cost analyses identified included estimates of cost-savings in traditional budget impact metrics such as per-member-per-month (PMPM) or per-member-per-year (PMPY), no papers evaluated the budget impact of PGx testing using more traditional approaches to budget impact modeling—that is, development of a patient funnel to identify eligible individuals, then estimating the cost of adopting the new technology assuming increased uptake over time (ie, increased market share) [74]. Such models provide useful insight for payers, who rely on budget impact models for short- and long-term financial planning and forecasting.

Limitations and Variability in Pharmacogenomic Test Specifications

Several of the model-based cost-effectiveness analyses reviewed did not explicitly specify the genes they evaluated, which presents significant limitations for interpreting and applying the findings clinically. Without clear identification of specific genes, it is challenging to assess the direct relevance or reproducibility of these studies in diverse clinical settings. Furthermore, among studies that did mention specific genes, many failed to identify the exact genetic variants evaluated. This omission is critical because genetic variants can vary widely in their impact on drug response, even within the same gene. Furthermore, omitting specific genetic variants relevant to the studied patient population could lead to increased *false-negative* results. For example, if critical variants are absent from a PGx test, individuals might incorrectly be classified as normal metabolizers when they may actually be ultrarapid, rapid, intermediate, or poor metabolizers if tested variants were comprehensive. Such inadequacies in test design, particularly variant selection, can significantly impact economic evaluations by influencing the accuracy of predicted clinical outcomes, thereby introducing heterogeneity and potentially skewing cost-effectiveness results [75]. Additionally, the majority of studies lacked detailed reporting on the genetic ancestry of the populations included in their models. Genetic ancestry significantly influences the distribution of genetic variants, and consequently, the clinical utility and cost-effectiveness of PGx testing may differ or not be applicable depending on which genes and/or specific variants are included in the model. We recommend that future pharmacogenomic economic analyses, especially those using a modeling approach, should explicitly identify the specific genes and variants assessed and clearly report on the genetic ancestry of the studied populations, if possible, to enhance clinical applicability and interpretability. This also provides clearer information for payers when developing policies around reimbursement for PGx testing.

All of the studies reviewed seem to be assessing the cost of genotyping, which is the most popular testing methodology for PGx at this time and is less expensive at present than sequencing-based methods. However, genetic testing technology continues to significantly advance and there is an increase in uptake and exploration of retrieving PGx results from whole genome/exome sequencing [76,77]. Therefore, future cost-effectiveness or cost-savings studies should consider the cost of these advanced technologies and the impact of cost-effectiveness for PGx moving forward. The anticipation is that whole genome/exome sequencing can provide individuals with a lot of health information (eg, genetic conditions, carrier status, PGx profile, etc) from a singular test. Although there is a cost associated with reanalysis, this approach may minimize the total cost of obtaining PGx information as compared to performing multiple different tests, which historically is done.

Clinical and Policy Considerations

PGx testing was found to be cost-effective or cost saving in nearly all situations except in studies focusing on warfarin and in 2 studies in psychiatry, though none of these papers were conducted from a United States payer perspective. Nonetheless, this implies that PGx testing may only be cost-effective for specific use cases; among those papers done in the United States, therapeutic areas included major depressive disorder, epilepsy disorder, polypharmacy, geriatrics, and acute coronary syndrome, all of which found PGx testing to be cost-effective or cost-saving.

Despite the adoption of PGx at different institutions across the United States, accessibility is still a significant barrier due to financial challenges including lack of insurance coverage of PGx testing [1]. In clinical practice, patients often come to appointments exhausted and hopeless having trialed so many medications without success, in hope of new information that can provide insight into how they might better tolerate, or respond to specific medications. PGx offers these individuals an opportunity to discover the cause of their response (or lack thereof) to a given medication. Unfortunately, many patients decline PGx testing due to cost and lack of insurance coverage. Currently available PGx panels can cost anywhere from the low hundreds to thousands of dollars, depending on the laboratory [78,79], which constitutes a large financial burden, particularly for those of lower socioeconomic status. While increasing testing volumes may marginally reduce per-sample costs in high-throughput settings, the major cost drivers in clinical pharmacogenomics remain personnel-related; including technical staff, regulatory oversight, and clinical interpretation. As PGx testing expands to encompass more complex technologies like whole genome sequencing, adequate reimbursement is essential to support the specialized expertise required for variant interpretation, particularly in undercharacterized or novel regions of the genome. In this context, future cost savings may be more dependent on innovations in automated analysis (machine learning) and decision support than on test volume alone.

Furthermore, although PGx testing improves health outcomes, payers also often rank cost as a major barrier to implementation in clinical practice, due to the perception that PGx test coverage may not necessarily reduce overall health care resource utilization; further, there is a high degree of variability in cost-effective models limiting the ability to generalize results for clinical adoption [80]. Payers are also more hesitant to cover PGx testing in the absence of strong language to support its use in Food and Drug Administration (FDA) labels and therapeutic guidelines (eg, National Comprehensive Cancer Network, American Heart Association) [81]. This can be detrimental for patient care, as updates to FDA labels depend not only on the pace of emerging PGx evidence but also on factors such as clarity in required evidence standards, regulatory decision-making processes, and alignment with clinical guideline recommendations, all of which can delay or complicate timely integration of PGx advances into routine practice. Despite numerous papers demonstrating the cost-savings and cost-effectiveness of PGx testing, advocates for PGx testing must continue to conduct retrospective and prospective cost analyses demonstrating the overall cost savings associated with PGx testing despite its upfront cost, in addition to cost-effectiveness analyses, where concepts such as QALYs may be difficult to interpret [82].

Additionally, though payers often cite a lack of evidence supporting PGx testing as the primary reason to deny coverage [83,84], they do not provide details regarding the types of studies that would be useful to support routine coverage of PGx testing. More high-quality studies (eg, randomized controlled trials) have been performed and showed the strong clinical utility of PGx, but in many cases payers remain reluctant and have still not made any changes or improvements to their policies. As discussed under Methodological Considerations, budget impact models from the payer perspective illustrating the potential PMPM or PMPY impact on a health plan's budget could provide additional useful information for payers developing policies around reimbursement.

Another consideration is perverse incentive mechanisms, such as capped payments for hospitalizations, which should be reevaluated to incorporate consideration of PGx testing into routine clinical care. Payers should consider alternate mechanisms of coverage for PGx testing, given the demonstrated downstream cost savings associated with both targeted and comprehensive testing. These policies could be tailored to specific therapeutic areas, drugs, or subgroups of individuals depending on clinical characteristics, and concurrent drug therapies and/or comorbid conditions.

CPIC has developed 28 peer-reviewed evidence-based guidelines for 28 genes and over 100 medications [3]. Yet, our review demonstrates that not all of these have been evaluated for cost-effectiveness or cost-savings, which is encouraged for future PGx economic studies. In the current clinical landscape, patients often receive PGx testing using comprehensive pharmacogenomic panels, which, in addition to providing the immediate benefit of a PGx result for a specific medication question, also contain results for multiple potential future therapeutic needs that can be referenced throughout the patient's life. Therefore, cost-effectiveness and savings are anticipated to accrue over an individual's lifetime. Based on current practices, it would be beneficial to see more economic modeling/studies showing the impact of preemptive panel-based PGx panel testing.

SUMMARY

Variability in individual drug responses can be influenced by multiple factors, with genetic variation playing a significant role in determining clinical outcomes. PGx testing guides medication selection to ensure optimal efficacy, reduce toxicity, and improve cost efficiency. As presented, evidence suggests that integrating PGx testing into clinical practice is for the most part cost-effective and cost-saving, though these findings may not be relevant for all therapeutic areas and all clinical scenarios. As payers remain reluctant to reimburse PGx testing, continued future collaboration between policymakers, clinicians, and the PGx community can further address research gaps to expand coverage of PGx testing, thus enhancing the quality and types of future studies conducted to provide relevant evidence for policymakers.

CLINICS CARE POINTS

- The adoption and coverage of PGx testing has the potential to vastly improve clinical care by providing tailored medication recommendations based on an individual's clinical characteristics. Nonetheless, substantial barriers to widespread implementation persist. Among these barriers is the limited availability of clinicians specializing in PGx, compounded by gaps in education and training among general health care professionals. Many clinicians are unfamiliar with the process of ordering PGx tests, interpreting complex genetic information, and translating this data into actionable prescribing decisions.
- Day-to-day clinical integration challenges include identifying which patients will benefit most from PGx testing, explaining the rationale and potential outcomes to patients, coordinating with genetic counseling services when needed, and addressing patient concerns about privacy and genetic information.
- Clinicians must also become proficient in recognizing when test results necessitate changes in medication regimens, including dose adjustments, medication substitutions, or more frequent monitoring.
- Efforts to overcome these implementation barriers are underway and include integrating PGx education into medical, pharmacy, and nursing curricula, as well as offering continuing education programs targeting current health care professionals.
- Additionally, the development of user-friendly clinical decision support tools integrated into electronic health records can guide clinicians through interpreting PGx results and applying them effectively in clinical practice.
- Finally, fostering multidisciplinary collaboration between geneticists, pharmacists, primary care providers, and specialists is crucial to fully harness the benefits of PGx testing and realize its promise of precision medicine in routine clinical practice.

DISCLOSURES

The authors have nothing to disclose. Dr C.L. Gong notes that this work was done independently of any past, current, or ongoing work at Curta; the views expressed here are Cynthia Gong's own and do not necessarily reflect the views of Curta.

REFERENCES

[1] McKinnon RA, Ward MB, Sorich MJ. A critical analysis of barriers to the clinical implementation of pharmacogenomics. Therapeut Clin Risk Manag 2007;3(5):751–9.
[2] Stanek EJ, Sanders CL, Taber KAJ, et al. Adoption of pharmacogenomic testing by US physicians: results of a nationwide survey. Clin Pharmacol Ther 2012;91(3): 450–8.

[3] Relling MV, Klein TE. CPIC: clinical pharmacogenetics implementation consortium of the pharmacogenomics research network. Clin Pharmacol Ther 2011;89(3):464–7.
[4] Arksey H, O'Malley L. Scoping studies: towards a methodological framework. Int J Soc Res Methodol 2005;8(1):19–32.
[5] Levac D, Colquhoun H, O'Brien KK. Scoping studies: advancing the methodology. Implement Sci 2010;5(1):69.
[6] Page MJ, McKenzie JE, Bossuyt PM, et al. The PRISMA 2020 statement: an updated guideline for reporting systematic reviews. BMJ 2021;372:n71.
[7] Rayyan. Rayyan: AI-powered systematic review management platform. Available at: https://www.rayyan.ai/. Accessed March 5, 2025.
[8] Fokoun C, Serrier H, Rabier H, et al. Pharmacogenetic-guided glimepiride therapy in type-2 diabetes mellitus: a cost-effectiveness study. Pharmacogenomics J 2021;21(5):559–65.
[9] Moretti ME, Lato DF, Berger H, et al. A cost-effectiveness analysis of maternal CYP2D6 genetic testing to guide treatment for postpartum pain and avert infant adverse events. Pharmacogenomics J 2018;18(3):391–7.
[10] Brixner D, Biltaji E, Bress A, et al. The effect of pharmacogenetic profiling with a clinical decision support tool on healthcare resource utilization and estimated costs in the elderly exposed to polypharmacy. J Med Econ 2016;19(3):213–28.
[11] Sugarman EA, Cullors A, Centeno J, et al. Contribution of pharmacogenetic testing to modeled medication change recommendations in a long-term care population with polypharmacy. Drugs Aging 2016;33(12):929–36.
[12] Chan SL, Ng HY, Sung C, et al. Economic burden of adverse drug reactions and potential for pharmacogenomic testing in Singaporean adults. Pharmacogenomics J 2019;19(4):401–10.
[13] Bain KT, Knowlton CH, Matos A. Cost avoidance related to a pharmacist-led pharmacogenomics service for the Program of All-inclusive Care for the Elderly. Pharmacogenomics 2020;21(10):651–61.
[14] Fragala MS, Keogh M, Goldberg SE, et al. Clinical and economic outcomes of a pharmacogenomics-enriched comprehensive medication management program in a self-insured employee population. Pharmacogenomics J 2024;24(5):30.
[15] Plumpton CO, Pirmohamed M, Hughes DA. Cost-effectiveness of panel tests for multiple pharmacogenes associated with adverse drug reactions: an evaluation framework. Clin Pharmacol Ther 2019;105(6):1429–38.
[16] Zhou Y, Krebs K, Milani L, et al. Global frequencies of clinically important HLA alleles and their implications for the cost-effectiveness of preemptive pharmacogenetic testing. Clin Pharmacol Ther 2021;109(1):160–74.
[17] Fagerness J, Fonseca E, Hess GP, et al. Pharmacogenetic-guided psychiatric intervention associated with increased adherence and cost savings. Am J Manag Care 2014;20(5):e146–56.
[18] Winner JG, Carhart JM, Altar CA, et al. Combinatorial pharmacogenomic guidance for psychiatric medications reduces overall pharmacy costs in a 1 year prospective evaluation. Curr Med Res Opin 2015;31(9):1633–43.
[19] Hornberger J, Li Q, Quinn B. Cost-effectiveness of combinatorial pharmacogenomic testing for treatment-resistant major depressive disorder patients. Am J Manag Care 2015;21(6):e357–65.
[20] Brown LC, Lorenz RA, Li J, et al. Economic utility: combinatorial pharmacogenomics and medication cost savings for mental health care in a primary care setting. Clin Ther 2017;39(3):592–602.e1.
[21] Groessl EJ, Tally SR, Hillery N, et al. Cost-effectiveness of a pharmacogenetic test to guide treatment for major depressive disorder. J Manag Care Spec Pharm 2018;24(8):726–34.
[22] Perlis RH, Mehta R, Edwards AM, et al. Pharmacogenetic testing among patients with mood and anxiety disorders is associated with decreased utilization and cost: a propensity-score matched study. Depress Anxiety 2018;35(10):946–52.
[23] Benitez J, Cool CL, Scotti DJ. Use of combinatorial pharmacogenomic guidance in treating psychiatric disorders. Per Med 2018;15(6):481–94.
[24] Girardin FR, Poncet A, Perrier A, et al. Cost-effectiveness of HLA-DQB1/HLA-B pharmacogenetic-guided treatment and blood monitoring in US patients taking clozapine. Pharmacogenomics J 2019;19(2):211–8.
[25] Sluiter RL, Janzing JGE, van der Wilt GJ, et al. An economic model of the cost-utility of pre-emptive genetic testing to support pharmacotherapy in patients with major depression in primary care. Pharmacogenomics J 2019;19(5):480–9.
[26] Tanner JA, Davies PE, Overall CC, et al. Cost-effectiveness of combinatorial pharmacogenomic testing for depression from the Canadian public payer perspective. Pharmacogenomics 2020;21(8):521–31.
[27] Jablonski MR, Lorenz R, Li J, et al. Economic outcomes following combinatorial pharmacogenomic testing for elderly psychiatric patients. J Geriatr Psychiatr Neurol 2020;33(6):324–32.
[28] Fabbri C, Kasper S, Zohar J, et al. Cost-effectiveness of genetic and clinical predictors for choosing combined psychotherapy and pharmacotherapy in major depression. J Affect Disord 2021;279:722–9.
[29] Ninomiya K, Saito T, Okochi T, et al. Cost effectiveness of pharmacogenetic-guided clozapine administration based on risk of HLA variants in Japan and the UK. Transl Psychiatry 2021;11(1):362.
[30] Ghanbarian S, Wong GWK, Bunka M, et al. Cost-effectiveness of pharmacogenomic-guided treatment for major depression. CMAJ (Can Med Assoc J) 2023;195(44):E1499–508.
[31] Lopez-Saavedra J, Abad-Santos F. Cost-effectiveness of pharmacogenetic screening in the management of major

depressive disorder in the Spanish Healthcare System. J Affect Disord 2024;365:597–605.
[32] Roe N, Passariello C, Brown L, et al. 170 prospective evaluation of the economic utility of combinatorial pharmacogenomics in generalized anxiety disorder and major depressive disorder. CNS Spectr 2018;23(1): 99–100.
[33] Najafzadeh M, Garces JA, Maciel A. Economic evaluation of implementing a novel pharmacogenomic test (IDgenetix®) to guide treatment of patients with depression and/or anxiety. Pharmacoeconomics 2017;35(12): 1297–310.
[34] GeneSight DNA test for psychiatric & depression medication. GeneSight. Available at: https://genesight.com/product/. Accessed March 6, 2025.
[35] YouScript. Tests. Genelex. 2014. Available at: http://genelex.jp/pharmacogenetic-tests/. Accessed March 6, 2025.
[36] IDgenetix. Castle biosciences. Available at: https://castlebiosciences.com/idgenetix. Accessed March 6, 2025.
[37] Chong HY, Saokaew S, Dumrongprat K, et al. Cost-effectiveness analysis of pharmacogenetic-guided warfarin dosing in Thailand. Thromb Res 2014 134(6):1278–84.
[38] Mitropoulou C, Fragoulakis V, Bozina N, et al. Economic evaluation of pharmacogenomic-guided warfarin treatment for elderly Croatian atrial fibrillation patients with ischemic stroke. Pharmacogenomics 2015;16(2): 137–48.
[39] Verhoef TI, Redekop WK, Langenskiold S, et al. Cost-effectiveness of pharmacogenetic-guided dosing of warfarin in the United Kingdom and Sweden. Pharmacogenomics J 2016;16(5):478–84.
[40] Eljilany I, Elewa H, Al-Badriyeh D. Cost-benefit analysis of genotype-guided interruption days in warfarin preprocedural management. Curr Probl Cardiol 2023; 48(6):101128.
[41] Anand A, Hegde NC, Chhabra P, et al. Pharmacogenetic guided versus standard warfarin dosing for routine clinical care with its pharmacoeconomic impact: a randomized controlled clinical trial. Ann Hematol 2024;103(6): 2133–44.
[42] Verhoef TI, Redekop WK, De Boer A, et al, EU-PACT Group. Economic evaluation of a pharmacogenetic dosing algorithm for coumarin anticoagulants in The Netherlands. Pharmacogenomics 2015;16(2):101–14.
[43] Hafeez A, Cipriano LE, Kim RB, et al. Cost-effectiveness analysis of pharmacogenomics (PGx)-based warfarin, apixaban, and rivaroxaban versus standard warfarin for the management of atrial fibrillation in Ontario, Canada. Pharmacoeconomics 2024;42(1):69–90.
[44] Koufaki MI, Fragoulakis V, Díaz-Villamarín X, et al. Economic evaluation of pharmacogenomic-guided antiplatelet treatment in Spanish patients suffering from acute coronary syndrome participating in the U-PGx PREPARE study. Hum Genom 2023;17(1):51.
[45] Jiang M, You JH. Cost-effectiveness analysis of personalized antiplatelet therapy in patients with acute coronary syndrome. Pharmacogenomics 2016;17(7):701–13.
[46] Fragoulakis V, Bartsakoulia M, Díaz-Villamarín X, et al. Cost-effectiveness analysis of pharmacogenomics-guided clopidogrel treatment in Spanish patients undergoing percutaneous coronary intervention. Pharmacogenomics J 2019;19(5):438–45.
[47] Kelley EF, Snyder EM, Alkhatib NS, et al. Economic evaluation of a pharmacogenomic multi-gene panel test to optimize anti-hypertension therapy: simulation study. J Med Econ 2018;21(12):1246–53.
[48] Geenen JW, Baranova EV, Asselbergs FW, et al. Early HTA in pharmacogenomics: a case example in cardiovascular drugs. Value Health 2016;19(7):A636.
[49] Mitchell D, Guertin JR, Dubois A, et al. A discrete event simulation model to assess the economic value of a hypothetical pharmacogenomics test for statin-induced myopathy in patients initiating a statin in secondary cardiovascular prevention. Mol Diagn Ther 2018;22(2): 241–54.
[50] Mitchell D, Guertin JR, Iliza AC, et al. Economic evaluation of a pharmacogenomic test for statin-induced myopathy in cardiovascular high-risk patients initiating a statin. Value Health 2015;18(7):A396.
[51] Iliza AC, Fanton Aita F, Mitchell D, et al. Development of a pharmacoeconomic model to assess the cost effectiveness of pharmacogenomics tests in chronic heart failure: the case of ivabradine. Value Health 2016; 19(3):A48–9.
[52] Dong OM, Wheeler SB, Cruden G, et al. Cost-effectiveness of multigene pharmacogenetic testing in patients with acute coronary syndrome after percutaneous coronary intervention. Value Health 2020;23(1):61–73.
[53] Butzke B, Oduncu FS, Severin F, et al. The cost-effectiveness of UGT1A1 genotyping before colorectal cancer treatment with irinotecan from the perspective of the German statutory health insurance. Acta Oncol 2016;55(3):318–28.
[54] Dionne F, Aminkeng F, Bhavsar AP, et al. An initial health economic evaluation of pharmacogenomic testing in patients treated for childhood cancer with anthracyclines. Pediatr Blood Cancer 2018;65(3). https://doi.org/10.1002/pbc.26887.
[55] Wei X, Sun H, Zhuang J, et al. Cost-effectiveness analysis of CYP2D6*10 pharmacogenetic testing to guide the adjuvant endocrine therapy for postmenopausal women with estrogen receptor positive early breast cancer in China. Clin Drug Invest 2020;40(1):25–32.
[56] Fragoulakis V, Roncato R, Bignucolo A, et al. Cost-utility analysis and cross-country comparison of pharmacogenomics-guided treatment in colorectal cancer patients participating in the U-PGx PREPARE study. Pharmacol Res 2023;197(106949):106949.
[57] Wei X, Cai J, Zhuang J, et al. CYP2D6*10 pharmacogenetic-guided SERM could be a cost-effective strategy in Chinese patients with hormone receptor-positive breast cancer. Pharmacogenomics 2019;21(1):43–53.
[58] Fuerte B, Burgos M, Cao V, et al. Budget impact analysis of TPMT and NUDT15 pharmacogenomic testing for

6-mercaptopurine in pediatric acute lymphoblastic leukemia patients. Pharmacogenet Genom 2025;35(2):73–80.
[59] Lo C, Nguyen S, Yang C, et al. Pharmacogenomics in Asian subpopulations and impacts on commonly prescribed medications. Clin Transl Sci 2020;13(5):861–70.
[60] Chen Z, Liew D, Kwan P. Real-world cost-effectiveness of pharmacogenetic screening for epilepsy treatment. Neurology 2016;86(12):1086–94.
[61] Ke CH, Chung WH, Wen YH, et al. Cost-effectiveness analysis for genotyping before allopurinol treatment to prevent severe cutaneous adverse drug reactions. J Rheumatol 2017;44(6):835–43.
[62] Plumpton CO, Yip VLM, Alfirevic A, et al. Cost-effectiveness of screening for HLA-A*31:01 prior to initiation of carbamazepine in epilepsy. Epilepsia (Cph) 2015;56(4): 556–63.
[63] Wang J, Pasternak AL, Maggo S, et al. CYP3A5 pharmacogenetic testing for tacrolimus in pediatric heart transplant patients: a budget impact analysis. Pharmacogenet Genom 2025;35(2):81–6.
[64] Fragoulakis V, Koufaki MI, Joefield-Roka C, et al. Cost-utility analysis of pharmacogenomics-guided tacrolimus treatment in Austrian kidney transplant recipients participating in the U-PGx PREPARE study. Pharmacogenomics J 2024;24(2):10.
[65] Sluiter RL, Van Marrewijk C, De Jong D, et al. Genotype-guided thiopurine dosing does not lead to additional costs in patients with inflammatory bowel disease. J Crohns Colitis 2019;13(7):838–45.
[66] Sluiter RL, Kievit W, van der Wilt GJ, et al. Cost-effectiveness analysis of genotype-guided treatment allocation in patients with alcohol use disorders using naltrexone or acamprosate, using a modeling approach. Eur Addctn Res 2018;24(5):245–54.
[67] Wu AC, Gay C, Rett MD, et al. Pharmacogenomic test that predicts response to inhaled corticosteroids in adults with asthma likely to be cost-saving. Pharmacogenomics 2015;16(6):591–600.
[68] Martes-Martinez C, Ḿndez-Seṕlveda C, Milĺn-Molina J, et al. Cost-utility study of warfarin genotyping in the VACHS affiliated anticoagulation clinic of Puerto Rico. Puert Rico Health Sci J 2017;36(3):165–72.
[69] Li X, Cao Y. Cost-effectiveness of Arg16Gly in ADRB2 pharmacogenomic-guided treatment for pediatric asthma. Expert Rev Pharmacoecon Outcomes Res 2023;23(8): 891–9.
[70] Rens NE, Uyl-de Groot CA, Goldhaber-Fiebert JD, et al. Cost-effectiveness of a pharmacogenomic test for stratified isoniazid dosing in treatment of active tuberculosis. Clin Infect Dis 2020;71(12):3136–43.
[71] Husereau D, Drummond M, Augustovski F, et al. Consolidated Health Economic Evaluation Reporting Standards 2022 (CHEERS 2022) statement: updated reporting guidance for health economic evaluations. BJOG 2022;129(3):336–44.
[72] Neumann PJ, Sanders GD, Russell LB, et al. Cost-effectiveness in health and medicine. 2nd edition. New York (NY): Oxford University Press; 2017. p. 496.
[73] PCORI's expanded mandate creates new opportunities for value assessment research. Am J Accountable Care 2021;9(3):19–21.
[74] Sullivan SD, Mauskopf JA, Augustovski F, et al. Budget impact analysis-principles of good practice: report of the ISPOR 2012 budget impact analysis good practice II task force. Value Health 2014;17(1):5–14.
[75] Hippman C, Nislow C. Pharmacogenomic testing: clinical evidence and implementation challenges. J Personalized Med 2019;9(3):40.
[76] Tafazoli A, Guchelaar HJ, Miltyk W, et al. Applying next-generation sequencing platforms for pharmacogenomic testing in clinical practice. Front Pharmacol 2021;12: 693453.
[77] Lanillos J, Carcajona M, Maietta P, et al. Clinical pharmacogenetic analysis in 5,001 individuals with diagnostic Exome Sequencing data. NPJ Genom Med 2022; 7(1):12.
[78] University of Florida health. Costs and insurance. University of Florida health. Available at: https://ufhealth.org/myrx/costs-insurance. Accessed March 5, 2025.
[79] GeneSight. Genetic testing cost. GeneSight. Available at: https://genesight.com/cost/. Accessed March 5, 2025.
[80] Virelli CR, Mohiuddin AG, Kennedy JL. Barriers to clinical adoption of pharmacogenomic testing in psychiatry: a critical analysis. Transl Psychiatry 2021;11(1):509.
[81] Shriver SP, Adams D, McKelvey BA, et al. Overcoming barriers to discovery and implementation of equitable pharmacogenomic testing in oncology. J Clin Oncol 2024;42(10):1181–92.
[82] Brower A. Is it time to take a harder look at the QALY? Biotechnol Healthc 2008;5(3):47–8.
[83] McKenny S. UHC will No longer cover pharmacogenetic panel tests for commercial and individual exchange plans. Telcor. 2024. Available at: https://telcor.com/uhc-will-not-cover-pharmacogenetic-panel-tests-for-commercial-and-individual-exchange-plans/. Accessed March 8, 2025.
[84] United Healthcare. Changes to genetic and molecular testing coverage and prior authorization requirements. Available at: https://www.uhcprovider.com/en/resource-library/news/2024/changes-genetic-molecular-testing-coverage-pa-requirements.html. Accessed March 8, 2025.

SECTION: INFECTIOUS DISEASE

Advances in Molecular Pathology 8 (2025) 113–129
ADVANCES IN MOLECULAR PATHOLOGY

A Beginner's Guide to Assay Development for Emerging Pathogens

Tristan R. Grams, PhD[a,b], Benjamin T. Bradley, MD, PhD[a,b,*]
[a]Department of Pathology, University of Utah, 500 Chipeta Way, Salt Lake City, UT 84108, USA; [b]ARUP Laboratories, MS115, 500 Chipeta Way, Salt Lake City, UT 84108, USA

KEYWORDS
• Emerging pathogen diagnostics • Assay development • Molecular diagnostics • Infectious disease testing • Disease outbreak diagnostics • Laboratory-developed tests • Clinical microbiology

KEY POINTS

- By addressing key preanalytical, analytical, and postanalytical considerations, this guide aims to provide laboratory professionals with a consolidated source of critical design aspects.
- Selecting appropriate specimen types, establishing robust internal controls, and optimizing testing platforms are critical for assay accuracy, scalability, and resilience during outbreaks or surges.
- Clear, standardized reporting with interpretative guidance tailored to clinical, public health, and administrative stakeholders enhances diagnostic reliability and facilitates timely clinical and epidemiologic decision-making.
- Proactive measures such as pooled testing, strategic reagent stockpiling, and continuous assay performance monitoring are essential to maintain testing capacity amid rapid increases in demand.

INTRODUCTION

Emerging pathogens present unique challenges for clinical laboratories. Unlike well-characterized infectious agents, newly identified or rapidly evolving pathogens require swift assay development and implementation to ensure timely detection, containment, and treatment. Because traditional assay validation and verification frameworks are not well suited for these pathogens, laboratories must adopt a flexible yet rigorous approach to assay design. Over the past decade, the urgency of developing clinical assays for emerging pathogens has been exemplified by responses to Zika virus, SARS-CoV-2, and, most recently, highly pathogenic avian influenza A (H5N1).

The emergence of Zika virus in the Americas revealed critical gaps in laboratory preparedness. Early diagnostic assays based on serology exhibited significant cross-reactivity with other flaviviruses, particularly dengue virus, complicating clinical interpretation and epidemiologic case tracking [1]. This underscored the necessity of rigorous target selection, robust analytical validation, and continuous performance monitoring of assays in affected regions. Similarly, the COVID-19 pandemic highlighted both the strengths and weaknesses of molecular diagnostics. While the rapid development of assays facilitated large-scale testing, laboratories faced challenges including supply chain disruptions, regulatory bottlenecks, and the absence of standardized protocols [2]. Despite these hurdles, institutions adapted quickly by developing laboratory-developed tests (LDTs) and leveraging high-throughput automation to meet unprecedented diagnostic demand.

At the time of this writing in early 2025, H5N1 has become a focal point in emerging pathogen diagnostics. Early laboratory assays for influenza A (H5) have

*Corresponding author. *E-mail address:* ben.bradley@hsc.utah.edu

https://doi.org/10.1016/j.yamp.2025.05.004 www.advancesinmolecularpathology.com
2589-4080/25/ © 2025 Elsevier Inc. All rights are reserved, including those for text and data mining, AI training, and similar technologies.

ABBREVIATIONS

BMBL	Biosafety in Microbiological and Biomedical Laboratories
CMS	Centers for Medicare & Medicaid Services
CLIA	Clinical Laboratory Improvement Amendments
Ct	cycle threshold
EUA	Emergency Use Authorization
ID	infectious disease
IVD	*in vitro* diagnostic
LDT	laboratory-developed test
PHE	public health emergency
PHL	public health laboratory
VTM	viral transport media

encountered multiple challenges, including limitations in acceptable specimen types, constraints on assay throughput, and complications arising from a newly evolving regulatory landscape for LDTs [3]. These obstacles highlight the continued need for adaptability in assay design and regulatory navigation.

This guide is intended for clinical pathologists, microbiologists, and molecular diagnostics professionals engaged in the development, validation, and implementation of diagnostic assays for emerging pathogens. It provides a structured framework to aid laboratories in designing assays tailored to their specific operational and clinical requirements. By addressing key preanalytical, analytical, and postanalytical considerations, this guide aims to provide laboratory professionals with a consolidated source of critical design aspects. As emerging infectious threats continue to arise, the ability to rapidly develop, validate, and deploy molecular assays will be critical in mitigating outbreaks and protecting public health.

Preanalytical considerations

The pathogen

Understanding the pathogen's characteristics is fundamental to assay design. A comprehensive literature review is necessary to evaluate prior diagnostic strategies, identify conserved and variable genomic regions, and cross-check available sequences in publicly available databases. The transmission route of the pathogen also dictates key aspects of the assay design and the threshold for triggering testing. Human-to-human transmission, as seen with SARS-CoV-2, typically necessitates rapid, high-sensitivity molecular assays to facilitate early detection and containment. In contrast, vector-borne pathogens, such as West Nile virus and dengue virus, often require a combination of molecular and serologic testing to assess for active or recent infection due to the transient viremia associated with these infections [4–6]. Zoonotic infections, like highly-pathogenic avian influenza, may require additional considerations for species barriers and cross-reactivity. For example, molecular assays for avian influenza should target unique, strain-specific regions while avoiding regions known for mutations following host adaptation. They should also minimize cross-reactivity with low-pathogenic strains and differentiate avian subtypes from circulating human influenza viruses. During the 2013 H7N9 avian influenza outbreak in China, early serologic and molecular assays faced cross-reactivity issues with other avian influenza subtypes, making it difficult to distinguish true H7N9 infections from background H7 influenza activity in poultry-exposed individuals [7]. To address this, assay designs were updated with subtype-specific primers and probes, improving specificity while reducing cross-reactivity [8].

Another key consideration in the preanalytical phase of test development is determining whether the pathogen is newly emerging, re-emerging, or experiencing antigenic shifts. Novel pathogens require *de novo* assay development, while re-emerging pathogens may benefit from modifications to existing assays. For viruses which have not adapted to mammalian or human hosts, the rate of acquiring mutations may initially be greater than once the virus becomes endemic [9]. Such mutations may be acquired through multiple transmission events or during prolonged infection of a single individual [10]. In cases of significant antigenic shift, as observed in influenza A viruses, continuous genomic surveillance is necessary to ensure that assays remain effective [11]. In both cases—whether dealing with a newly emerging virus or significant antigenic shift—the use of primers and probes targeting multiple genomic regions can help safeguard assay performance by reducing the risk of target dropout caused by genetic variability in a single region. Finally, choosing between molecular and serologic testing depends on the pathogen's characteristics and diagnostic objectives. While molecular assays allow for direct detection of pathogen nucleic acids and are generally favored for diagnosing acute infections, serologic testing plays a crucial role in assessing past exposure and conducting surveillance, particularly for infections with a short window for molecular detection, such as Zika or dengue virus [6].

The patient

Patient-related factors play a vital role in assay development, as the intended use of test results can vary significantly depending on the clinical and public health context. Diagnostic assays should be designed with clear objectives, whether for identifying active infections, guiding treatment decisions, assessing disease prognosis, or supporting epidemiolcgic surveillance and containment efforts. In certain situations, molecular testing is essential for rapid decision-making in patient care, while in others, pooled testing approaches offer a practical solution for large-scale screening efforts. Assessing assay performance in pooled versus individual sample testing is critical, as sensitivity and limit of detection can vary between these approaches. For example, during the COVID-19 pandemic, some real-time polymerase chain reaction (RT-PCR) assays required higher cycle threshold (Ct) cutoffs for pooled testing to account for dilution effects, ensuring that low viral load cases were still detected [12]. Surveillance strategies must be flexible enough to address constraints in testing capacity and supply shortages. In resource-limited environments, pooling samples can improve efficiency and reduce reagent consumption, allowing broader population screening.

Special populations introduce additional considerations in test design and implementation. Children, pregnant women, and vulnerable populations may present unique diagnostic challenges because of physiologic differences, health care access, or ethical and legal concerns surrounding testing. For example, maternal-fetal transmission of pathogens like Zika virus necessitates highly sensitive and specific assays capable of detecting low viral loads in amniotic fluid or placental tissues [13]. Acquiring appropriate specimen matrices for validation studies can be challenging, particularly when targeting specific populations. Ensuring accurate and effective pathogen detection in these groups may require collaboration with peer institutions, reference laboratories, or public health agencies to obtain necessary validation materials and establish robust testing frameworks. Pediatric testing may require alternative specimen collection methods to enhance compliance and minimize discomfort [14]. In the case of vulnerable populations, logistical barriers such as limited health care access, language differences, and concerns over medical privacy can impact the success of testing programs [15].

Specimen collection

Selecting the right specimen type is essential for accurate diagnostics. The choice depends on the pathogen's tropism and the stage of infection. If preferred specimen types are unavailable due to supply shortages or the need for an invasive collection procedure, less invasive matrices such as saliva or urine may provide a viable alternative solution if they demonstrate adequate sensitivity. Flexibility is a key in this area as emerging pathogens may present in nontypical fashion, as seen with H5N1 influenza virus and the need for conjunctival specimens [16].

Redundancy in the supply chain is critical to preventing disruptions in specimen collection and processing. Resiliency to supply chain issues can be met by validating multiple specimen types at the time of assay development or examining nontraditional transport media (eg, saline or buffered salt solutions). In the event of an acute shortage of a critical component, bridging studies may provide the necessary stopgap measure to continue patient testing [17]. Alternatively, as demonstrated during the SARS-CoV-2 pandemic, the laboratory also possesses the capability to produce media such as viral transport media (VTM) [18]. Extraction-free methods can streamline workflows and reduce dependency on specific reagents, which may become scarce during outbreaks [19].

Proper collection, storage, and shipping protocols are essential for preserving specimen integrity. VTM is specifically designed for preserving viral particles from mucosal swabs, where the sample matrix has low cellularity and nuclease activity. In contrast, blood and urine require collection systems tailored to stabilize nucleic acids and prevent cellular degradation, as these specimens contain higher levels of enzymes and cellular components that can compromise sample integrity and affect downstream molecular testing. Adherence to biosafety regulations, including Centers for Disease Control and Prevention (CDC) guidelines, the Biosafety in Microbiological and Biomedical Laboratories (BMBL), and select agent regulations, is essential for the safe transport of infectious samples. Proper classification of the sample—such as BSL containment requirements or designation as a select agent—dictates the necessary packaging, labeling, and transport conditions to mitigate biosafety risks. Temperature control and regulatory compliance ensure sample integrity while preventing potential exposure during transit. By standardizing these processes, laboratories can minimize errors and enhance diagnostic reliability.

When to go live

In the United Sates, regulatory frameworks significantly influence the timeline for launching diagnostic assays. Emergency Use Authorization (EUA) is a crucial mechanism that accelerates access to diagnostic testing during declared public health emergencies (PHEs). By allowing expedited approval based on available data, the EUA pathway enables laboratories to respond swiftly to emerging threats. However, the shortened validation timeline under EUA can introduce challenges, as tests may receive approval with limited performance data. The greatest number of tests to be submitted under EUA occurred during the SARS-CoV-2 pandemic. This greatly expanded access to testing but also allowed for the deployment of suboptimal assays and fraudulent testing practices [20]. Additionally, evolving regulatory requirements may necessitate further validation as more clinical data becomes available over the course of a PHE.

It is important to recognize that prior FDA clearance or approval of an assay does not necessarily ensure optimal performance. Emerging pathogens can undergo genetic mutations that reduce the effectiveness of previously approved tests, requiring continuous evaluation and potential modifications. This was evident during the SARS-CoV-2 pandemic when in January 2021, the FDA published a letter titled, "SARS-CoV-2 Viral Mutations: Impact on COVID-19 Tests." The letter addressed concerns about SARS-CoV-2 viral mutations and their potential effects on molecular tests. This was subsequently followed by another FDA document outlining the FDA's concerns about the impact of viral mutations and recommendations for evaluating molecular, antigen and serology in vitro diagnostic (IVD) tests accordingly. Moreover, differences in specimen types, assay platforms, and laboratory workflows can impact real-world test accuracy. Laboratories must remain proactive in monitoring assay efficacy and be prepared to make necessary adjustments to maintain reliable diagnostic results.

Following the March 31, 2025, decision in *American Clinical Laboratory Association v. FDA*, the US District Court for the Eastern District of Texas vacated the FDA's 2024 Final Rule that sought to regulate LDTs as medical devices. The court concluded that LDTs constitute professional laboratory services rather than "devices," thereby affirming that regulatory oversight remains with the Centers for Medicare & Medicaid Services (CMS) under the Clinical Laboratory Improvement Amendments of 1988 (CLIA), rather than with the FDA. The ruling nullifies FDA jurisdiction over LDTs as "medical devices," thereby exempting LDTs from premarket clearance or approval, device-quality system requirements, and EUA provisions of the FDA leaving oversight solely with CMS under CLIA. The EUA framework continues to apply only to commercially manufactured test kits, allowing clinical laboratories to independently develop and implement their own assays during PHEs. In the immediate term, this ruling restores critical flexibility for laboratories to rapidly design, validate, and deploy diagnostics thereby avoiding the delays and regulatory hurdles that would have accompanied FDA oversight. However, regulatory uncertainty persists as the FDA weighs a potential appeal and legislative efforts to clarify LDT oversight continue in Congress.

Public health laboratories (PHLs) play a critical role in the early detection and surveillance of emerging pathogens, but their ability to meet testing demands depends on factors such as testing volume, turnaround time, and the intended use of results. One of the first considerations is whether PHLs can support the necessary testing volume. While they are well-equipped for outbreak investigations and surveillance, they may not have the infrastructure for high-throughput clinical diagnostics, making it crucial to determine at what point their capacity would be overwhelmed. Widespread community transmission or policy shifts requiring routine screening can quickly exceed their surge capacity, particularly if resources such as reagents, trained personnel, and instrumentation are limited. Additionally, the urgency of test results depends on their clinical implications. If testing is used primarily for surveillance, longer turnaround times are acceptable, but if results guide clinical management, delays can have significant consequences. Another important consideration is whether the result from the PHL can be documented in the patient's medical record or if it is solely intended for epidemiologic surveillance.

Certain pathogen characteristics can further strain PHL capacity. If a virus shifts from zoonotic to human-to-human transmission, the resulting surge in cases can create an immediate demand for broader testing. Similarly, pathogens with increased pathogenicity require faster turnaround times to guide treatment and infection control measures, making reliance on PHLs alone insufficient. National policy changes, such as mandates for universal testing of hospitalized patients, can also overwhelm PHLs by significantly increasing the required testing volume. In these scenarios, early collaboration between PHLs, clinical laboratories, and regulatory agencies is essential to expand testing capacity before bottlenecks occur. By identifying key pathogen features and anticipating shifts in policy, stakeholders can ensure a timely and effective laboratory response to emerging infectious threats.

Ultimately, determining the right time to launch an assay for an emerging pathogen requires careful consideration of regulatory requirements, clinical demand, and test performance. Balancing these factors is essential to ensuring timely, effective, and reliable diagnostic solutions in rapidly evolving public health situations. For a structured overview of key preanalytical considerations, refer to Table 1.

TABLE 1
Preanalytical considerations

Category	Feature	Key considerations
Pathogen characteristics	Literature review	Which published assays are currently available in the literature? Are certain genetic regions or genes better to target? Is there a database of sequenced isolates to inform assay design? Do other pathogens have a similar clinical presentation to the intended target?
	Transmission route	How is the virus acquired and how effectively does it transmit between humans? Vector borne: is the vector present in my region? Is transmission via fomites a risk and what is the stability *ex vivo*?
	Novel vs Re-emerging pathogens	Novel pathogens require *de novo* assay development, re-emerging pathogens may be adapted from existing assays Continuous genomic surveillance ensures assays remain effective against potential antigenic shifts or mutations acquired during host adaptation
	Molecular vs Serologic Testing	Is the pathogen detectable by molecular methods while the patient is symptomatic? How long is the window for molecular detection and does serology provide enhanced detection?
Patient considerations	Test purpose	How will testing affect patient diagnosis, treatment, prognosis, or epidemiologic surveillance?
	Pooled vs ndividual testing	Will large groups of asymptomatic patients need to be screened for infection? Or is testing reserved to individuals with clear exposure risk for the disease?
	Special Populations	Will testing focus on any patient group (e.g., children, pregnant patients, immunocompromised)? Do any of these groups require alternative specimen collection methods?
Specimen collection	Specimen type	Which specimens are appropriate given pathogen tropism and infection stage? Should alternative less invasive matrices (eg, saliva or urine) be validated for enhanced testing capacity?
	Supply chain redundancy	What are the current supplier obligations to provide testing reagents? Should extraction-free methods be developed? Is there sufficient on site storage for reagents and consumables, including freezer space?
	Collection, storage, and transport	Does onsite capacity exist for media or reagent preparation? Does the pathogen risk assessment necessitate additional control measures to mitigate risk to laboratory staff and health care workers?

(*continued on next page*)

TABLE 1 (continued)

Category	Feature	Key considerations
Regulatory considerations	Emergency use authorization (EUA)	Is the pathogen associated with a currently declared PHE or has a EUA been issued for test development?
	FDA-approved assay limitations	Does the assay design fit with the laboratory's operational practices and available testing equipment? If primer and probe sequences are available, are these good matches to the currently circulating strain? Will some part of the procedure need to be modified? If so, would this then require assay validation?
	Laboratory-Developed Tests (LDTs)	Does the laboratory have the technical expertise and resources available to perform validation studies?

Analytical considerations

Target selection

Selecting the appropriate target is a fundamental step in developing an accurate and reliable diagnostic assay. The choice between detecting DNA or RNA typically depends on the nature of the pathogen and testing platform. Additionally, the decision to use one or multiple targets impacts assay sensitivity and specificity. Multiplex assays can improve detection rates and mitigate the risk of false negatives, but they also introduce challenges such as cross-reactivity and competition among targets. Another important consideration is the trade-off between highly sensitive versus highly specific targets. For example, in *Bordetella pertussis* detection, some assays utilize *IS481*, a highly sensitive target present in multiple copies, which increases the likelihood of detection but also raises the risk of cross-reactivity with *Bordetella holmesii* which contains the identical sequence at a lower copy number [21]. Conversely, single-copy gene targets (eg, the promoter region of *ptxP*) provide higher specificity but may reduce sensitivity, potentially leading to false negatives in low-burden infections [22]. It is critical that assay performance characteristics be relayed to the ordering providers such that if the clinical suspicion of a false positive or negative result is high, these concerns will be communicated back to the laboratory for investigation. Following the prior example, if a clinician reaches out about a positive *B. pertussis* result in a patient with incompatible exposure history and the laboratory observes a very late CT value for the specimen, then the sample may have been contaminated by nucleic acid at the collection site. This has been observed when vaccination for *B. pertussis* and testing occurred in the same room [23].

When designing a test, laboratories must consider whether to follow existing protocols (eg, from the CDC) or develop an in-house assay tailored to specific needs. CDC-endorsed targets often provide a standardized approach for pathogen detection; however, they may not always reflect regional variation in circulating strains. In addition, implementation of FDA-cleared CDC assays can be challenging for clinical laboratories due to requirements for specific instrumentation that may not be widely available or supported. Many of these assays were developed with manual workflows such as separate extraction and plating steps, and utilize single target wells, requiring multiple reactions per sample to detect all necessary analytes. This design increases labor and resource burden, which can be prohibitive for high throughput clinical environments. Automation is essential in modern clinical laboratories to ensure efficiency, consistency, and scalability. As such, future assay development and regulatory frameworks should consider broader definitions of substantial equivalence, accounting for variations in extraction platforms and real-time PCR instrumentation, to better align with the operational realities of diverse laboratory settings. In contrast to existing protocols, in-house development allows for greater flexibility and responsiveness to local epidemiology but carries the added need for validation.

Poor target selection has led to significant diagnostic challenges in past outbreaks. For example, the loss of the mpox clade I target in the newly emerging clade Ib strain led to false negative results when orthopoxvirus subtyping was performed [24]. Similarly, some existing influenza A(H5) assays are not optimized for the 2.3.4.4b clade, resulting in decreased sensitivity [3]. Oropouche virus testing presents another challenge, as the most sensitive target, the S gene, is shared by 2 other orthobunyaviruses, leading to potential misidentifications [25]. Outdated dengue virus targets have also struggled to differentiate between serotypes, highlighting the need for continuous reassessment of assay designs [26].

Lastly, the target selection must also align with the technology and testing platform used, as different platforms, such as real-time PCR, digital PCR, and next-generation sequencing, have varying requirements for primer and probe design, sensitivity thresholds, and throughput capabilities. The selected target must be compatible with the assay format to ensure optimal performance and reproducibility.

Platform selection

Selecting an appropriate testing platform and extraction method is crucial for optimizing molecular assay performance, efficiency, and scalability. The extraction method directly impacts assay sensitivity, turnaround time, and overall workflow efficiency. Automated extraction systems are favored in high-throughput environments due to their ability to enhance reproducibility and reduce labor costs. However, manual extraction may still be necessary in resource-limited settings or when working with specific sample matrices that require specialized handling. In some cases, manual extraction can also improve assay performance and nucleic acid yield [27].

When evaluating for testing throughput, traditional real-time PCR instruments require separate nucleic acid extraction, which can be labor-intensive and increase the risk of contamination and pipetting errors. While these systems offer high analytical sensitivity and flexibility, they may not be ideal for large-scale testing during outbreaks. During the SARS-CoV-2 pandemic, for example, the testing capacity of a 96-well RT-PCR instrument varied depending on the assay and workflow, with laboratories processing anywhere from 96 to 372 samples within an 8-hour shift [28].

To improve efficiency, laboratories could transition to automated platforms with open-channel access, including but not limited to those offered by Hologic (Panther Fusion), BD (BD MAX), Abbott (AlinityM), and Roche (cobas 58/68/8800 platforms). These systems streamline workflow by integrating extraction, amplification, and reporting steps thereby reducing the risk of contamination and improving time to result. However, differences in chemistry between platforms must be considered. For example, Hologic's chemistry is similar to traditional real-time PCR, while Roche platforms require O-methyl group modifications to probes, impacting assay design and reagent compatibility [29]. Another key consideration when transitioning to an automated platform is the minimum specimen volume required for testing. This requirement varies by manufacturer and instrument, and platforms that demand larger sample volumes may leave insufficient remaining specimen for repeat testing or confirmatory testing at PHLs. In addition, differences in extraction volume and the amount of eluate used for amplification can significantly impact assay sensitivity and overall performance, necessitating careful evaluation prior to clinical implementation [30].

A comparison of available open channel diagnostic platforms reveals distinct performance characteristics suited to different testing demands. The Hologic Panther Fusion with Aptima system can process up to 500 samples in an 8-hour shift (around 10,000 per week), making it ideal for mid-to-high throughput laboratory settings. In contrast, the Roche Cobas 8800 system can process up to 1056 samples in an 8-hour shift thus enabling a weekly throughput exceeding 22,000 samples. These high-throughput capabilities position automation as essential tools for large-scale diagnostic efforts, particularly in PHEs where rapid and widespread testing is required. Knowing the anticipated testing volume may also help laboratories select the most appropriate instrument for open channel development. Examples of open channel assay design for emerging infections include mpox, influenza, and SARS-CoV-2 [29,31,32].

Repurposing an existing FDA-cleared or approved test can be an effective strategy for rapid deployment. For instance, point-of-care or rapid influenza assays could be adapted for conjunctival swab testing to investigate cases of influenza A(H5) conjunctivitis, reducing reliance on more resource-intensive methods. However, because the intended specimen type was modified, a validation study must be completed prior to clinical testing.

Internal controls

The inclusion of internal controls in molecular assays is essential for ensuring the accuracy and reliability of test results. Internal controls help detect assay failures, monitor sample quality, and variation in reagent lots. Laboratories must decide between endogenous and exogenous controls, each with distinct advantages and potential limitations.

Endogenous controls derived from the patient sample (eg, RNAseP, ß-actin) can serve as built-in quality checks to confirm proper specimen collection and nucleic acid integrity [33]. However, their use may lead to an increased number of indeterminate or repeat results due to poor specimen collection practices. For example, in populations that are more challenging to sample such as children, there may be insufficient detection of the host target requiring repeat testing or recollection. In low prevalence settings, such as mpox testing in children, an endogenous control may lead to greater testing expense with minimal impact on case detection [34]. Furthermore, a recent research study suggested that while endogenous controls are commonly used as quality control measures, they may not always accurately reflect the true quality of specimen collection [35].

Exogenous controls, on the other hand, are artificially introduced into the sample after collection. As these controls can be added at any step during the process, they provide a more standardized quality assessment and can help identify issues related to extraction, amplification, or reagent performance. For instance, stool samples, which contain high levels of inhibitors, can benefit from exogenous internal controls to ensure accurate pathogen detection. Examples of exogenous controls include MS2 bacteriophage RNA, phocine herpesvirus 1 DNA/RNA, and equine arteritis virus RNA, among others [36]. However, the inclusion of exogenous material increases test complexity and may require additional optimization to prevent interference with target detection.

Understanding the trade-offs between endogenous and exogenous controls, as well as optimizing control selection based on sample type, is critical for improving diagnostic accuracy and minimizing repeat testing burdens in clinical laboratory and PHL.

Validation for an emerging virus

Validating diagnostic assays for emerging viruses requires a structured approach that balances regulatory guidance with the practical challenges posed by limited reference materials. Lessons learned from COVID-19 provide a valuable framework for evaluating accuracy, analytical specificity, limit of detection, and reproducibility to ensure robust assay performance in real-world settings.

One of the primary challenges in assay validation is acquiring positive control material. This may be due to the relative paucity of clinical samples or due to strict handling requirements necessitating a select agent license or BSL-3 containment. For example, during the early stages of COVID-19 pandemic, the FDA recommended 25 positive SARS-CoV-2 samples be used for accuracy studies despite only 14 cases identified nationally [37]. In such cases, alternatives material, such as synthetic ssDNA, Armored RNA, and gBlocks, serve as viable surrogates for live virus testing. In addition, laboratories can source control materials from public repositories including BEI resources, IRR, and veterinary diagnostic laboratories, which play a crucial role in supporting assay validation efforts. The use of inactivated pathogens allows laboratories to perform validation studies using material without the prerequisite of a select agent license or BSL-3 handling practices. A comparison of commonly used positive control materials can be found in Table 2.

Bridging studies are another key component of validation, particularly when adapting an existing test to detect a novel strain or variant. These studies evaluate whether modifications to primers, probes, or reaction conditions impact the test's sensitivity and specificity. Ensuring that an assay maintains its analytical performance across different strains is critical for maintaining diagnostic reliability. These considerations are of greatest importance when an assay originally granted EUA is transitioned to an FDA-cleared or approved IVD. Laboratories must ensure that their validation or verification studies are thorough and complete at this stage [17].

For molecular assays, establishing appropriate Ct cutoffs is critical for ensuring accurate result interpretation. For emerging pathogens, adjustments to Ct cutoffs must be guided by clinical relevance and epidemiologic data to minimize false positives and negatives. For example, during the COVID-19 pandemic, there was significant debate over what constituted a meaningful Ct value for clinical decision-making [2,38]. While a lower Ct value generally correlated with higher viral loads and potential infectivity, high Ct values (eg, above 35) raised questions about whether the detected viral RNA represented active infection or residual nonviable genetic material. Late Ct values may also indicate potential cross-contamination from high-titer specimens processed simultaneously. This issue became particularly evident with assays detecting mpox virus, which is known to present with high viral loads in clinical samples. Specimens with very low Ct values posed a risk of contaminating adjacent wells, leading to false-positive results for nearby samples. Due to this concern, the CDC issued guidance recommending retesting for samples with Ct values ≥ 34 [39]. Subsequent studies demonstrated that adopting a more conservative approach by lowering the Ct threshold for repeat testing helped reduce false positives, particularly in high-consequence cases such as pediatric samples [40].

Issues surrounding SARS-CoV-2 and mpox virus testing underscored the need to interpret Ct values in

TABLE 2
Different types of positive control materials: pros and cons

Control type	Description	Pros	Cons
Live virus	Cultured virus used as a positive control	Most representative of actual infection; allows full workflow validation	May require BSL-3 containment or select agent license; biohazard risk; limited capacity for viral culture in most laboratories
Inactivated virus	Chemically or heat-inactivated virus	Safer alternative to live virus; maintains viral structure for assay validation	May not fully mimic live virus nucleic acid integrity; requires careful inactivation validation
Synthetic RNA/DNA	Artificially synthesized viral nucleic acid	Highly specific; easily customizable; noninfectious	Lacks full virion complexity; does not assess sample extraction efficiency; limited stability
Armored® RNA/DNA	RNA/DNA encapsulated in a protective shell	Protects against degradation; mimics true virus structure; stable across conditions; can customize genetic sequence	More expensive than standard synthetic controls; requires specialized production
Plasmid controls	Recombinant plasmids carrying target sequences	Stable and easy to produce in large quantities; cost-effective	Lacks true viral structure; may not mimic RNA viruses well, requires technical knowledge of plasmid design; potential for cross-contamination
Whole genome controls	Full-length viral genome (synthetic or extracted)	Enables full assay validation, including sequencing applications	Expensive; requires specialized synthesis and handling
Cell-based controls	Cell line which stably expresses pathogen DNA/RNA	Closely mimics clinical samples; ensures integrity of extraction and amplification processes	Requires cell culture expertise; biohazard risks; potential for genetic drift over time

the context of clinical symptoms, timing of infection, and epidemiologic factors rather than relying solely on numerical thresholds. Similar considerations must be made when designing assays for newly identified pathogens, as overly stringent Ct thresholds may lead to underreporting, while overly lenient cutoffs can increase false-positive rates. Optimizing Ct values based on pathogen kinetics, specimen type, and assay performance is crucial for ensuring diagnostic reliability and clinical utility. Table 3 offers a comprehensive summary of key analytical considerations.

Postanalytical considerations

Developing a rational report

Effective reporting of diagnostic results is critical for ensuring accurate clinical interpretation and public

TABLE 3
Analytical considerations

Category	Features	Key considerations
Target selection	DNA vs RNA	What is the composition of the virus and its replication cycle? Does the replication process involve DNA intermediates that could be targeted, or is detection limited to RNA-based approaches? Detection of RNA transcripts may be used to indicate pathogen is actively replicating Genomic DNA or RNA may be detected after a patient is no longer infectious
	Multiplexing vs Single target	Would multiplexing different pathogens provide a more robust solution (eg, co-testing for HSV and mpox)? Given the genomic instability of RNA viruses, does the pathogen require multiple targets? Should additional targets for clade or strain-level identification be included?
	Published design vs In-house development	If using a published assay, is there any new data or novel pathogen mutations that may affect assay performance? Should existing primer or probes be modified to create shorter amplicons or include mixed bases to improve assay robustness?
Platform selection	Manual vs Automated systems	What is the anticipated testing volume for an assay? Are there clinical scenarios in which testing volumes may spike on short notice? If using an FDA-cleared assay, how long are the test reagents stable? Is there anticipated reagent waste?
	Open-channel access (LDT)	How familiar is my laboratory with development of open channel assays? Are analyte-specific reagents available and compatible with the instrument? Have other groups published on open channel assays for this pathogen or closely related pathogens?
	Extraction platforms	Are the sample matrices suitable for automated extraction? Are the samples viscous, nonhomogenous, or cause a high rate of instrument errors? Are pretreatment, lysis, or homogenization steps available to improve automated specimen handling?
Internal controls	Endogenous vs Exogenous	Endogenous controls verify sample integrity but may increase repeat testing in low-prevalence settings. Exogenous controls, introduced before processing, help monitor assay performance and extraction efficiency but require careful design to prevent interference with target detection
	Sample-specific considerations	Is the matrix tested known for a high presence of inhibitors (eg, stool)? Are processes in place to monitor for suboptimal collection practices (eg, monitoring Ct values of endogenous positive control)?
Validation for emerging viruses	Positive control materials	Select agents/BSL-3 restrictions may necessitate synthetic alternatives like ssDNA, Armored® RNA, and gBlocks

(*continued on next page*)

TABLE 3
(continued)

Category	Features	Key considerations
		Are control materials available through commercial vendors or repositories? (eg, BEI resources, IRR, veterinary diagnostic laboratories)
	Bridging studies	Required when modifying assays for new variants What is the assay performance over time? Have mutations emerged since initial development that requires modifications to the assay? Have clinical syndromes shifted such that new sample types are clinically relevant?
	Ct threshold determination	What is an appropriate Ct value threshold for detection? What is the typical Ct value for a clinical sample? For infections with high burden and low Ct values, are extra quality control steps needed to monitor for contamination? Is a repeat algorithm needed for specimens with late Ct values?

health decision-making. The structure of a report should clearly convey results while minimizing ambiguity or misinterpretation. One of the fundamental considerations in postanalytical reporting is the distinction between "Detected" and "Positive" results. "Detected" indicates that the target nucleic acid was identified in the specimen but does not necessarily confirm active infection or clinical disease. "Positive" is often interpreted as clinically significant and may imply active infection requiring medical intervention. Laboratories should use precise language to ensure that clinicians understand the implications of each term, particularly for pathogens with prolonged shedding or intermittent detection.

In cases where an assay detects multiple related targets, such as influenza A and influenza A(H5), reports must be structured to clearly differentiate between broad classifications and specific subtypes. For example, detecting influenza A may indicate a common seasonal strain, whereas detecting influenza A(H5) suggests a more concerning avian influenza variant. To prevent confusion, reports should include interpretative comments explaining the significance of each detected target and its potential clinical and public health implications. For assays detecting high-consequence pathogens, a process for immediate provider notification of critical results should be implemented to ensure results are not lost to follow-up [41]. Policies and procedures should also be established to ensure timely reporting to public health agencies based on state or local guidelines.

Diagnostic reports are interpreted by a diverse group of health care providers and public health officials. Key stakeholders include infectious disease (ID) teams, general physicians, hospital epidemiologists, and public health authorities. The laboratory director should create a report that is interpretable by all end users while accounting for the needs of individual groups. General physicians often rely on summary interpretations and clinical guidance within the report. In contrast, health care providers well-versed in management of infectious conditions may ask for more granular genotypic data or Ct values to aid in patient management. Hospital epidemiologists and infection prevention teams utilize reports for outbreak monitoring and hospital infection control measures, while public health authorities may require reporting of specific pathogens to track disease incidence, particularly for emerging infections and reportable diseases.

Understanding the needs of these various stakeholders ensures that reports provide the necessary information tailored to each audience while maintaining clarity and clinical relevance. A standardized reporting format, along with appropriate interpretative comments, can improve communication and enhance the utility of diagnostic testing in patient care and public health interventions.

Sharing "extra" data

Beyond standard reporting, laboratory results often contain additional metadata that can provide deeper insights into the disease state. A crucial aspect of postanalytical data sharing is determining whom this data should be shared with and why. For example, Ct values must be carefully interpreted, as differences in assay platforms, sample types, and collection timing can influence results [42]. Laboratories should ensure a policy for sharing nonchartable information exists. This may take the form of educating laboratory staff to direct physician questions to the director. More robust options include building test information dashboards with restricted access or involving a laboratory utilization committee for policy making [43].

Early during an outbreak, the range of clinical presentations for a particular pathogen may be poorly defined. As such, providers may request testing of nonvalidated specimen types out of curiosity or nascent research interests. For example, in mpox diagnosis, there has been interest in testing nonlesional sites to detect subclinical infections. Studies have identified mpox infections in individuals without visible lesions, prompting discussions about expanding screening efforts [44]. However, the current EUA for mpox diagnostic assay development is only indicated for lesions specimens. Understanding the full spectrum of disease is crucial for defining appropriate testing indications and selecting suitable sample types. While testing nonlesional sites could improve disease surveillance and provide insights into transmission dynamics, it also introduces challenges in result interpretation and regulatory compliance. Laboratories must clearly communicate these limitations when reporting results from specimen types that have not been validated for diagnostic use.

Working with public health and other stakeholders

Collaboration between clinical laboratories, public health agencies, and administrative stakeholders is essential for optimizing the response to emerging pathogens. In the public health setting, one of the key aspects of this collaboration is sharing specimens [45]. Setting up a structured framework for specimen sharing is essential for effective public health monitoring. This framework should define clear guidelines on specimen selection, storage, transport, and data sharing while ensuring compliance with regulatory standards. While these policies are critical during the emergence of a novel pathogen, such policies can be instituted prior to an outbreak. For example, if a laboratory were to establish a policy sharing a subset of influenza A positive samples with their state or local public health laboratory as part of routine seasonal surveillance, this policy could be leveraged or expanded during the emergence of a novel influenza A virus.

Another critical element is communicating laboratory needs to hospital administrators, particularly during PHEs. Laboratories must proactively engage with hospital leadership, supply chain managers, and funding bodies to secure necessary reagents, staffing, and infrastructure. Determining when to engage with administrative stakeholders should begin early and may follow a Health Alert Network message from the CDC, relevant notification by state or local public health agency, or when monitoring positivity rates at the hospital level. Early engagement should focus on summarizing the pathogen risk and determining which trigger events (eg, positivity rates, documented community spread, and availability of commercial assays) may cause a laboratory to bring testing on site.

Additionally, laboratories play a vital role in stewarding testing resources during high-demand or low-incidence settings. During surges in testing demand, prioritizing specimens based on clinical urgency and public health impact can help maximize laboratory efficiency [46]. The COVID-19 pandemic highlighted the importance of triaging specimens based on clinical urgency, such as prioritizing hospitalized patients, high-risk individuals, and health care workers [47]. Implementing tiered testing protocols ensures that the most urgent cases receive timely results while maintaining overall laboratory efficiency. Conversely, in periods of low incidence, maintaining assay performance and ensuring continued surveillance require strategic planning to prevent supply shortages and testing gaps. Laboratories should collaborate with public health agencies to align testing strategies with epidemiologic trends, ensuring that resources are allocated effectively to support both patient care and broader disease control efforts.

Dealing with testing surges

Managing sudden increases in testing demand requires strategic planning to ensure timely and accurate diagnostics. One effective approach in low-incidence settings is pooled testing, which allows laboratories to conserve resources by combining multiple specimens into a single test. This method is particularly useful for surveillance and screening programs where the expected positivity rate is low. If a pooled sample tests negative, all individual specimens are considered negative, reducing reagent usage and workload. However, when a pooled sample tests positive, individual testing must be performed, which may introduce delays [48].

In the event of an outbreak involving a reemerging pathogen such as measles virus, laboratories must be prepared to rapidly scale up testing. Ensuring an

TABLE 4
Postanalytical considerations

Category	Features	Key considerations
Developing a rational report	Detected vs Positive	How should results be reported to health care providers? "Detected" often indicates that the target nucleic acid was identified in the specimen but does not confirm active infection or clinical disease "Positive" is often interpreted as clinically significant or may imply active infection
	Reporting related targets	Ensure clarity by differentiating broad classifications (eg, influenza A) from specific subtypes (eg, H5) to prevent ambiguous reporting and misinterpretation Will the director or appropriately trained individual be available to assist with interpreting reports?
	Key stakeholders	Who will be interpreting these reports? Are additional comments necessary to assist in results interpretation? If the assay will be shared with public health or epidemiologists, have they been included in reporting discussions? ID teams, general physicians, epidemiologists, and public health authorities can provide subject matter expertise and identify critical data fields for reports to contain
Sharing "extra" data	Ct values	Interpretation depends on assay platform, sample type, and infection stage. Will the audience understand the nuance for reporting? Who should this be shared with and under what circumstances?
	Nonvalidated specimen testing	What literature is available to suggest that the requested testing is appropriate? What is the volume of these requests? Does a new specimen validation need to be performed? If testing is performed on nonvalidated specimens, how will this affect interpretation of results? How will results be communicated on nonvalidated specimens for organisms that are reportable to public health officials? Is this testing being performed as part of a research study or being used for clinical diagnosis?
Working with public health and stakeholders	Sample Sharing Framework	Can standardized guidelines for specimen selection, storage, transport, and data sharing be instituted prior to an outbreak?

(*continued on next page*)

TABLE 4
(continued)

Category	Features	Key considerations
	Communicating with administrators	Are there Health Alert Network messages and/or communications from state or local public health agencies that could be used to request additional resources? Have administrators been involved in discussions as to what events may trigger a change in testing? Are administrators aware of current staffing and laboratory capacity?
	Resource stewardship	Will there be stewardship of the assay? Will other stakeholders help with laboratory stewardship?
Dealing with testing surges	Pooled testing	Has the assay been validated on pooled specimen sources? Does pooled testing make sense based on positivity rate? How will pooled testing affect turnaround time?
	Outbreak response	Can a greater volume of reagents be ordered for pathogens that may have volume surges? If supplies are unavailable, can extended stability studies be performed to utilize reagents that may be past the manufacturer's expiration date? Are backup sources available in case of reagent shortage? What is the validation plan for the backup reagent?
	Specimen triage	Are plans in place for laboratory testing during surges in testing demand? Does there need to be prioritization of specimens based on patient population or clinical scenarios? Are stakeholders in agreement of specimen triage plans?

adequate stock of reagents is critical, and laboratories should work closely with manufacturers to anticipate demand surges. Early communication with suppliers allows for proactive adjustments in production and distribution, preventing shortages. Identifying backup reagent sources and alternate supply chains can further safeguard against disruptions. Laboratories may consider keeping a greater amount of reagents on hand (eg, keeping 6 months vs 3 months) for pathogens with the potential for volume surges and performing extended reagent stability studies past the manufacturer's expiration date.

By adopting proactive strategies such as pooled testing, securing reagent supply chains, and prioritizing specimen processing, laboratories can enhance their resilience and responsiveness during testing surges. These measures help ensure continuity of diagnostic services while optimizing resource utilization in both routine and emergency settings. Refer to Table 4 for a structured overview of key postanalytical considerations.

SUMMARY

Unfortunately, no one-size-fits-all approach exists for responding to emerging pathogens. However, by taking a stepwise approach to evaluate the preanalytical, analytical, and postanalytical considerations unique to each pathogen, laboratories can develop an evidence-based response plan. Laboratories must balance regulatory requirements, assay design, validation, and public health collaboration to ensure timely and effective diagnostic solutions. From specimen collection to report generation and data sharing, every stage of the diagnostic pipeline plays a crucial role in outbreak response and disease surveillance.

Key insights from previous sections underscore the need for adaptable assay development to address emerging and evolving pathogens, strategic resource planning to mitigate supply chain disruptions and testing surges, and strong collaboration with public health agencies to facilitate disease surveillance and response. Additionally, standardized and transparent reporting practices are essential to ensure accurate clinical interpretation and effective epidemiologic tracking. As laboratory medicine continues to advance, the capacity to swiftly develop, validate, and deploy diagnostic assays remains critical for identifying and controlling infectious threats.

The emergence of infectious pathogens poses increasingly complex challenges to public health on a worldwide scale. Viruses such as Nipah, Oropouche, and Hendra continue to raise concerns due to their potential for zoonotic transmission and outbreak unpredictability. Recent cases of Nipah virus in South Asia, Oropouche virus outbreaks in South America, and Hendra virus spillover events in Australia highlight the urgent need for improved diagnostic capabilities [49–51]. Rapid detection, molecular subtyping, and surveillance strategies are essential for monitoring viral evolution, assessing interspecies transmission risks, and mitigating potential public health threats.

Several previously controlled or declining diseases have experienced a resurgence, necessitating heightened surveillance and improved diagnostic strategies. Measles outbreaks continue to occur due to declining immunization rates in some regions, making early detection through molecular and serologic assays critical for containment efforts [52]. *B. pertussis*, responsible for pertussis, has seen increasing cases in recent years, partly due to waning immunity and bacterial adaptations [53]. Enhanced PCR-based detection methods can support timely diagnosis and outbreak management. The detection of vaccine-derived polioviruses in wastewater from New York City in 2022 further highlights the need for continued diagnostic capacity even for pathogens believed to be eradicated [54].

Preparing for the next major epidemic or pandemic threat requires an engaged laboratory director. During the announcement of a new or re-emerging threat, reviewing the questions in Tables 1, 3, and 4 can help assess the laboratory's preparedness and response capabilities. If gaps are identified, steps should be taken to determine how best to proactively address them. If appropriately prepared, timely deployment of testing resources can significantly reduce patient morbidity and mortality.

CLINICS CARE POINTS

- There are limited resources available for diagnosing emerging infections at the point of care.
- Assays developed in response to an emerging pathogen for point of care devices may be labeled as moderate or high-complexity. In this situation the assay must be performed in the appropriate laboratory and not at the point of care.
- Testing of non-approved sources on an FDA-cleared or approved device requires validation studies.

DISCLOSURE

The authors have nothing to disclose.

REFERENCES

[1] Rabe IB, Staples JE, Villanueva J, et al. Interim guidance for interpretation of zika virus antibody test results. MMWR Morb Mortal Wkly Rep 2016;65:543–6.

[2] Binnicker MJ. Challenges and controversies to testing for COVID-19. J Clin Microbiol 2020;58. https://doi.org/10.1128/jcm.01695-01620.

[3] Pinsky BA, Bradley BT. Opportunities and challenges for the U.S. laboratory response to highly pathogenic avian influenza A(H5N1). J Clin Virol 2024;174:105723.

[4] Paz-Bailey G, Rosenberg ES, Doyle K, et al. Persistence of zika virus in body fluids - final report. N Engl J Med 2018;379:1234–43.

[5] Hunsperger EA, Muñoz-Jordn J, Beltran M, et al. Performance of dengue diagnostic tests in a single-specimen diagnostic algorithm. J Infect Dis 2016;214:836–44.

[6] Sharp TM, Fischer M, Muñoz-Jordn JL, et al. Dengue and zika virus diagnostic testing for patients with a clinically compatible illness and risk for infection with both viruses. Morb Mortal Wkly Rep, Recomm Rep 2019;68:1–10.

[7] Guo L, Wang D, Zhou H, et al. Cross-reactivity between avian influenza A (H7N9) virus and divergent H7 subtypic- and heterosubtypic influenza A viruses. Sci Rep 2016;6:22045.

[8] Zhang J, Feng Y, Hu D, et al. Rapid and sensitive detection of H7N9 avian influenza virus by use of reverse transcription-loop-mediated isothermal amplification. J Clin Microbiol 2013;51:3760–4.

[9] Sparrer MN, Hodges NF, Sherman T, et al. Role of spillover and spillback in SARS-CoV-2 transmission and the importance of one health in understanding the dynamics of the COVID-19 pandemic. J Clin Microbiol 2023;61:e0161022.

[10] Truong TT, Ryutov A, Pandey U, et al. Increased viral variants in children and young adults with impaired humoral immunity and persistent SARS-CoV-2 infection: a consecutive case series. EBioMedicine 2021;67: 103355.

[11] Jernigan DB, Lindstrom SL, Johnson JR, et al. Detecting 2009 pandemic influenza A (H1N1) virus infection: availability of diagnostic testing led to rapid pandemic response. Clin Infect Dis 2011;52:S36–43.

[12] Abdalhamid B, Bilder CR, McCutchen EL, et al. Assessment of specimen pooling to conserve SARS CoV-2 testing resources. Am J Clin Pathol 2020;153:715–8.

[13] Mercado M, Ailes EC, Daza M, et al. Zika virus detection in amniotic fluid and Zika-associated birth defects. Am J Obstet Gynecol 2020;222:610.e611–3.

[14] Miller JM, Binnicker MJ, Campbell S, et al. Guide to utilization of the microbiology laboratory for diagnosis of infectious diseases: 2024 update by the infectious diseases society of America (IDSA) and the American society for microbiology (ASM. Clin Infect Dis 2024. https://doi.org/10.1093/cid/ciae104.

[15] Limaye N, Ninesling B, Marcelin F, et al. COVID-19 pandemic response in a migrant farmworker community: excess mortality, testing access and contact tracing in immokalee, Florida. Ann Glob Health 2022;88:77.

[16] Garg S, Reed C, Davis CT, et al. Outbreak of highly pathogenic avian influenza A(H5N1) viruses in U.S. Dairy cattle and detection of two human cases - United States, 2024. MMWR Morb Mortal Wkly Rep 2024;73:501–5.

[17] Peaper DR, Rhoads DD, Sullivan KV, et al. Considerations from the college of American pathologists for implementation of an assay for SARS-CoV-2 testing after a change in regulatory status. J Clin Microbiol 2021;59: e0116721.

[18] Smith KP, Cheng A, Chopelas A, et al. Large-scale, inhouse production of viral transport media to support SARS-CoV-2 PCR testing in a multihospital health care Network during the COVID-19 pandemic. J Clin Microbiol 2020;58.

[19] Jayaprakasam M, Aggarwal S, Mane A, et al. RNA-extraction-free diagnostic method to detect SARS-CoV-2: an assessment from two states, India. Epidemiol Infect 2021;149.

[20] Zuckerman DM. Emergency use authorizations (EUAs) versus FDA approval: implications for COVID-19 and public health. Am J Public Health 2021;111:1065–9.

[21] Reischl U, Lehn N, Sanden GN, et al. Real-time PCR assay targeting IS481 of Bordetella pertussis and molecular basis for detecting Bordetella holmesii. J Clin Microbiol 2001;39:1963–6.

[22] Tatti KM, Wu KH, Sanden GN, et al. Molecular diagnosis of Bordetella pertussis infection by evaluation of formalin-fixed tissue specimens. J Clin Microbiol 2006;44:1074–6.

[23] Salimnia H, Lephart PR, Asmar BI, et al. Aerosolized vaccine as an unexpected source of false-positive Bordetella pertussis PCR results. J Clin Microbiol 2012;50:472–4.

[24] Srivastava S, Laxmi SK, Sridhar SB, et al. Clade Ib: a new emerging threat in the Mpox outbreak. Front Pharmacol 2024;15:1504154.

[25] Lambert AJ, Lanciotti RS. Consensus amplification and novel multiplex sequencing method for S segment species identification of 47 viruses of the *Orthobunyavirus*, *Phlebovirus*, and *Nairovirus* Genera of the family *Bunyaviridae*. J Clin Microbiol 2009;47:2398–404.

[26] Sekaran SD, Soe HJ. Issues in contemporary and potential future molecular diagnostics for dengue. Expert Rev Mol Diagn 2017;17:217–23.

[27] Knepp JH, Geahr MA, Forman MS, et al. Comparison of automated and manual nucleic acid extraction methods for detection of enterovirus RNA. J Clin Microbiol 2003; 41:3532–6.

[28] Mannonen L, Kallio-Kokko H, Loginov R, et al. Comparison of two commercial platforms and a laboratory-developed test for detection of severe acute respiratory syndrome coronavirus 2 (SARS-CoV-2) RNA. J Mol Diagn 2021;23:407–16.

[29] Nïrz D, Hoffmann A, Aepfelbacher M, et al. Clinical evaluation of a fully automated, laboratory-developed multiplex RT-PCR assay integrating dual-target SARS-CoV-2 and influenza A/B detection on a high-throughput platform. J Med Microbiol 2021;70.

[30] Kogoj R, Kmetĭ P, Oštrbenk Valeňak A, et al. Real-life head-to-head comparison of performance of two high-throughput automated assays for the detection of SARS-CoV-2 RNA in nasopharyngeal swabs: the alinity m and cobas 6800 SARS-CoV-2 assays. J Mol Diagn 2021;23:920–8.

[31] Nïrz D, Tang HT, Emmerich P, et al. Rapid adaptation of established high-throughput molecular testing infrastructure for monkeypox virus detection. Emerg Infect Dis 2022;28:1765–9.

[32] Villa RD, Pentella MA, Benfer JL. A laboratory-developed assay for clade II human mpox virus on the panther fusion open access system. J Infect Dis 2023;229: S132–6.

[33] Mostafa HH. Importance of internal controls to monitor adequate specimen collection: the case of orthopoxvirus real-time PCR. J Clin Virol 2022;156:105294.

[34] Ma A, Bradley BT. Clinical testing of pediatric mpox specimens: unique features and challenges in a low prevalence population. J Clin Virol 2023;163:105447.

[35] Crawford KHD, Baniecki ML, Dushin EG, et al. Specimen adequacy assay controls in nucleic acid amplification tests do not correlate with nasopharyngeal swab collection method. J Clin Microbiol 2024;62:e0097524.

[36] Okuyama T, Ohtsuka K, Ogura W, et al. Establishing an internal quality control method for the stable extraction of nucleic acids of severe acute respiratory syndrome

coronavirus 2 and RT-PCR-based detection. J Clin Lab Anal 2021;35:e23998.

[37] Greninger AL, Jerome KR. The first quarter of SARS-CoV-2 testing: the university of Washington medicine experience. J Clin Microbiol 2020;58.

[38] Christensen BB, Azar MM, Turbett SE. Laboratory diagnosis for SARS-CoV-2 infection. Infect Dis Clin North Am 2022;36:327–47.

[39] Prevention CfDCa. Lab Advisory: monkeypox virus testing considerations to prevent false positive test results, on CDC's Laboratory Outreach Communication System. 2022. Available at: https://www.cdc.gov/locs/2022/08-23-2022-Lab-Advisory-Monkeypox_Virus_Testing_Considerations_Prevent_False_Positive_Test_Results.html.

[40] Shean RC, Hymas WC, Klein J, et al. Repeat testing of mpox specimens with late CTs improves detection of potential false positive cases. J Clin Microbiol 2024;62: e01223–75.

[41] Genzen JR, Tormey CA, Education Committee of the Academy of Clinical Laboratory Physicians and Scientists. Pathology consultation on reporting of critical values. Am J Clin Pathol 2011;135:505–13.

[42] Rhoads D, Peaper DR, She RC, et al. College of American pathologists (CAP) microbiology committee perspective: caution must Be used in interpreting the cycle threshold (Ct) value. Clin Infect Dis 2020;72: e685–6.

[43] White TE, Wong WB, Janowiak D, et al. Strategies for laboratory professionals to drive laboratory stewardship. Pract Lab Med 2021;26:e00249.

[44] Edouard S, Boschi C, Colson P, et al. Incidental diagnosis of mpox virus infection in patients undergoing sexually transmitted infection screening—findings from a study in France. Int J Infect Dis 2024;143: 107009.

[45] Marinissen MJ, Chandrasekera R, Simpson J, et al. Sharing of biological samples during public health emergencies: challenges and opportunities for national and International action, p 155-173. In: Halabi SF, Katz R, editors. Viral sovereignty and technology transfer: the changing global system for sharing pathogens for public health research. Cambridge: Cambridge University Press; 2020. https://doi.org/10.1017/9781108676076.011.

[46] World Health O. Laboratory testing strategy recommendations for COVID-19: interim guidance, 21 March 2020. Geneva: World Health Organization; 2020.

[47] Peaper DR, Doern CD, Sharp S, et al. Proceedings of the Clinical Microbiology Open 2022—assessing clinical laboratory and industry responses to COVID-19 pandemic testing capacity challenges (part 1). J Clin Microbiol 2024;62:e00923–41.

[48] Grobe N, Cherif A, Wang X, et al. Sample pooling: burden or solution? Clin Microbiol Infection 2021;27: 1212–20.

[49] Khan S, Akbar SMF, Mahtab MA, et al. Twenty-five years of Nipah outbreaks in Southeast Asia: a persistent threat to global health. IJID Reg 2024;13:100434.

[50] Guagliardo SAJ, Connelly CR, Lyons S, et al. Reemergence of Oropouche virus in the Americas and risk for spread in the United States and its territories, 2024. Emerg Infect Dis 2024;30:2241–9.

[51] Eby P, Peel AJ, Hoegh A, et al. Pathogen spillover driven by rapid changes in bat ecology. Nature 2023;613: 340–4.

[52] Harris E. Measles outbreaks grow amid declining vaccination rates. JAMA 2023;330:2242.

[53] Mooi FR, Van Der Maas NA, De Melker HE. Pertussis resurgence: waning immunity and pathogen adaptation - two sides of the same coin. Epidemiol Infect 2014;142: 685–94.

[54] Ryerson AB, Lang D, Alazawi MA, et al, 2022 U.S. Poliovirus Response Team. Wastewater testing and detection of poliovirus type 2 genetically linked to virus isolated from a paralytic polio case - New York, March 9-October 11, 2022. MMWR Morb Mortal Wkly Rep 2022;71: 1418–24.

Advances in Molecular Pathology 8 (2025) 131–144
ADVANCES IN MOLECULAR PATHOLOGY

Current State of Metagenomics for Infectious Diseases Diagnosis

Limitations and Future Directions

LingHui David Su, BSc[a], Patrick Benoit, MD, FRCPC[b], Evann E. Hilt, M(ASCP)[CM], PhD, D(ABMM)[c,d], Catherine A. Hogan, MD, MSc, FRCPC[a,e,*]

[a]Public Health Laboratory, BC Centre for Disease Control, Vancouver, British Columbia, Canada; [b]Department of Laboratory Medicine, University of California, San Francisco, San Francisco, CA, USA; [c]Department of Laboratory Medicine and Pathology, University of Minnesota, Minneapolis, MN, USA; [d]Infectious Diseases Diagnostic Laboratory, M Health Fairview, Minneapolis, MN, USA; [e]Department of Pathology and Laboratory Medicine, University of British Columbia, Vancouver, British Columbia, Canada

KEYWORDS

- Metagenomic next-generation sequencing (mNGS) • Precision medicine • Clinical impact
- Immunocompromised • Pediatric • Infectious diseases diagnostic • Challenging diagnoses • Future directions

KEY POINTS

- Metagenomic next-generation sequencing (mNGS) largely does not rely on prior hypotheses and can identify a wide range of pathogens from patient samples including rare and unexpected organisms.
- Clinically validated, commercially available mNGS assays are accessible in North America most commonly for plasma and cerebrospinal fluid samples.
- There is substantial opportunity for standardization and guideline development for mNGS wet laboratory, bioinformatics, and clinical result interpretation.
- Collaborative consortia and working groups are essential to advocate for optimized use of mNGS testing.
- Future efforts that integrate diagnostic and antimicrobial stewardship efforts with mNGS will help move the field forward for enhanced clinical and public health use.

INTRODUCTION

In the past decade, metagenomic next-generation sequencing (mNGS) has evolved from a research-focused tool into a diagnostic method directly applicable in the clinical microbiology setting. The principle behind mNGS testing is compelling as it is based on sequencing all the nucleic acid in a sample to pinpoint sequences associated with potential pathogens. This enables an approach that can detect a wide range of microorganisms, providing unique diagnostic value for unusual, emerging, and/or unexpected infections. Despite the substantial advancements in sequencing technology, several challenges remain including limited availability of clinically validated assays, high costs, heterogeneity of sample types, test performance variability, and the need for specialized bioinformatics support. We have witnessed great strides in the investigation of test performance and clinical impact of mNGS testing in the last few years, starting from isolated case reports on actionability to studies including cohorts of several thousand individuals for plasma and cerebrospinal fluid (CSF) mNGS [1,2]. In this

*Corresponding author. BC Centre for Disease Control, 655 W 12th Avenue, Room 2054, Vancouver, British Columbia V5Z4R4. *E-mail address:* catherine.hogan@bccdc.ca

https://doi.org/10.1016/j.yamp.2025.05.005
2589-4080/25/ © 2025 Elsevier Inc. All rights are reserved, including those for text and data mining, AI training, and similar technologies.

ABBREVIATION	
AMR	antimicrobial resistance
BAL	bronchoalveolar lavage
CNS	central nervous system
CSF	cerebrospinal fluid
FN	febrile neutropenia
IE	infective endocarditis
IFI	invasive fungal infection
mNGS	metagenomic next-generation sequencing
NAAT	nucleic acid amplification test
NPV	negative predictive value
PPA	positive percent agreement

article, we propose a brief review of mNGS testing availability by sample type, describe current challenges in the fields, and highlight potential ways forward to continue building meaningful evidence for clinical implementation.

THE CURRENT STATE OF TESTING AND ITS CLINICAL IMPACT

Currently, a handful of specialized reference laboratories and academic centers in North America perform in-house mNGS testing for clinical application, and a key consideration is sample type. While CSF and plasma are the most commonly performed mNGS tests for clinical application in North America, additional sample types including bronchoalveolar lavage, ocular samples, synovial fluid, urine, and tissue biopsy samples have also been tested in pilot studies [1–6]. Each sample type poses distinct challenges and potential biases, such as host DNA contamination, variation in pathogen load, and high commensal bacteria background. These factors underscore the importance of using standardized workflows tailored to each specimen, as depicted in Fig. 1. The following section will examine the testing method and performance characteristics for each sample type and briefly review mNGS testing availability. Testing availability constantly evolves, and reference to the most up-to-date test menu and laboratory services is recommended.

BLOOD/PLASMA

A limited number of mNGS tests for bloodstream infection have been developed and evaluated for clinical use. Currently, the commercially available Karius test (Karius, Redwood City, CA) is the most commonly reported plasma mNGS test in the United States. This testing approach analyzes cell-free microbial DNA in plasma and can detect over 1200 pathogens [7]. Several studies have demonstrated the promise and complexity of using the Karius test in the clinical setting. Earlier laboratory validation data demonstrated that the Karius test presented a sensitivity of 92.9% for positive samples by composite diagnostic methods (culture, serology, nucleic acid amplification test [NAAT], and clinical adjudication; $n = 350$) and 62.7% specificity for negative samples by composite diagnostic methods ($n = 166$) [7].

Several studies have since examined the assay's clinical impact, using variable definitions and interpretations with limited comparability of findings across the field. In an early cohort of 82 patients, the positivity rate of the Karius test was 61%, with 7.3% of tests resulting in positive clinical impact and 3.7% negative clinical impact [8]. In a smaller study of 41 participants, the positivity was 49%, and there was no demonstrable positive impact. Furthermore, *Rothia mucilaginosa*, *Prevotella melaninogenica,* and other mucosal commensal organisms were detected. Clinical relevance of these detections is particularly challenging to ascertain, especially in certain patient populations and clinical contexts where there is high biological plausibility for pathogenicity including graft-versus-host-disease-associated mucosal damage [9]. Other studies have demonstrated a higher proportion of clinical impact in immunocompromised hosts, especially for results defined as clinically relevant and based on antimicrobial management changes [10–12]. More recently, a much larger retrospective evaluation of 1000 plasma mNGS test results documented positivity of 58.3%, with 82.2% of tests resulting in no clinical impact, 16.2% in positive impact, and 1.6% in negative impact [1]. Additionally, the Karius test is able to detect certain antimicrobial resistance (AMR) markers, including mecA, VanA, KPC, and ESBL; analytical test performance data have been published, and real-world utilization will require further study [13]. Of note, mNGS testing can miss significant pathogens including *Mycobacterium tuberculosis* and *Aspergillus* spp. [9,14]. With current technology, plasma mNGS is far from a *one-for-all* solution and cannot be relied on solely to rule out infections. With appropriate diagnostic stewardship, mNGS testing can yield additional insights that supplement—but do not currently replace—conventional microbiology testing (CMT) methods. Thus, conventional diagnostic approaches and empiric treatment remain essential.

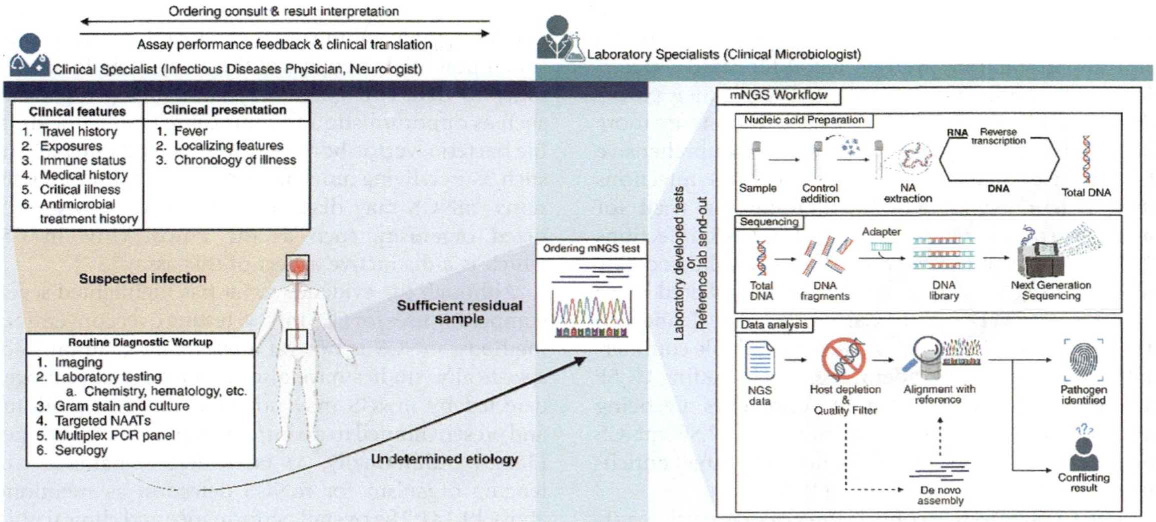

FIG. 1 Overview of the mNGS workflow [98].This figure demonstrates the full workflow for mNGS testing for infectious disease applications. The importance of communication between clinical and laboratory specialists is emphasized. PCR, polymerase chain reaction; NA, nucleic acid. (*Adapted from* Su LD, et al. Clinical metagenomic next-generation sequencing for diagnosis of central nervous system infections: advances and challenges. Mol Diagn Ther 2024:28:513–23.)

BRONCHOALVEOLAR LAVAGE

Pulmonary infections are challenging to diagnose due to the limited sensitivity of conventional testing and the need for numerous ancillary tests (eg, beta-D-glucan, serum and/or urine antigen, and others) [15–19]. The potential hypothesis-free nature of mNGS testing is compelling for use in diagnosing pulmonary infections, but differentiating between infection and colonization can still be challenging in complex samples with a high commensal background such as bronchoalveolar lavage (BAL) and may lead to false-positive results [20,21]. The availability of mNGS tests designed specifically for lung infections is limited; however, multiple studies have been conducted to evaluate its utility to support this diagnosis. In a pilot study of 128 BAL samples, mNGS testing could provide same-day results for 85.9% of respiratory samples with 93% agreement to conventional culture and detect clinically relevant pathogens in 19% of culture-negative samples including *M. tuberculosis*, *Tropheryma whipplei*, *Legionella pneumophila*, and cytomegalovirus [22,23]. Furthermore, in a US study that included 201 BAL samples, a targeted mNGS workflow yielded similar accuracy to an untargeted mNGS workflow for respiratory pathogen detection; however, the study suggested that both mNGS workflows could not fully replace conventional testing due to the high limit of detection (10^3 to 10^4 CFU/mL) and missed diagnoses on clinically significant filamentous molds including *Aspergillus*, *Rhizopus*, *Fusarium*, and *Cladosporium* species [5].

While mNGS has shown promise to improve pathogen detection, its clinical utility has varied across studies. In the above-mentioned study by Charalampous and colleagues, mNGS not only provided accurate results with fast turnaround time but was also able to contribute to 80% of prescribing decisions in the study [22,23]. In contrast, other studies have shown that despite the higher detection rate of mNGS assay compared to conventional testing, mNGS test results infrequently led to antibiotic de-escalation, mainly due to the difficulty in interpreting results especially in differentiating colonization from infection. Nonetheless, patients in the mNGS group were noted to have fewer empiric antiviral prescriptions and a lower antibiotic escalation rate due to physicians' confidence in mNGS results [24]. Respiratory mNGS may prove valuable in other respiratory sample types such as pleural fluid or upper respiratory samples to diagnose rare or emerging infections.

CEREBROSPINAL FLUID

CSF represents one of the first specimens used for clinical mNGS testing due to the particular challenges of central nervous system (CNS) infection management, including broad differential diagnosis, overlapping clinical presentations, and potential for rapid progression. Furthermore, the normal sterility of CSF is particularly suitable for mNGS testing as detections are more likely to be clinically relevant. Despite comprehensive diagnostic evaluations, the cause of CNS infections often remains unknown, highlighting the need for more effective diagnostic assays for CNS infections [25]. In North America, most clinically validated CSF mNGS testing has been performed and offered since 2016 at University of California San Francisico (UCSF) [26]. CSF mNGS is currently available commercially and in selected academic centers including UCSF and the Mayo Clinic. Different approaches are being evaluated to enhance the sensitivity of CSF mNGS including novel host depletion methods, target enrichment, and long-read sequencing [27–30].

A 2019 prospective cohort study of 204 participants demonstrated that CSF mNGS could detect an infectious etiology in 13/58 (22%) that were missed by traditional diagnostic methods, with 8 of these diagnoses leading to a clinical effect [31]. Furthermore, a 7-year retrospective review of 1164 CSF mNGS tests conducted at UCSF showed that the overall sensitivity was 63.1%, which was higher than serologic testing (28.8%) and combined direct detection methods on CSF (45.9%), including culture, antigen detection, and nucleic acid amplification testing. These test performance estimates may vary depending on the comparator method used across different settings. As with other sample types, mNGS testing can detect a broad range of pathogens including fastidious organisms and novel pathogens [2]. Other studies have reported similar findings, indicating that CSF mNGS results in better diagnostic yield particularly for viruses [29,32]. CSF mNGS also holds the potential to identify AMR genes directly from specimens and as a complementary tool in outbreak investigation [33,34].

One advantage of mNGS testing is that the approach is agnostic, enabling the diagnosis of unexpected, rare, and/or fastidious pathogens such as recently with an outbreak of *Fusarium solani* meningitis [35]. In a large cohort of patients with CNS infections, CSF mNGS successfully identified pathogens that CMT missed for various reasons: (1) the treating clinician had not considered the diagnosis, (2) there was no available reference diagnostic assay for the pathogen, (3) conventional microbiology yielded a false-negative result due to prior effective antimicrobial treatment before CSF collection or low sensitivity [2]. This illustrates how mNGS proves valuable when the clinical presentation involves overlapping infectious causes, and the sample volume is constrained for testing. Additional potential strengths of the assay include its capability to detect diagnostically challenging organisms, such as opportunistic and dimorphic Fungi, unculturable bacteria, vector-borne pathogens, and rare parasites such as free-living amebae [2,36]. In certain rare situations, mNGS may diagnose a novel or newly recognized organism, such as the Potosi virus in CSF, which is a distinctive aspect of this assay [37].

Although the evidence so far has highlighted several compelling uses for CSF mNGS testing over conventional methods, mNGS is not yet a *one-for-all* solution. More specifically, studies have also identified that pathogens detected by mNGS may not bear clinical significance and present limited to no impact on patient management [38,39]. Additionally, *M tuberculosis* remains a challenging organism for mNGS detection as mentioned above [9,14]. The overall performance and clinical utility of CSF mNGS likely depend on multiple factors, such as the patient population, clinical syndrome, and pathogen type, and this area will benefit from ongoing study [2].

OTHER SAMPLE TYPES

In addition to the previously mentioned sample type, mNGS has been applied to ocular, joint, and tissue samples to address diagnostic gaps where conventional microbiological testing may suffer from low-sensitivity, prolonged turnaround time, limited sample volume, and limited pathogen coverage, further complicated by complex etiologies and atypical presentations in immunocompromised patients [40–47]. There are currently no reference laboratories that provide mNGS testing for these sample types and most studies are conducted with research use only-protocols.

The utility of the mNGS assay was assessed using synovial fluid to diagnose prosthetic joint infections. In multiple studies, mNGS was shown to detect 90.2% to 96.5% of the pathogens in culture-positive cases and may be especially helpful in culture-negative cases; however, the interpretation of organisms as true pathogens versus contamination may be a challenge [6,48]. In tissue samples, mNGS reached 51% to 85% sensitivity and contributed to new diagnoses in 49.5% of cases, though many studies involve small sample sizes or isolated reports, and the nonsterile nature of some tissue samples may lead to false-positive results [49–57]. Multiple studies have investigated the potential of intraocular fluid mNGS testing with promising results based on the high positivity rate of mNGS especially for rare organisms. However, at present, there is only very limited literature on the positive impact of intraocular fluid mNGS testing [4,58–64].

THE UTILITY OF METAGENOMIC NEXT-GENERATION SEQUENCING ACROSS PATIENT POPULATIONS AND CLINICAL SYNDROMES

Immunocompromised Hosts

The proportion of immunosuppressed hosts in North America has increased over the last decade, and infections remain a major cause of morbidity and mortality in this group [65,66]. These individuals may present with atypical and/or nonspecific symptoms, and the differential diagnosis may be very broad. For these reasons, the hypothesis-free potential of mNGS testing may be particularly well-suited for this patient population. However, determining whether a detected organism is clinically relevant represents a stronger concern in this patient population.

Retrospective cohort studies evaluating the performance of mNGS assays across various sample types frequently include immunocompromised hosts as part of the study cohort, reflecting the current diagnostic gaps and ordering practices in this patient group. Overall, the evidence base has aligned to show a higher diagnostic yield of mNGS compared to conventional testing methods in immunocompromised hosts [2,31,67–72]. Few studies have selectively assessed mNGS test performance in immunocompromised populations, and most of these are based on plasma mNGS testing [73]. A single-center study including 100 samples found that plasma mNGS diagnostic testing yielded clinically significant pathogens in 61% of immunocompromised hosts versus 35% in immunocompetent patients [10]. In a prospective study using mNGS as a second-line test on various specimens, mNGS testing yield was higher in immunocompromised patients [74]. Studies have shown that mNGS delivers a higher clinical impact; for example, ranging from 6.6% to 25.8%, in immunocompromised populations including patients with hematologic malignancies, solid-organ transplant recipients. and individuals undergoing immunosuppressive therapy [49,75,76].

One notable condition in immunocompromised patients is invasive fungal infection (IFI). Diagnosis of IFIs is often complicated by the lack of sensitivity, long turnaround time, and the potential need for invasive sampling. Plasma mNGS testing may be useful in certain settings as a noninvasive alternative for the diagnosis of IFI especially for organisms other than *Aspergillus* where biomarkers are lacking [77,78]. However, the usefulness of plasma mNGS for diagnosing IFI remains a challenge, as a recent study showed that plasma mNGS presented lower sensitivity than galactomannan testing, which is performed routinely in high-risk individuals [67]. For CNS infections, CSF mNGS can identify a variety of fungi that are frequently challenging to detect, including *Histoplasma capsulatum*, *M. tuberculosis*, and *Coccidioides* spp. However, compared to CSF antigen testing, a recent study showed that mNGS missed 2 cases of *Cryptococcus* spp. and *Coccidioides* spp. infection (23 cases vs 25 cases) [2]. This discrepancy may be attributed to positive testing for *Cryptococcus* spp. and *Coccidioides* spp. antigens, while mNGS testing was negative in samples collected after the initiation of empiric antifungal treatment. Timing of sample collection relative to initiation of empiric antifungal treatment may be an important consideration [78].

Another notable condition is febrile neutropenia (FN), a frequent complication of chemotherapy, which is frequently driven by an infectious process [79]. Compared with conventional microbiological testing, current studies indicate that plasma mNGS testing can shorten result turnaround time by 87% and lead to early antimicrobial optimization in 47% of patients [80]. Importantly, the yield of plasma mNGS is unaffected by previous antimicrobial therapy in FN whereas blood culture positivity significantly declined [81]. However, negative predictive value of a negative plasma mNGS test for excluding bacterial infections remains uncertain. Interpreting plasma mNGS results in FN patients with disrupted mucosal barriers is complex given the high rate of polymicrobial detection with ambiguous significance [82]. One study noted positive plasma mNGS results in 18% of asymptomatic cancer patients, emphasizing the concern that mNGS results lead to unnecessary antimicrobial treatment and highlighting the important role of diagnostic and antimicrobial stewardship in mNGS result interpretation [83].

Immunocompromised populations represent a heterogeneous group, and it is unclear if certain types of immunosuppression are better candidates for mNGS testing. One study involving immunocompromised children has shown that the positive percent agreement (PPA) of plasma mNGS was lower than anticipated compared to the validation study in adults with sepsis (50% vs 85%), with low overall clinical impact [82]. This highlights the variable performance and utility across diverse indications and populations. Positive results also need to be carefully evaluated in immunocompromised hosts with mucosal barrier injury, as the significance of such results is often unclear [84]. Although the use of mNGS in immunocompromised patients may be particularly relevant, the optimal patient population, ordering providers, and use cases continue to be the focus of research attention to help leverage optimal use (Fig. 1).

Pediatrics

Comprehensive assessments of diagnostic performance and the clinical impacts of mNGS among large pediatric cohorts are limited as most studies have been focused on adults [85]. A large retrospective study found that among 1493 blood, CSF, BAL, and sputum samples in pediatric patients, mNGS testing showed higher PPA than conventional microbiological testing compared to clinical diagnosis (53.1% vs 25.8%) [71]. In this extensive study, mNGS testing proved particularly useful in CSF samples, immunocompromised children, and those under 6 years of age. Furthermore, most cases of *Streptococcus pneumoniae, Streptococcus agalactiae, M. tuberculosis* complex, and *Pneumocystis jirovecii* infection were diagnosed by mNGS alone. The use of mNGS for the diagnosis of lower respiratory tract infections has shown greater sensitivity than CMT in diagnosing lower respiratory tract infections (LRTI) [86]. Interestingly, co-detection of potential pathogens occurred in 52% of cases, and incidentally, the carriage of potentially pathogenic microorganisms was observed in 68% of children without LRTI in 1 study [87]. These findings underscore the challenges in interpreting mNGS results in this population. Additionally, several studies have evaluated CSF mNGS for diagnosing viral meningoencephalitis in children and have reported increased yield with mNGS [30,88].

OTHER INFECTIONS AND/OR CLINICAL SYNDROMES

Parasitic Infections

mNGS has been employed in various specimens to detect rare parasitic diseases, including neurocysticercosis, leishmaniasis, free-living amebiasis, and angiostrongyliasis [2,89–91]. Diagnosing these conditions can be difficult due to limited testing options for parasites, the frequent false-negative results from microscopy—the gold standard for many parasitic infections—and the frequent necessity of invasive testing [2]. Nonetheless, there is a lack of large-scale studies that evaluate mNGS performance compared to traditional microbiological testing for parasitic infections, especially since parasites are among the least commonly detected organisms in plasma and CSF [2,36]. Additionally, the high cost of mNGS assays limits their widespread adoption, especially in resource-limited settings where the incidence of parasitic infections is highest.

Blood Culture-Negative Endocarditis

Approximately 10% of infective endocarditis (IE) cases are blood culture-negative [92]. This occurrence often results from the inability to cultivate bacteria due to previous antimicrobial treatment or the presence of organisms that standard culture methods cannot identify. Research indicates that plasma or cardiac valve mNGS can identify as many or more IE cases than traditional diagnostic approaches [93–95]. Some instances were diagnosed even after extended antibiotic therapy. One study found a positive impact from mNGS testing in cases of blood culture-negative endocarditis (BCNE) [1]. Additionally, a study found that shotgun mNGS demonstrated detection rates similar to targeted next-generation sequencing in IE cases, including BCNE. These findings contributed to the 2023 revision of the modified Duke Criteria, incorporating plasma mNGS detection of *Coxiella burnettii, Bartonella* spp., or *Trophyrema whipplei* as a major microbiologic criterion and the detection of other IE-compatible organisms as a minor microbiologic criterion [92].

Use as a Complementary Rule-Out Test

The use of mNGS assays has been investigated as a complementary diagnostic tool to rule out infections. A retrospective review at a tertiary center indicated that the most common reason for physician to order CSF mNGS (in 47% of cases) was to rule out infections in complex cases. However, the overall diagnostic yield was considerably low; pathogens were detected in only 15% of cases, and 9% of tests produced false-positive results [39]. Most studies regarding mNGS indicate that false-negative results are common, with a negative predictive value (NPV) that is insufficient to rely solely on mNGS for ruling out infections [85]. In a single study where CSF mNGS is regularly employed as a rule-out test for CNS infections, the NPV was 92.3% [2]. False-negative outcomes predominantly occurred in instances with high backgrounds of human DNA in samples, which diminished CSF mNGS sensitivity, or when diseases lacked detectable nucleic acids in CSF at collection, and also when pathogens were only identifiable in samples other than CSF. Overall, given the imperfect sensitivity of mNGS, the current literature does not support routine mNGS test use to exclude infections; however, future studies may help confirm in what clinical contexts and patient populations it could be advantageous (see Fig. 1).

Integration with Stewardship

Several variables must be considered to maximize the yield of mNGS testing for infectious diseases including clinical features/presentation, residual sample volume and consultation with laboratory specialists (Fig. 2). In addition, false-positive results from mNGS testing present clinical challenges and may lead to unnecessary treatment [39]. Regular and open dialogue between laboratory specialists and clinical teams is essential to fully understand the test performance characteristics, limitations, and potential harms of mNGS testing. Additionally, mNGS represents one of the costliest diagnostic testing strategies in microbiology laboratories. Consequently, efforts that focus on enhancing mNGS testing clinical relevance and value are needed. Positive results tend to have a greater impact; therefore, diagnostic stewardship prioritizes identifying high-yield indications or populations. For instance, higher mNGS yields have been correlated with conditions like high pretest probability for infection, immunocompromised hosts, BCNE, and pneumonia in various studies [1,10,74–76]. To select patients with an elevated pretest probability of infection more effectively, the involvement of infectious diseases specialists and/or clinical microbiologists before test ordering may be crucial [70,96]. One study indicated that reviewing all plasma mNGS orders led to a 37% reduction in tests conducted without impacting microbiological or clinical outcomes for patients [9]. Another study assessed a committee-based approach to limit mNGS test usage in a children's hospital and found that the clinical impact of their mNGS assay was 55% for approved testing cases, outpacing studies without diagnostic stewardship interventions [97]. These studies lay the groundwork for evaluating and implementing diagnostic stewardship strategies for mNGS testing, but additional research is essential. There is a need to better characterize factors linked to positive and clinically impactful results, alongside economic analyses, to determine for which populations and clinical indications mNGS testing is cost-effective (see Fig. 2).

CURRENT CHALLENGES AND FUTURE AVENUES

While clinical metagenomics for infectious disease diagnostics has made significant progress over the past decade, many challenges remain and are outlined as follows.

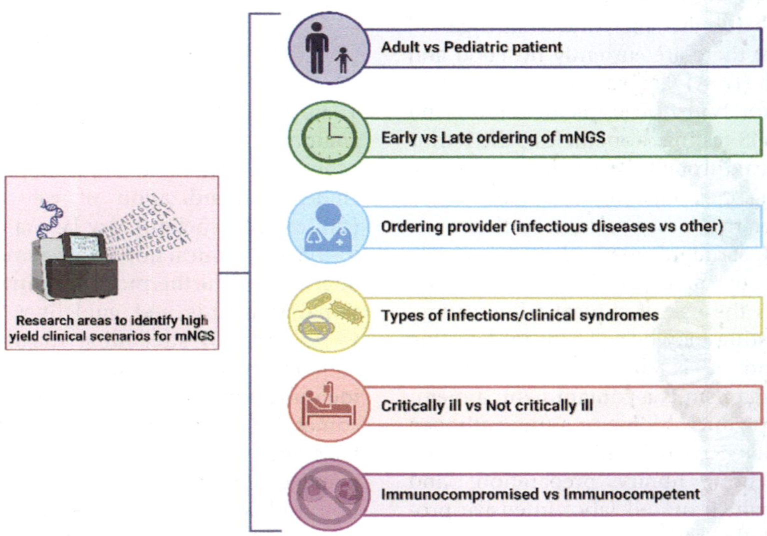

FIG. 2 Possible research areas to identify applications with highest clinical utility of mNGS testing. This figure illustrates an overview of the key comparators used in mNGS assessment. Each subsection highlights the strategic area for assessing assays' clinical utility, offering clear directions for future research and clinical studies.

LABORATORY CHALLENGES

Laboratory challenges can be grouped into 3 phases: preanalytical, analytical, and postanalytical phases. Regarding preanalytical challenges, one key challenge is determining the appropriate time to order mNGS testing. Currently, mNGS testing is frequently ordered when conventional microbiologic testing has been negative or in severely immunocompromised or critically ill patients [98]. Several institutions have championed diagnostic stewardship workflows to optimize the timing of mNGS testing relative to laboratory testing available in-house. Recently, one group has shown the advantage of this type of diagnostic stewardship for the Karius test to improve clinical utility [1]. Specifically, they showed that increased oversight in ordering of the Karius test enhanced clinical impact of the test [1]. Additional research in this field will help inform policies for enhanced diagnostic stewardship efforts. Another preanalytical challenge is the proximity of the ordering hospital to the laboratory that performs the mNGS test. Due to the low number of the laboratories that offer mNGS testing, the test accessibility is limited and poses challenges on cost and turnaround times, which needs to be incorporated for local workflow planning [32,99,100]. In-house mNGS testing efforts are being developed, but their generalizability is limited by the significant expertise and resources available for the development, implementation, and sustainability of such services.

The major theme for the analytical challenges of mNGS testing is that there are currently no Food and Drug Administration (FDA)-cleared options for testing and no guidelines for both the implementation and performance of mNGS testing; nonetheless, the Karius has received FDA Breakthrough Device designation for diagnosis and management of lung infections, which may expedite further regulatory review. Furthermore, the lack of a gold standard method to accurately compare the results of mNGS testing may be challenging and requires the use of clinical adjudication, given that mNGS testing may be superior in detecting microorganisms, and it is difficult to determine whether the microorganism is a contaminant, a member of the sample type microbiome or a true pathogen [101]. Accuracy of mNGS testing can also be affected by nucleic acid extraction, library preparation, and sequencer loading, which are all labor-intensive processes that require skilled technologists.

Finally, the major postanalytical challenges of mNGS testing are the bioinformatics analysis, reporting, and interpretation of the results. The development, validation, and clinical implementation of bioinformatics pipelines require considerable time and expertise, not only with regard to coding and computing but also for accurate and clinically relevant result interpretation. Differentiating pathogen versus commensal organisms can be challenging and sample-dependent, as sterile samples should not have any contending microbiome [7,102–104]. Even in samples normally considered sterile, bacterial DNA can be found in healthy individuals [105], such that future research in this area, such as prospective clinical trials to assess what is the *expected* background in the different source types will be beneficial to move the field forward. Another challenge in bioinformatics analysis relates to the detection of other nucleic acid sources (contaminants), such as the *kit-ome* of reagents used for mNGS [106–110]. This contamination with extraneous DNA can unfavorably impact the results of samples, particularly in low-biomass samples, highlighting the need for result interpretation support by physicians and providers familiar with the techniques and methods used in mNGS testing. Many institutions have implemented precision medicine teams comprising representatives from the microbiology laboratory, infectious disease providers, and computational biologists [20,111]. These teams discuss the results and provide an interpretation of the mNGS results so that proper actions can be taken based on clinically relevant data. They also represent a useful approach to bolster stewardship efforts to ensure the high relevance of mNGS testing.

FUTURE AVENUES

There is currently substantial opportunity for standardization in the field of mNGS workflows and evidence generation across the continuum of testing. This includes standardization of wet laboratory methods (full mNGS pipeline), dry laboratory methods (bioinformatics), clinical impact assessment, and stewardship approaches. Furthermore, the integration of international standards and guidelines into mNGS testing workflows can streamline diagnostic processes and enhance the accuracy and reproducibility of organism identification, which in turn can optimize patient outcomes [112]. Several national and global standards have been developed to facilitate an integrated quality management approach for mNGS clinical implementation and workflows, and others are in development. For example, the ISO20397 standard published in 2022 specifies requirements and provides guidance for nucleic acid, library preparations, and quality assessments [113]. Similarly, the ISO24420 standard published in 2023 illustrates the workflow of shotgun metagenomics sequence data processing [113]. Furthermore, the National Institute of Standards and Technology has developed an entire suite of reference materials to provide measurement assurance for mNGS testing [114]. These efforts are crucial to build quality assurance efforts and to enhance intralaboratory and interlaboratory reproducibility [115]. Additionally, proficiency testing programs are also in development, and several guideline development efforts are in the pipeline.

Collaborative consortia and working groups are vital for knowledge dissemination and integrated advocacy. One example of such a group is the Consortium for Clinical Metagenomics in Infectious Diseases, a collaborative group of microbiologists, clinicians, and scientists established in 2022. This group conducts needs assessments, shares experiences from different institutes, and bridges industry and academia. Within this framework, there is a great opportunity to engage with diverse and complementary stakeholders to draft consensus opinions, reviews and guidelines that will serve as references for mNGS testing. For example, a recent commentary uses an *operational value* framework to evaluate test performance by its result quality, utility, and cost-effectiveness, which contributes to the effort on standardization of mNGS test utility assessments [116].

Several new and emerging applications of mNGS testing are also in development and carry great potential to improve clinical impact in the future. For example, direct AMR detection by mNGS, which is crucial for treatment optimization in culture-negative cases, has been explored across several applications in clinical and public health [13,117,118] and will grow in use in the future. Another exciting potential of mNGS testing is the analysis of the host response using transcriptomics via RNA sequencing [119–122]. This would be advantageous in the more microbiome-rich sites, such as the respiratory tract, to help determine the difference between true pathogens and the commensal respiratory microbiome [120]. Future work that compares different modalities in a head-to-head fashion will also be instrumental to fully understanding the pros and cons of mNGS-based testing approaches. Finally, novel applications for rapid and sensitive use of mNGS in outbreak investigation and pathogen detection and surveillance have been increasingly used, as highlighted recently by the announcement of mNGS-based public health surveillance by the United Kingdom Health Security Agency Health [123].

SUMMARY

In conclusion, in the past decade, we have directly witnessed the translation of mNGS testing from research to clinical settings for a range of sample types, most commonly plasma and CSF in the North American setting. The evidence base supporting the use of mNGS has expanded considerably over the last decade; however, several challenges remain, including its high cost, heterogeneity of sample types, test performance limitations, and the need for specialized bioinformatics support. The evidence so far has highlighted the importance of patient selection, testing timing, and integration with diagnostic, and antimicrobial stewardship to enhance the clinical impact of mNGS testing. Future research work to standardize evidence generation and protocols, enhance comparability of research findings across settings, and confirm the highest yield clinical use scenarios will continue moving the field forward, in addition to several other areas of opportunities for mNGS to positively impact patient care and public health surveillance as outlined in this article.

CLINICS CARE POINTS

- metagenomic next-generation sequencing (mNGS) testing can offer unique diagnostic insights, particularly for immunocompromised populations and investigation of unusual clinical syndromes with high suspicion of infection in the central nervous system and bloodstream.
- Several laboratory-developed mNGS assays are available for clinical use in North America.
- mNGS is not a *one-for-all* solution and providers need to consider the possibility of contamination and colonization when interpreting the results.
- Consulting with infectious disease specialists and/or clinical microbiologists for test ordering and result interpretation optimizes clinical impact and diagnostic stewardship.

DISCLOSURE

The authors have nothing to disclose. C.A.H. is a steering committee member of the Consortium for Clinical Metagenomics in Infectious Diseases.

REFERENCES

[1] Kaur I, Shaw B, Multani A, et al. Real-world clinical impact of plasma cell-free DNA metagenomic next-generation

sequencing assay. Infect Control Hosp Epidemiol 2025; 1–8. https://doi.org/10.1017/ice.2024.242.
[2] Benoit P, Brazer N, de Lorenzi-Tognon M, et al. Seven-year performance of a clinical metagenomic next-generation sequencing test for diagnosis of central nervous system infections. Nat Med 2024;30:3522–33.
[3] Han D, Li Z, Li R, et al. mNGS in clinical microbiology laboratories: on the road to maturity. Crit Rev Microbiol 2019;45:668–85.
[4] Doan T, Acharya NR, Pinsky BA, et al. Metagenomic DNA Sequencing for the diagnosis of intraocular infections. Ophthalmology 2017;124:1247–8.
[5] Gaston DC, Miller HB, Fissel JA, et al. Evaluation of metagenomic and targeted next-generation sequencing workflows for detection of respiratory pathogens from bronchoalveolar lavage fluid specimens. J Clin Microbiol 2022;60:e0052622.
[6] Ivy MI, Thoendel MJ, Jeraldo PR, et al. Direct detection and identification of prosthetic joint infection pathogens in synovial fluid by metagenomic shotgun sequencing. J Clin Microbiol 2018;56:e00402–18.
[7] Blauwkamp TA, Thair S, Rosen MJ, et al. Analytical and clinical validation of a microbial cell-free DNA sequencing test for infectious disease. Nat Microbiol 2019;4:663–74.
[8] Hogan CA, Yang S, Garner OB, et al. Clinical impact of metagenomic next-generation sequencing of plasma cell-free DNA for the diagnosis of infectious diseases: a multicenter retrospective cohort study. Clin Infect 2021;72:239–45.
[9] Graf EH, Bryan A, Bowers M, et al. One size fits small: the narrow utility for plasma metagenomics. J Appl Lab Med 2025;10:171–83.
[10] Rossoff J, Chaudhury S, Soneji M, et al. Noninvasive diagnosis of infection using plasma next-generation sequencing: a single-center experience. Open Forum Infect Dis 2019;6:ofz327.
[11] Shishido AA, Noe M, Saharia K, et al. Clinical impact of a metagenomic microbial plasma cell-free DNA next-generation sequencing assay on treatment decisions: a single-center retrospective study. BMC Infect Dis 2022;22:372.
[12] Wu J, Song W, Yan H, et al. Metagenomic next-generation sequencing in detecting pathogens in pediatric oncology patients with suspected bloodstream infections. Pediatr Res 2024;95:843–51.
[13] Christians FC, Akhund-Zade J, Jarman K, et al. Analytical and clinical validation of direct detection of antimicrobial resistance markers by plasma microbial cell-free DNA sequencing. J Clin Microbiol 2024;62:e0042524.
[14] Niles DT, Wijetunge DSS, Palazzi DL, et al. Plasma metagenomic next-generation sequencing assay for identifying pathogens: a retrospective review of test utilization in a large children's hospital. J Clin Microbiol 2020;58. https://doi.org/10.1128/jcm.00794-20.
[15] Tarrand JJ, Lichterfeld M, Warraich I, et al. Diagnosis of invasive septate mold infections. a correlation of microbiological culture and histologic or cytologic examination. Am J Clin Pathol 2003;119:854–8.
[16] White PL, Backx M, Barnes RA. Diagnosis and management of Pneumocystis jirovecii infection. Expert Rev Anti Infect Ther 2017;15:435–47.
[17] Suneja M, Beekmann SE, Dhaliwal G, et al. Diagnostic delays in infectious diseases. Diagn Berl Ger 2022;9: 332–9.
[18] Quinton LJ, Walkey AJ, Mizgerd JP. Integrative physiology of pneumonia. Physiol Rev 2018;98:1417–64.
[19] Jain S, Self WH, Wunderink RG, et al. Community-acquired pneumonia requiring hospitalization among U. S. adults. N Engl J Med 2015;373:415–27.
[20] Simner PJ, Miller S, Carroll KC. Understanding the promises and hurdles of metagenomic next-generation sequencing as a diagnostic tool for infectious diseases. Clin Infect 2018;66:778–88.
[21] Dulanto Chiang A, Dekker JP. From the pipeline to the bedside: advances and challenges in clinical metagenomics. J Infect Dis 2020;221:S331–40.
[22] Lydon E, Langelier CR. Respiratory metagenomics: ready for prime time? Am J Respir Crit Care Med 2024;209:124–6.
[23] Chen Y, Feng W, Ye K, et al. Application of metagenomic next-generation sequencing in the diagnosis of pulmonary infectious pathogens from bronchoalveolar lavage samples. Front Cell Infect Microbiol 2021;11:541092.
[24] Yan M, Zou X, Wang Y, et al. Impact of metagenomic next-generation sequencing of bronchoalveolar lavage fluid on antimicrobial stewardship in patients with lower respiratory tract infections: a retrospective cohort study. J Infect Dis 2024;229:223–31.
[25] Glaser CA, Honarmand S, Anderson LJ, et al. Beyond viruses: clinical profiles and etiologies associated with encephalitis. Clin Infect Dis 2006;43:1565–77.
[26] Miller S, Naccache SN, Samayoa E, et al. Laboratory validation of a clinical metagenomic sequencing assay for pathogen detection in cerebrospinal fluid. Genome Res 2019;29:831–42.
[27] Ji X-C, Zhou LF, Li CY, et al. Reduction of human DNA contamination in clinical cerebrospinal fluid specimens improves the sensitivity of metagenomic next-generation sequencing. J Mol Neurosci 2020;70:659–66.
[28] Sung YH, Ju YK, Lee HJ, et al. Clinical performance of real-time nanopore metagenomic sequencing for rapid identification of bacterial pathogens in cerebrospinal fluid: a pilot study. Sci Rep 2025;15:3493.
[29] Piantadosi A, Mukerji SS, Ye S, et al. Enhanced virus detection and metagenomic sequencing in patients with meningitis and encephalitis. mBio 2021;12:e0114321.
[30] Carbo EC, Buddingh EP, Karelioti E, et al. Improved diagnosis of viral encephalitis in adult and pediatric hematological patients using viral metagenomics. J Clin Virol 2020;130:104566.
[31] Wilson MR, Sample HA, Zorn KC, et al. Clinical metagenomic sequencing for diagnosis of meningitis and encephalitis. N Engl J Med 2019;380:2327–40.

[32] Klontz EH, Solomon IH, Turbett SE, et al. Cerebrospinal fluid metagenomics has greatest added value as a test for Powassan virus among patients in New England with suspected central nervous system infection. Diagn Microbiol Infect Dis 2024;108:116169.
[33] Tian Y, Xia H, Zhang L, et al. Detection of multidrug-resistant acinetobacter baumannii by metagenomic next-generation sequencing in central nervous system infection after neurosurgery: a case report. Front Public Health 2022;10:1028920.
[34] Griffin IS, Smith DJ, Annambhotla P, et al. Outcomes in solid organ transplant recipients receiving organs from a donor with Fusarium solani species complex meningitis. Transpl Infect Dis 2024;26:e14331.
[35] Chiu CY, Servellita V, de Lorenzi-Tognon M, et al. Metagenomic identification of fusarium solani strain as cause of US fungal meningitis outbreak associated with surgical procedures in Mexico, 2023. Emerg Infect Dis 2025;31:948–57.
[36] Park SY, Chang EJ, Ledeboer N, et al. Plasma microbial cell-free DNA sequencing from over 15,000 patients identified a broad spectrum of pathogens. J Clin Microbiol 2023;61:e0185522.
[37] Chiu CY, Godasi RR, Hughes HR, et al. Two human cases of fatal meningoencephalitis associated with potosi and lone star virus infections, United States, 2020-2023. Emerg Infect Dis 2025;31:215–21.
[38] Shean RC, Garrett E, Malleis J, et al. A retrospective observational study of mNGS test utilization to examine the role of diagnostic stewardship at two academic medical centers. J Clin Microbiol 2024;62: e0060524.
[39] Rodino KG, Toledano M, Norgan AP, et al. Retrospective review of clinical utility of shotgun metagenomic sequencing testing of cerebrospinal fluid from a U.S. tertiary care medical center. J Clin Microbiol 2020;58: e01729-20.
[40] Taravati P, Lam D, Van Gelder RN. Role of molecular diagnostics in ocular microbiology. Curr Ophthalmol Rep 2013;1.
[41] Gomez-Urena EO, Tande AJ, Osmon DR, et al. Diagnosis of prosthetic joint infection: cultures, biomarker and criteria. Infect Dis Clin 2017;31:219–35.
[42] Berbari EF, Marculescu C, Sia I, et al. Culture-negative prosthetic joint infection. Clin Infect Dis 2007;45: 1113–9.
[43] Tobin EH, Tristram D. Tuberculosis overview. In: StatPearls. Treasure Island (FL): StatPearls Publishing; 2025.
[44] Hope W, Natarajan P, Goodwin L. Invasive fungal infections. Clin Med Lond Engl 2013;13:507–10.
[45] Schafer KR, Shah N, Almira-Suarez MI, et al. Disseminated balamuthia mandrillaris infection. J Clin Microbiol 2015;53:3072–6.
[46] Noor A, Khetarpal S. Anaerobic infections. In: StatPearls. Treasure Island (FL): StatPearls Publishing; 2025.
[47] Doan T, Wilson MR, Crawford ED, et al. Illuminating uveitis: metagenomic deep sequencing identifies common and rare pathogens. Genome Med 2016;8:90.
[48] Huang Z, Li W, Lee GC, et al. Metagenomic next-generation sequencing of synovial fluid demonstrates high accuracy in prosthetic joint infection diagnostics: mNGS for diagnosing PJI. Bone Jt Res 2020;9:440–9.
[49] Tang H, Chen Y, Tang X, et al. Yield of clinical metagenomics: insights from real-world practice for tissue infections. EBioMedicine 2025;111:105536.
[50] Flurin L, Wolf MJ, Mutchler MM, et al. Targeted metagenomic sequencing-based approach applied to 2146 tissue and body fluid samples in routine clinical practice. Clin Infect Dis 2022;75:1800–8.
[51] Zhang X, Liu Y, Zhang M, et al. Case report: diagnosis of visceral leishmaniasis using metagenomic next-generation sequencing and bone marrow smear. Front Cell Infect Microbiol 2022;12:1095072.
[52] Tang C, He S, Wang N, et al. A case report and literature review: diagnosis and treatment of human immunodeficiency virus coinfected with visceral leishmania by metagenomic next-generation sequencing in China. Ann Transl Med 2022;10:497.
[53] Li E, Zhu Q, Lv Z, et al. Visceral leishmaniasis: a case confirmed by metagenomic next-generation sequencing from Northwestern China. Infect Drug Resist 2024;17: 3153–8.
[54] Han N, Yu J, Wang M, et al. The value of metagenomic next-generation sequencing in leishmaniasis diagnosis: a case series and literature review. Open Forum Infect Dis 2022;9:ofac511.
[55] Yang H, Xu N, Yan M, et al. Comparison of metagenomic next-generation sequencing and conventional culture for the diagnostic performance in febrile patients with suspected infections. BMC Infect Dis 2024;24:350.
[56] Wang Q, Miao Q, Pan J, et al. The clinical value of metagenomic next-generation sequencing in the microbiological diagnosis of skin and soft tissue infections. Int J Infect Dis 2020;100:414–20.
[57] Rodriguez C, Jary A, Hua C, et al. Pathogen identification by shotgun metagenomics of patients with necrotizing soft-tissue infections. Br J Dermatol 2020;183: 105–13.
[58] Qian Z, Zhang Y, Wang L, et al. Application of metagenomic next-generation sequencing in suspected intraocular infections. Eur J Ophthalmol 2023;33:391–7.
[59] Pan X-Y, Wang M, Xu Y-D, et al. Application of metagenomic next-generation sequencing in the diagnosis of infectious keratitis. J Ophthalmol 2024; 2024:9911979.
[60] Scharf SA, Friedrichs L, Bock R, et al. Oxford nanopore technology-based identification of an acanthamoeba castellanii endosymbiosis in microbial keratitis. Microorganisms 2024;12:2292.
[61] Fan W, Li P, Wei Q, et al. Metagenomic next-generation sequencing-assisted diagnosis of a rare case of primary

cutaneous acanthamoebiasis in an HIV patient: a case report. Front Cell Infect Microbiol 2024;14:1356095.

[62] Dong G, Hao Z, Zhang C, et al. Unveiling challenging corneal infections: a comprehensive etiological diagnosis through metagenomic next-generation sequencing (mNGS) of corneal tissue samples. Int Ophthalmol 2024;44:246.

[63] Seitzman GD, Thulasi P, Hinterwirth A, et al. Capnocytophaga keratitis: clinical presentation and use of metagenomic deep sequencing for diagnosis. Cornea 2019;38:246–8.

[64] Zhu J, Xia H, Tang R, et al. Metagenomic next-generation sequencing detects pathogens in endophthalmitis patients. Retina Phila PA 2022;42:992–1000.

[65] Linden PK. Approach to the immunocompromised host with infection in the intensive care unit. Infect Dis Clin 2009;23:535–56.

[66] Martinson ML, Lapham J. Prevalence of immunosuppression among US adults. JAMA 2024;331:880–2.

[67] Bergin SP, Chemaly RF, Dadwal SS, et al. Plasma microbial cell-free DNA sequencing in immunocompromised patients with pneumonia: a prospective observational study. Clin Infect Dis 2024;78:775–84.

[68] Zinter MS, Dvorak CC, Mayday MY, et al. Pulmonary metagenomic sequencing suggests missed infections in immunocompromised children. Clin Infect Dis 2019;68:1847–55.

[69] Azar MM, Schlaberg R, Malinis MF, et al. Added diagnostic utility of clinical metagenomics for the diagnosis of pneumonia in immunocompromised adults. Chest 2021;159:1356–71.

[70] Vissichelli NC, Morales MK, Kolipakkam B, et al. Cell-free next-generation sequencing impacts diagnosis and antimicrobial therapy in immunocompromised hosts: a retrospective study. Transpl Infect Dis 2023;25:e13954.

[71] Zhu Y, Gan M, Ge M, et al. Diagnostic performance and clinical impact of metagenomic next-generation sequencing for pediatric infectious diseases. J Clin Microbiol 2023;61:e0011523.

[72] Parize P, Muth E, Richaud C, et al. Untargeted next-generation sequencing-based first-line diagnosis of infection in immunocompromised adults: a multicentre, blinded, prospective study. Clin Microbiol Infect 2017;23:574.e1–6.

[73] Casto AM, Fredricks DN, Hill JA. Diagnosis of infectious diseases in immunocompromised hosts using metagenomic next generation sequencing-based diagnostics. Blood Rev 2022;53:100906.

[74] Fourgeaud J, Regnault B, Ok V, et al. Performance of clinical metagenomics in France: a prospective observational study. Lancet Microbe 2024;5:e52–61.

[75] Lee RA, Al Dhaheri F, Pollock NR, et al. Assessment of the clinical utility of plasma metagenomic next-generation sequencing in a pediatric hospital population. J Clin Microbiol 2020;58:e00419–20.

[76] Niles DT, Revell PA, Ruderfer D, et al. Clinical impact of plasma metagenomic next-generation sequencing in a large pediatric cohort. Pediatr Infect Dis J 2022;41:166–71.

[77] Park SY, Ardura MI, Zhang SX. Diagnostic limitations and challenges in current clinical guidelines and potential application of metagenomic sequencing to manage pulmonary invasive fungal infections in patients with haematological malignancies. Clin Microbiol Infect 2024;30:1139–46.

[78] Hill JA, Dalai SC, Hong DK, et al. Liquid biopsy for invasive mold infections in hematopoietic cell transplant recipients with pneumonia through next-generation sequencing of microbial cell-free DNA in plasma. Clin Infect Dis 2021;73:e3876–83.

[79] Freifeld AG, Bow EJ, Sepkowitz KA, et al. Clinical practice guideline for the use of antimicrobial agents in neutropenic patients with cancer: 2010 update by the infectious diseases society of america. Clin Infect Dis 2011;52:e56–93.

[80] Benamu E, Gajurel K, Anderson JN, et al. Plasma microbial cell-free DNA next-generation sequencing in the diagnosis and management of febrile neutropenia. Clin Infect Dis 2022;74:1659–68.

[81] Feng S, Rao G, Wei X, et al. Clinical metagenomic sequencing of plasma microbial cell-free DNA for febrile neutropenia in patients with acute leukaemia. Clin Microbiol Infect 2024;30:107–13.

[82] Lehman AC, Goren LR, Evans MD, et al. Clinical performance of plasma metagenomic sequencing in immunocompromised pediatric patients. J Pediatr Infect Dis Soc 2024;13:276–81.

[83] Goggin KP, Gonzalez-Pena V, Inaba Y, et al. Evaluation of plasma microbial cell-free DNA sequencing to predict bloodstream infection in pediatric patients with relapsed or refractory cancer. JAMA Oncol 2020;6:552–6.

[84] Castejon-Ramirez S, Glasgow HL, Ferrolino JA, et al. Plasma metagenomic sequencing in immunocompromised children: a call for caution in the interpretation of results. J Pediatr Infect Dis Soc 2024;13:334–5.

[85] Edward P, Handel AS. Metagenomic next-generation sequencing for infectious disease diagnosis: a review of the literature with a focus on pediatrics. J Pediatr Infect Dis Soc 2021;10:S71–7.

[86] Dworsky ZD, Lee B, Ramchandar N, et al. Impact of cell-free next-generation sequencing on management of pediatric complicated pneumonia. Hosp Pediatr 2022;12:377–84.

[87] Tsitsiklis A, Osborne CM, Kamm J, et al. Lower respiratory tract infections in children requiring mechanical ventilation: a multicentre prospective surveillance study incorporating airway metagenomics. Lancet Microbe 2022;3:e284–93.

[88] Castellot A, Camacho J, Fernńdez-García MD, et al. Shotgun metagenomics to investigate unknown viral etiologies of pediatric meningoencephalitis. PLoS One 2023;18:e0296036.

[89] Pedrosa DA, Bruniera Peres Fernandes G, Filipe de Souza Godoy L, et al. Neurocysticercosis: diagnosis

via metagenomic next-generation sequencing. Pract Neurol 2023;23:509–11.
[90] Wang C, Li A, Shi Q, et al. Metagenomic next-generation sequencing clinches diagnosis of leishmaniasis. Lancet Lond Engl 2021;397:1213.
[91] Zhao R, He G, Xiang L, et al. Metagenomic next-generation sequencing assists in the diagnosis of visceral leishmaniasis in non-endemic areas of China. Front Cell Infect Microbiol 2025;15:1517046.
[92] Fowler VG, Durack DT, Selton-Suty C, et al. The 2023 duke-international society for cardiovascular infectious diseases criteria for infective endocarditis: updating the modified duke criteria. Clin Infect Dis 2023;77: 518–26.
[93] To RK, Ramchandar N, Gupta A, et al. Use of plasma metagenomic next-generation sequencing for pathogen identification in pediatric endocarditis. Pediatr Infect Dis J 2021;40:486–8.
[94] Eichenberger EM, Degner N, Scott ER, et al. Microbial cell-free DNA identifies the causative pathogen in infective endocarditis and remains detectable longer than conventional blood culture in patients with prior antibiotic therapy. Clin Infect Dis 2023;76:e1492–500.
[95] Haddad SF, DeSimone DC, Chesdachai S, et al. Utility of metagenomic next-generation sequencing in infective endocarditis: a systematic review. Antibiot Basel Switz 2022;11:1798.
[96] Parrish NF, Gaston DC. Metagenomics in infectious disease diagnostics: toward best-use practices to optimize actionable results. Transpl Infect Dis 2023;25:e13959.
[97] Allen BS, Kidd M, Sue PK, et al. A committee-based diagnostic stewardship model for pathogen metagenomic sequencing in children. J Appl Lab Med 2025; 10:59–65.
[98] Su LD, Chiu CY, Gaston D, et al. Clinical metagenomic next-generation sequencing for diagnosis of central nervous system infections: advances and challenges. Mol Diagn Ther 2024;28:513–23.
[99] Afshinnekoo E, Chou C, Alexander N, et al. Precision metagenomics: rapid metagenomic analyses for infectious disease diagnostics and public health surveillance. J Biomol Tech 2017;28:40–5.
[100] Greninger AL, Naccache SN, Federman S, et al. Rapid metagenomic identification of viral pathogens in clinical samples by real-time nanopore sequencing analysis. Genome Med 2015;7:99.
[101] Chiu CY, Miller SA. Clinical metagenomics. Nat Rev Genet 2019;20:341–55.
[102] Naccache SN, Federman S, Veeraraghavan N, et al. A cloud-compatible bioinformatics pipeline for ultrarapid pathogen identification from next-generation sequencing of clinical samples. Genome Res 2014;24: 1180–92.
[103] Pendleton KM, Erb-Downward JR, Bao Y, et al. Rapid pathogen identification in bacterial pneumonia using real-time metagenomics. Am J Respir Crit Care Med 2017;196:1610–2.
[104] Zhou Y, Wylie KM, El Feghaly RE, et al. Metagenomic approach for identification of the pathogens associated with diarrhea in stool specimens. J Clin Microbiol 2016;54:368–75.
[105] Gosiewski T, Ludwig-Galezowska AH, Huminska K, et al. Comprehensive detection and identification of bacterial DNA in the blood of patients with sepsis and healthy volunteers using next-generation sequencing method - the observation of DNAemia. Eur J Clin Microbiol Infect Dis 2017;36:329–36.
[106] Simner PJ, Salzberg SL. The human 'contaminome' and understanding infectious disease. N Engl J Med 2022;387:943–6.
[107] Eisenhofer R, Minich JJ, Marotz C, et al. Contamination in low microbial biomass microbiome studies: issues and recommendations. Trends Microbiol 2019; 27:105–17.
[108] Salter SJ, Cox MJ, Turek EM, et al. Reagent and laboratory contamination can critically impact sequence-based microbiome analyses. BMC Biol 2014;12:87.
[109] Laurence M, Hatzis C, Brash DE. Common contaminants in next-generation sequencing that hinder discovery of low-abundance microbes. PLoS One 2014; 9:e97876.
[110] Chrisman B, He C, Jung JY, et al. The human 'contaminome': bacterial, viral, and computational contamination in whole genome sequences from 1000 families. Sci Rep 2022;12:9863.
[111] Price TK, Realegeno S, Mirasol R, et al. Validation, implementation, and clinical utility of whole genome sequence-based bacterial identification in the clinical microbiology laboratory. J Mol Diagn 2021;23: 1468–77.
[112] Kan C-M, Tsang HF, Pei XM, et al. Enhancing clinical utility: utilization of international standards and guidelines for metagenomic sequencing in infectious disease diagnosis. Int J Mol Sci 2024;25:3333.
[113] ISO - international organization for standardization. ISO Available at: 2025. https://www.iso.org/home.html (Accessed 20 May 2025).
[114] J Kralj, S Servetas, SP Forry, et al., Standards for metagenomics. NIST Available at: https://www.nist.gov/programs-projects/standards-metagenomics (Accessed 20 May 2025).
[115] Graf EH. We all know standardization is key, but how do we get there with clinical metagenomics? Clin Chem 2023;69:948–50.
[116] Gaston DC. Clinical metagenomics for infectious diseases: progress toward operational value. J Clin Microbiol 2023;61:e0126722.
[117] Markkanen MA, Haukka K, Pärnänen KMM, et al. Metagenomic analysis of the abundance and composition of antibiotic resistance genes in hospital wastewater in Benin, Burkina Faso, and Finland. mSphere 2023; 8:e0053822.
[118] Lott MEJ, Norfolk WA, Dailey CA, et al. Direct wastewater extraction as a simple and effective method for

SARS-CoV-2 surveillance and COVID-19 community-level monitoring. FEMS Microbes 2023;4:xtad004.

[119] Gliddon HD, Herberg JA, Levin M, et al. Genome-wide host RNA signatures of infectious diseases: discovery and clinical translation. Immunology (Oxf) 2018;153:171–8.

[120] Langelier C, Kalantar KL, Moazed F, et al. Integrating host response and unbiased microbe detection for lower respiratory tract infection diagnosis in critically ill adults. Proc Natl Acad Sci USA 2018;115:E12353–62.

[121] Bouquet J, Soloski MJ, Swei A, et al. Longitudinal transcriptome analysis reveals a sustained differential gene expression signature in patients treated for acute lyme disease. mBio 2016;7:e00100–16.

[122] Ramchandar N, Coufal NG, Warden AS, et al. Metagenomic next-generation sequencing for pathogen detection and transcriptomic analysis in pediatric central nervous system infections. Open Forum Infect Dis 2021;8:ofab104.

[123] UKHSA launches new metagenomic surveillance for health security. GOV.UK. Available at: https://www.gov.uk/government/news/ukhsa-launches-new-metagenomic-surveillance-for-health-security.

Advances in Molecular Pathology 8 (2025) 145–161
ADVANCES IN MOLECULAR PATHOLOGY

Molecular Detection of Antimicrobial Resistance Markers, Clinical Application, and Limitations

Drew T. Dickinson, PharmD, MPH[a], Dan Ilges, PharmD[a], Andrew Bryan, MD, PhD[b,*]
[a]Department of Pharmacy, Mayo Clinic Arizona, 5777 E Mayo Boulevard, Phoenix, AZ 85054, USA; [b]Department of Laboratory Medicine and Pathology, Mayo Clinic Arizona, 5777 E Mayo Boulevard, Phoenix, AZ 85054, USA

KEYWORDS
• Antimicrobial resistance • Molecular • Antimicrobial stewardship • Diagnostic stewardship
• Rapid molecular diagnostic testing • FDA-approved • mRDT

KEY POINTS

- Molecular detection of antimicrobial resistance determinants can inform both the escalation and de-escalation of antimicrobial therapy and the implementation of infection control measures.
- Detection of carbapenemase genes facilitates timely appropriate therapy compared to traditional susceptibility testing alone due to treatment differences based on specific resistance determinants.
- Blood cultures are the most common application of rapid molecular resistance panels and may reduce all-cause mortality, especially when paired with active stewardship.
- We recommend a multidisciplinary approach to implementing rapid molecular diagnostic testing that includes microbiology, antimicrobial stewardship/pharmacy, infectious diseases, infection prevention, and information technology.

INTRODUCTION

The combination of Food and Drug Administration (FDA)-approved rapid molecular assays and important pathogens with strong genotypic-phenotypic relationships to antimicrobial resistance has led to the current era of widespread adoption of molecular rapid diagnostic tests (mRDTs) for clinical use. This collective group of assays has the potential for significant medical impact with results in 1 to 3 hours compared to 1 to 3 days for most standard phenotypic susceptibility testing. Herein, we review the common molecular resistance determinants and commercial FDA-approved mRDTs, including practical aspects of implementation from laboratory, clinical/antimicrobial stewardship, and infection control perspectives to maximize impact.

FRAMEWORK FOR CLINICAL APPLICATION OF RAPID MOLECULAR DIAGNOSTICS

The goal of a clinical assay that aims to detect antimicrobial resistance is to improve patient outcomes or implement infection prevention and control measures. As mRDTs for diagnostic purposes must typically be followed by conventional phenotypic testing, the optimal indication for use narrows to when the turn-around-time is clinically relevant. We distill this into 3 categories: (1) escalation of therapy, (2) de-escalation of

*Corresponding author. *E-mail address:* Bryan.Andrew@mayo.edu

https://doi.org/10.1016/j.yamp.2025.07.002 www.advancesinmolecularpathology.com
2589-4080/25/ © 2025 Elsevier Inc. All rights are reserved, including those for text and data mining, AI training, and similar technologies.

ABBREVIATIONS	
CoNS	coagulase-negative staphylococci
CPE	carbapenemase-producing Enterobacterales
CRAB	carbapenem-resistant *Acinetobacter baumannii*
CRE	carbapenem-resistant Enterobacterales
CRPA	carbapenem-resistant *Pseudomonas aeruginosa*
ESBLs	extended-spectrum beta-lactamases
FDA	Food and Drug Administration
LIS	laboratory information system
MBLs	metallo-beta-lactamases
MDR	multidrug-resistant
mRDTs	molecular rapid diagnostic tests
MRSA	methicillin-resistant *Staphylococcus aureus*
PCR	polymerase chain reaction
ROI	return-on-investment

therapy, and/or (3) screening for resistance for infection control purposes (Table 1). Establishing a framework around the goals of these assays is critical to all phases of implementation, from performance verification to antimicrobial stewardship.

For an mRDT result to lead to escalation, the presence of the gene or allele must indicate resistance to empiric therapy. In most cases with current FDA-approved tests, this means the presence of a single gene/allele is adequate to indicate resistance, as methods to detect multifactorial resistance mechanisms are more challenging to design and validate. Institution-specific antibiograms and empiric therapy guides may aid front-line clinicians in decision-making and influence the impact of a mRDT. For example, detecting *CTX-M* from an Enterobacterales bloodstream isolate should lead to escalation from ceftriaxone to meropenem, but may not be particularly helpful for escalation in a patient with febrile neutropenia already empirically treated with meropenem. To maximize effectiveness, a test for escalation should be (1) straightforward to run and result, (2) have a clear and concise result in the electronic health record that is easily seen and interpreted by any clinician, (3) have an active push notification (phone or electronic) to the treating team, and (4) have clear institutional treatment guidance—all of these ideally available at all hours. Gaps in any one of these factors may reduce the utility of running the assay during off hours.

For a test to lead to de-escalation, the variables can be more complex and the treatment risk differs as there is the potential for narrowing to an ineffective agent if the genotype is not captured by the assay. While the factors important for escalation still apply, there may be additional emphasis on (1) microbiology/epidemiology, (2) test design and validation, (3) patient acuity, and (4) staffing of clinical expertise and confidence to de-escalate across shifts. First, the genotypic-phenotypic association must be strong with well-defined epidemiology. For example, not detecting *CTX-M* may be adequate to de-escalate an *Escherichia coli* bacteremia in some populations, but not in others that have high rates of non-*CTX-M* extended-spectrum beta-lactamases (ESBLs). Second, the test design must emphasize sensitivity and/or be performed only on cultures. For example, a nucleic acid amplification-based method is typically more sensitive than probe-based or array-based methods. Third and fourth, the patient acuity and clinical expertise and confidence: This is where the laboratory and patient-facing workflows, particularly antimicrobial stewardship, converge at the point of diagnostic stewardship at the individual patient level. That is, general treatment guidelines may be adequate for escalation, but a more detailed individual patient review by antimicrobial stewardship may be necessary to confidently de-escalate. As such, staffing the laboratory to run the test on night shift may facilitate escalation, but may not make a patient impact for de-escalation if adequate clinical expertise is not available. Lastly, because mRDTs are not entirely comprehensive in their ability to detect resistance, there must be robust workflows to follow conventional phenotypic testing results.

The last bin of direct of mRDT resistance applications we address are screening tests for infection prevention and control (eg, contact precautions). Certain tests, such as screening the nares for methicillin-resistant *Staphylococcus aureus* (MRSA), may be deployed concurrently to consider de-escalation of empiric anti-MRSA therapy for pneumonia and assess for the need of contact precautions. Even if the same test can be used both therapeutically and for infection control precautions, it can be useful to cognitively separate these 2 different applications. In this MRSA example, and assuming empiric vancomycin coverage, the medically actionable result is either the negative result (de-escalation) or the positive result (contact precautions). Similarly, the care team members taking the action are different: The treating team or antimicrobial stewardship for de-escalation versus the patient's nurse or infection control. These different patient-facing workflows may dictate different resulting and reporting workflows

TABLE 1
Example Impact of Test Result

Resistance Determinant	Host Organism(s)	Notable Phenotypic Resistance	Example Escalation (Pos Result)	Example De-escalation (Neg Result)	Infection Control
mecA	*Staphylococcus* spp	Beta-lactam (except ceftaroline and ceftobiprole)	Start/continue vancomycin	Discontinue vancomycin; Start cefazolin or antistaphylococcal penicillin	Contact precautions, current admission
vanA/B	*E faecium*, *E faecalis*	Vancomycin	Switch to daptomycin	Continue vancomycin for *E faecium*/de-escalate to ampicillin for *E faecalis*	
CTX-M	Enterobacterales	Third-generation cephalosporins; variable in vitro resistance to piperacillin-tazobactam and cefepime	Escalate to meropenem	Continue cefepime (organism high-risk for AmpC[a]) or de-escalate to ceftriaxone (low-risk for AmpC), assuming known epidemiology and low incidence of non-*CTX-M* ESBLs	
KPC	Enterobacterales; rarely *P aeruginosa* and *A baumanni* complex	Penicillins, cephalosporins, carbapenems, and aztreonam	Escalate to meropenem-vaborbactam		Contact precautions, current and potentially future admission(s)
NDM IMP VIM		Penicillins, cephalosporins, carbapenems, ceftazidime-avibactam, meropenem-vaborbactam, and imipenem-relebactam	Escalate to ceftazidime-avibactam plus aztreonam or cefiderocol		
OXA-48		Penicillins, cephalosporins, carbapenems, aztreonam, meropenem-vaborbactam, and imipenem-relebactam	Escalate to ceftazidime-avibactam		

Actions assume patient is on vancomycin and either piperacillin-tazobactam or cefepime for blood stream infection.

Abbreviations: CPE, carbapenemase producing Enterobacterales; CRE, carbapenem-resistant Enterobacterales; ESBL, extended-spectrum beta-lactamase.

[a] Organisms high-risk for clinically significant expression of AmpC: *Enterobacter cloacae* complex, *Klebsiella aerogenes*, *Citrobacter freundii*, ± *Hafnia alvei*.

from the laboratory. Whereas the tendency from the laboratory is to emphasize positive results, it may be the negative result that is actionable for treatment purposes.

Another distinction between tests intended to manage an individual patient versus infection control becomes apparent when considering the interplay of test sensitivity, cost, and pretest probability. Implementing a costly higher sensitivity test for only the high-risk patients may be preferred. However, when the pretest probability based on screening questions or patient history is less apparent, a cheaper and less-sensitive test that could be deployed for all admissions may be more cost-effective and identify a greater number of patients across an institution.

Herein, we dive into the specific resistance determinants most widely available on FDA-approved test systems, which include *mecA*, *vanA/B*, *CTX-M*, and the "big 5" carbapenemases (KPC, NDM, VIM, IMP, and OXA). We also consider *rpoB* for rifampin resistance in *Mycobacterium tuberculosis* in the respiratory section.

SPECIFIC RESISTANCE DETERMINANTS

mecA/C

Current mRDTs typically detect methicillin (oxacillin) resistance through the presence of the *mecA* gene from the staphylococcal cassette chromosome *mec* element (SCC*mec*). Some assays also detect *mecC*. The SCC*mec* cassette encodes for the altered penicillin-binding protein, PBP2a, which has reduced binding affinity for beta-lactam antibiotics, thereby conferring resistance to all beta-lactam apart from ceftaroline and ceftobiprole. The clinical relevance of methicillin resistance relies on the staphylococcal species detected. Coagulase-negative staphylococci (CoNS) demonstrate a high rate of oxacillin resistance, but in contrast to *S aureus* and *Staphylococcus lugdunensis*, their detection often represents contamination in specimen collection [1,2]. When *mecA/C* is detected in pathogenic staphylococci, therapy is often escalated to include highly active empiric agents such as vancomycin, daptomycin, or linezolid. Given a strong genotypic-phenotypic relationship, in the absence of molecular detection of *mecA/C*, therapy can often be de-escalated or adjusted to optimally target *methicillin-susceptible staphylococcus aureus* (MSSA) [3].

A diagnostic challenge and risk of false-positive MRSA result can occur by 2 main mechanisms: (1) drop-out mutants of *mecA* from the SCC*mec* cassette and (2) polymicrobial samples with MSSA and oxacillin-resistant CoNS. To limit false-positives from drop-out mutants, most assays have incorporated separate targets for *mecA* and the SSC*mec* cassette. To address polymicrobial samples, methods have been developed to differentiate *mecA* in *S aureus* from CoNS by the detection of a SCC*mec* target where it has integrated into the *S aureus* chromosome [4]. The *SCCmec* cassette integrates at the *attB* site of the *S aureus* chromosome at the 3′ end of *rlmH* (formerly *orfX*), the so-called right extremity junction (MREJ) [5]. While the performance of proprietary primers and terminology may vary by vendor (MREJ, SCC*mec-orfX*, detection of SCC*mec* at *attB*, and so forth), the intent is as mentioned earlier, to limit false-positive MRSA results. Although uncommon, even assays with multiple targets could result in phenotypic mismatch if the MSSA isolate has a drop-out mutant of SSC*mec* concomitant with oxacillin-resistant CoNS [4].

vanA/B

Nearly one-third of all health care–associated enterococcal infections are resistant to vancomycin [6]. In the United States, the majority of vancomycin-resistant enterococci are *Enterococcus faecium*, containing a mobile genetic element with *vanA* and less commonly *vanB* [7]. Rarely, *Enterococcus faecalis* can contain both *vanA/B*. *Enterococcus casseliflavus* and *Enterococcus gallinarum* display chromosomally-mediated vancomycin resistance through *vanC*. The resulting action upon detection of *vanA or vanB* from a clinical isolate depends on the infecting pathogen, specimen source, and patient acuity. The detection of *vanA/B* in conjunction with *E faecium* from a sterile site often necessitates escalation of therapy to include daptomycin, linezolid, or a glycylcycline as these agents are unaffected by the cell wall modifications mediated by *vanA/B*. The lack of detection of *vanA/B* in conjunction with *E faecium* allows for vancomycin use until phenotypic confirmation of susceptibility. The detection of *vanA/B* within *E faecalis* is often not clinically actionable as therapy can be narrowed to an aminopenicillin since nearly all *E faecalis* isolates are susceptible to ampicillin according to the SENTRY Antimicrobial Surveillance Program (https://sentry-mvp.jmilabs.com/).

CTX-M

The detection of *CTX-M* generally means escalation of therapy to a carbapenem for severe infections or use of non–beta-lactam agents appropriate for the infection [8]. De-escalation of therapy when *CTX-M* is not detected comes with higher risk, as it depends on the local epidemiology and the patient's acuity. To unpack this, a primer on ESBLs is helpful. ESBLs are a heterogenous group of enzymes classically characterized by their ability to hydrolyze extended-spectrum cephalosporins (eg, ceftriaxone) and monobactams (eg, aztreonam), but not carbapenems or cephamycins (eg, cefotetan) and are inhibited by clavulanate in vitro [9,10]. *CTX-M* variants are currently the most widely distributed genetic mechanism, although ESBLs were originally described as variants of TEM and SHV [9,11]. Other less common ESBLs include GES, PER, VEB, while some OXA beta-lactamases (Ambler class D) can display similar phenotypes to ESBLs [9,10]. Clinically, the term ESBL typically refers to these enzymes in Enterobacterales, although they can occur in *Pseudomonas* and *Acinetobacter*. In vitro phenotypic antimicrobial susceptibility testing yields variable rates of resistance to cefepime and piperacillin-tazobactam, but various evidence suggests worse outcomes to these agents compared to treatment with a carbapenem [8,12–14]. Guidelines generally suggest treatment of ESBL Enterobacterales with a carbapenem for severe infections outside of the urinary tract [8].

Carbapenemases (KPC, IMP, VIM, NDM, and OXA)

Carbapenem resistance represents a critically important world health problem and can result in dismal patient outcomes if not rapidly identified and appropriately managed [15,16]. Carbapenemases are beta-lactamases that catalyze carbapenems, thereby conferring phenotypic resistance to carbapenems and most other traditional beta-lactam [17]. Thus, the detection of carbapenemases in true pathogens nearly always necessitates escalation of both antibiotic therapy and infection control measures. Molecular detection of carbapenemases is of most importance in carbapenem-resistant Enterobacterales (CRE), carbapenem-resistant *Pseudomonas aeruginosa* (CRPA), and carbapenem-resistant *Acinetobacter baumannii* (CRAB) [8]. Carbapenem resistance is complex, with wide epidemiologic variability in the proportion of carbapenem-resistant isolates possessing a carbapenemase, which is dependent on the specific organism/organism group and region. While the molecular detection of a carbapenemase gene rules in carbapenem resistance with high specificity and therefore can inform escalation practices, the absence of carbapenemase gene detection does not rule out carbapenem resistance.

In the United States, carbapenemase detection in CRPA is rare (~2%) as most carbapenem resistance in *P aeruginosa* is not enzymatically mediated, although the rate of carbapenemase detection in CRPA in certain regions of the world is as high as 67% [18,19]. Carbapenem resistance in CRAB is complex; however, OXA carbapenemases (eg, OXA-23-like, OXA-24/40-like, and OXA-58-like) are the most common determinants of carbapenem resistance [20,21]. Depending on local epidemiology, the detection of *A baumanii* complex, even without resistance determinants, can be sufficient to change therapy, as nearly half of *A baumanii* complex isolates in the United States are carbapenem resistant [22]. Overall, Enterobacterales are most relevant to the discussion of carbapenemases in the United States. CRE are defined as having resistance to at least one carbapenem antibiotic or producing a carbapenemase enzyme and are categorized as either carbapenemase-producing Enterobacterales (CPE) or non–carbapenemase-producing Enterobacterales [8]. Approximately 35% to 85% of CRE in the United States are carbapenemase-producing, and the overall incidence of CRE is increasing [23,24].

Detection of specific carbapenemase determinants, whether genotypic or phenotypic, is superior to generic phenotypic tests that just detect carbapenem inactivation (eg, modified carbapenem inactivation method) as treatment regimens vary by specific carbapenemases (see Table 1). New laboratory guidance is included in the 2025 CLSI M100 35th Edition [25]. For example, meropenem-vaborbactam or ceftazidime-avibactam is effective for treating KPC-producing isolates but ineffective against metallo-beta-lactamases (MBLs). While historically KPC has been the predominant carbapenemase in the United States, recent epidemiologic data suggest that the incidence of MBLs, and NDM in particular, is increasing, with some regions of the United States now recognized as endemic for NDM [24]. Ideally, notification of detection should be paired with treatment recommendations tailored to the specific enzyme detected and informed by current recommendations [8]. An example of our institutional antimicrobial stewardship recommendations for molecular detection of carbapenemases and other resistance determinants in bloodstream isolates is included in Fig. 1. The full guidance document is included in the supplementary information (Appendix 1).

When No Specific Resistance Determinants Are Detected

In many instances, mRDT platforms will identify bacteria in the absence of specific molecular determinants for resistance. As noted earlier, the ability to which these negative results can rule out resistance varies by species and target. For this reason, de-escalation recommendations should be performed by individuals

If any of the following resistance genes are detected with any of the organisms listed above, refer to the following recommendations:.

****When there are multiple resistance targets detected, select regimen with broadest coverage (i.e., the lowest detected option on this table)****

Resistance Gene	Preferred Therapy[a]	Comments
Gram-Negative Resistance Genes (apply to any gram-negative organism listed above)		
CTX-M (only)	Ertapenem 1g IV q24h or Meropenem 1-2g IV q8h (if critically ill in the ICU)	Marker for most common extended-spectrum beta-lactamase (ESBL) found in gram-negative pathogens; meropenem should be recommended for critically ill patients in the ICU. Cefepime and piperacillin/tazobactam are NOT appropriate.
KPC	Meropenem/vaborbactam 4g IV q8h	**RECOMMEND ID CONSULT. Indicates carbapenem resistance.** Alternative: ceftazidime/avibactam 2.5g IV q8h
OXA-48-like	Ceftazidime/avibactam 2.5g IV q8h	**RECOMMEND ID CONSULT. Indicates carbapenem resistance.**
IMP	Ceftazidime/avibactam 2.5g IV q8h (infused over 3 hours) PLUS aztreonam 2g IV q8h (infused over 3 hours)	**RECOMMEND ID CONSULT. Indicates carbapenem resistance.** Schedule both agents simultaneously. Use NDM order panel. They are Y-site compatible.
NDM	Ceftazidime/avibactam 2.5g IV q8h (infused over 3 hours) PLUS aztreonam 2g IV q8h (infused over 3 hours)	**RECOMMEND ID CONSULT. Indicates carbapenem resistance.** Schedule both agents simultaneously. Use NDM order panel. They are Y-site compatible.
VIM	Ceftazidime/avibactam 2.5g IV q8h (infused over 3 hours) PLUS aztreonam 2g IV q8h (infused over 3 hours)	**RECOMMEND ID CONSULT. Indicates carbapenem resistance.** Schedule both agents simultaneously. Use NDM order panel. They are Y-site compatible.

FIG. 1 Example excerpt from institutional guidance for rapid blood culture diagnostics for gram-negative resistance determinants. The document provides clear direction to pharmacists to reference when acting on blood culture PCR results 24/7. The document is updated as needed by a multidisciplinary team and is located in a shared drive for pharmacy services. The full document is available in the supplementary materials (Appendix 1). [a]All doses are based on normal renal function; some doses may need adjustment for augmented renal clearance.

trained in infectious diseases and/or antimicrobial stewardship and who have a firm understanding of institutional epidemiology or in accordance with an updated institutional guidance document. Additionally, there are several instances for which detection of the species alone will be sufficient to warrant early change in therapy. Examples of this include narrowing to ampicillin with the detection of *Enterococcus faecalis* (regardless of detection of *vanA/B*, as mentioned earlier) or escalating to trimethoprim/sulfamethoxazole and/or cefiderocol with the detection of *Stenotrophomonas maltophilia*.

BLOOD CULTURE TEST SYSTEMS

Rapid molecular assays for positive blood cultures are the most common applications for these test systems due to the clear potential for patient impact and marketability. However, the road to successful impact on medical decision-making, that is, escalation or de-escalation of therapy, is often murkier and relies on a number of factors as outlined earlier. Despite the allure of a rapid blood culture diagnostic, minimal patient impact may be observed without thoughtful implementation within a stewardship framework [26].

Patient population and epidemiology, as foundational factors to consider when implementing mRDT panels, were discussed earlier in the framework and resistance determinant sections; however, they may interplay with which available test system has the potential for the greatest impact at a given institution. Three of the most common currently available multianalyte panels with FDA approval include the Biofire BCID2, cobas ePlex BCID (GP and GN), and Verigene (GP and GN; Table 2). Cobas and Verigene split their panels between gram-negative and gram-positive, creating more reliance on the Gram stain. Lumping GP and GN together, the number of organism targets vary between systems, with the ePlex having the most targets and Verigene the fewest. Additional panels include offerings from iCubate and more targeted *S aureus*/MRSA assays from Cepheid and Great Basin Scientific. While this review is focused on the resistance determinants, the full list of pathogens included on each panel is also critical to review for escalation and de-escalation of therapy, for example, *S maltophilia*, which may be particularly pertinent for a hospital with cystic fibrosis and bone marrow transplant units. Each panel's included organism targets also become important to understand the reporting of resistance targets, since resistance determinants are only reported if there is a corresponding organism genus or species target detected.

As we examine the distinctions between molecular resistance determinants across panels, a few themes appear. First is the earlier issue of requiring specific organism genus or species targets for reporting of resistance, with some nuances between manufacturers. For example, both the ePlex gram-positive panel and Biofire FilmArray include genus-level targets for *Staphylococcus*,

TABLE 2
Rapid Molecular Blood Culture Diagnostics

		Resistance Determinants						
Panel	**Manufacturer**	**Staphylococci**	**Enterococci**	**Enterobacterales**	***P aeruginosa***	***A baumanii* Complex**	**Analytical Turn-Around-Time**	**FDA Submission**
Biofire BCID2	Biomerieux (formerly Biofire)	mecA/C and MREJ: S. aureus, *S epidermidis*, *S lugdunensis* only.	vanA/B: *E faecium* and *E faecalis* only	*CTX-M*, KPC, NDM, VIM, IMP, OXA-48-like: Any Enterobacterales detected. mcr-1 for limited species[a]	*CTX-M*, KPC, NDM, VIM, and IMP		~1 h	K193519 and K243759
cobas ePlex BCID-GP	Roche (formerly GenMark)	mecA, mecC: Any *Staphylococcus* spp	vanA, vanB: Any *Enterococcus* spp	—	—	—	~1.5 h	K181663
cobas ePlex BCID-GN	Roche (formerly GenMark)	—	—	*CTX-M*, KPC, NDM, VIM, IMP, OXA (OXA-23/48)[b]			~1.5 h	K213236 and K182619
Verigene gram-positive	Diasorin (formerly Nanosphere, Luminex)	mecA: *S aureus*, *S epidermidis*, *S lugdunensis* only.	vanA, vanB: *E faecium* only.	—	—	—	~2 h	K122514
Verigene gram-negative	Diasorin (formerly Nanosphere, Luminex)		—	*CTX-M*, KPC, NDM, VIM, IMP, OXA: *E coli*, K pneumoniae, *Klebsiella oxytoca* only	—	—	~2 h	K132843
iC-GPC	iCubate	mecA: *S aureus* and *S epidermidis* only	vanA/B: *E faecium* and *E faecalis* only	—	—	—	~2 h	K163390/ S001

(continued on next page)

TABLE 2
(continued)

		Resistance Determinants						
Panel	**Manufacturer**	**Staphylococci**	**Enterococci**	**Enterobacterales**	***P aeruginosa***	***A baumanii* Complex**	**Analytical Turn-Around-Time**	**FDA Submission**
iC-GN	iCubate	—	—	*CTX-M* group 1, KPC, NDM: *E cloacae* complex, *E coli*, *K oxytoca*, *K pneumoniae*, *Proteus* spp, *Serratia marcescens*	*CTX-M* group 1y, KPC, NDM		~2 h	K190341
Xpert MRSA/SA blood culture	Cepheid	mecA: *S aureus* only	—	—	—	—	~1 h	K190771
VERIGENE Staphylococcus Blood Culture Nucleic Acid Test (BC-S)	Diasorin (formerly Nanosphere, Luminex)		—	—	—	—	—	K112424
Staph ID/R blood culture	Great Basin Scientific	mecA: Any *Staphylococcus* spp	—	—	—	—	~1 h	K152470/ S001

mecA/C, vanA/B, and OXA-23/48 imply reported as single target. mecA, mecC and vanA, vanB imply separately reported targets.

[a] Reported for *E cloacae* complex, *E coli*, *K aerogenes*, *K oxytoca*, *K pneumoniae* group, *Salmonella* spp.

[b] Reported for *A baumanni*, *Citrobacter* spp, *E cloacae* complex, *Enterobacter* spp, *E coli*, *K oxytoca*, *K pneumoniae* group, *Morganella morganii*, *Proteus* spp, *P mirabilis*, *Salmonella*, *Serratia* spp, and *S marcescens*. Only KPC reported for *Cronobacter sakazakii* and only *CTX-M* reported for *S maltophilia*.

but only the ePlex will report *mecA/C* if that is the only organism target detected (Biofire requires *S aureus*, *S lugdunensis*, or *Staphylococcus epidermidis*). Thus, the ePlex could theoretically report *mecA/C* on *Staphylococcus hominis* (reported as *Staphylococcus* species), but not the Biofire. Inversely, for the gram-negatives, only the Biofire FilmArray panel includes an Order-level Enterobacterales target. A *CTX-M* from a *Providencia stuartii*, which does not have its own discrete target, could potentially be reported on the Biofire as an Enterobacterales, but not on the ePlex. The clinical significance of these distinctions may depend on institutional guidance for CoNS or the frequency of less commonly encountered Enterobacterales.

Two other distinctions between panels arise related to how the resistance markers are methodologically detected. For staphylococci, the Biofire FilmArray harnesses MREJ with the *mecA/C* and organism targets to help determine if *mecA/C* is associated with *S aureus* or not; this is particularly helpful in mixed staphylococcal populations. For the enterococci, the Verigene and ePlex distinguish between *vanA* and *vanB*, while the Biofire reports them as a combined target. This is primarily relevant when therapy with dalbavancin or telavancin are being considered, as these agents are primarily effective against the less-common *vanB*-mediated resistance [27].

Mixed populations present at least some challenges for most assays [28–32]. With the exception of MREJ, most molecular assays are unable to attribute a resistance determinant to a specific species if it is detected concurrently with 2 organisms on a panel. A second issue for mixed populations is technical sensitivity. Overall, the amplification effect of in vitro growth in a blood culture bottle mitigates subtle differences in technical sensitivity for monomicrobial cultures. However, for mixed populations with a minor population of a resistance determinant, array-based technologies (eg, Verigene) may be less sensitive than amplification-based technologies. The polymerase chain reaction (PCR)-based assays are not immune to the challenges of mixed populations, however, and both the ePlex and Biofire package inserts disclaim they may not identify all organisms in mixed cultures. It may not be practical for manufacturers or individual laboratories to evaluate every organism-determinant combination in a range of different dilutions given the relative sensitivity of the assays and low numbers of mixed cultures in most populations. Extensive head-to-head comparisons of mixed populations are scant, and laboratories may choose to educate or add disclaimers relating to reduced sensitivity for mixed bacterial populations.

Beyond the earlier microbiologic/technical distinctions, some differences in analytical turn-around-time exist (see Table 2), although they are small compared to the larger gains of traditional phenotypic methods. The cumulative impact of analytical time, ease of setup of each system, staffing, and the laboratory information system (LIS) build can impact the ability to run a test on all shifts.

A key component to 24/7 reporting is the LIS build, including building all or most organism-determinant combinations, appropriate comments, and interface to the electronic health record (EHR) [33]. The time required for such a build is often a significant investment but may make the difference in the clinical utility. The resource return-on-investment (ROI) may also differ whether a given result is primarily used for escalation of therapy (likely to occur on all shifts) versus de-escalation of therapy, which may only occur during the day when primary teams, infectious disease, and antimicrobial stewardship/pharmacy are more fully staffed. For the test systems that split targets between panels, the complexities of the builds and ROI for medical impact may differ between gram-positive and gram-negative organisms. The decision to build the rapid molecular result incorporated into the blood culture workup in the microbiology module of an LIS versus a separate build within a general laboratory module should be deliberate. LIS systems and their interface to the EHR may vary, but building and reporting the molecular result within the original blood culture can optimize the ability to integrate the final culture result with the rapid diagnostic. In contrast, building and reporting the rapid molecular result as a separate test in a general LIS module could facilitate programmatic reporting rules, interfacing, and flags or push notifications, as well as enhance visibility within the medical record. See Fig. 2 and supplemental information (Appendix 1), for example, reports in the EHR.

It is also important to acknowledge the practicalities of laboratory/hospital resources, space constraints, and existing capital equipment may outweigh both the microbiologic and workflow distinctions between the assays. Administrative/budgetary leadership buy-in is key, given the reagent costs of these diagnostics primarily performed in the inpatient setting under capitated diagnosis-related group billing. Several vendors offer limited panels primarily for the detection of MRSA/MSSA for laboratories unable to bring on the larger panels (see Table 2). Diagnostic stewardship of blood culture orders, monitoring contamination rates, and careful reflexive rules of when to perform the molecular tests may reduce waste [34,35]. For example, only

Blood Culture Supplemental PCR (Anaerobic Bottle) Order: 2222005521756

Collected **3/22/2024 22:02** Status: **Final result**

Test Result Released: **No (inaccessible in Patient Online Services)**

Component Ref Range & Units	
Specimen Source	Blood Culture
Enterobacterales Undetected	**Detected !**
Klebsiella aerogenes Undetected	**Detected !**
OXA-48-like Undetected	**Detected !**
Interpretation	Presumptive Klebsiella aerogenes. Presumptive carbapenemase-producing organism. Likely resistant to penicillins, cephalosporins, and carbapenems.

Comment:
----ADDITIONAL INFORMATION----
Test is considered supplemental, always refer to standard blood culture results. Not all species, strains, or variants of the below targets may be detected (rare). Additional organisms and/or resistance determinants may be present and not detected or distinguished by this assay. Panel includes: 11 targets for Gram-positive bacteria (Enterococcus faecalis, E. faecium, Listeria monocytogenes, Staphylococcus aureus, S. epidermidis, S. lugdunensis, Staphylococcus (other, genus-only ID), Streptococcus agalactiae, S. pneumoniae, S. pyogenes, Streptococcus (other, genus-only ID)); 15 targets for Gram-negative bacteria (includes Acinetobacter calcoaceticus-baumannii complex, Bacteroides fragilis, Haemophilus influenzae, Neisseria meningitidis (encapsulated), Pseudomonas aeruginosa, Stenotrophomonas maltophilia, Enterobacter cloacae complex, Escherichia coli, Klebsiella aerogenes, Klebsiella oxytoca, Klebsiella pneumoniae group, Proteus spp., Salmonella spp., Serratia marcescens, Bacteria of the Order Enterobacterales (not otherwise determined)); 7 targets for yeast (Candida albicans, Candida auris, Candida glabrata, Candida krusei, Candida parapsilosis, Candida tropicalis, Cryptococcus neoformans/gattii); and 10 antimicrobial resistance determinants (mecA/C, mecA/C and MREJ, vanA/B, KPC, CTX-M, IMP, mcr-1, VIM, NDM, OXA-48-like).

FIG. 2 Example result of an interfaced blood culture mRDT in the EHR based on rules built in the laboratory information system. No manual reporting is required, facilitating 24/7 reporting of complicated results and comments, as well as push notifications to a pharmacist-monitored inbox. Suppression of targets that are not detected reduce the noise in the EHR, while an integrative interpretation of the targets detected is provided. In this example, the OXA-48 target detection supersedes an AmpC comment, which would be appended if no other resistance determinants were detected. Additional screenshots are provided in the supplementary materials (Appendix 1). (© 2024 Epic Systems Corporation.)

performing the mRDT when time-to-positivity is less than 48 hours (less likely contaminant) and Gram stain morphology is compatible with on-panel organisms could reduce resource consumption.

The implementation of mRDTs in patients with bloodstream infections has been shown to decrease mortality risk, reduce length of stay, shorten time to effective therapy, and even reduce health care costs [16,36–40]. Thoughtful implementation, however, including automated routing and reporting, ideally with real-time prospective audit and feedback, is critical to harnessing the greatest impact from these panels. Indeed, a recent meta-analysis found that while mRDTs for bloodstream infections improved mortality overall with a number needed to treat of 20, the impact was more pronounced in studies with an active antimicrobial stewardship component. The subanalysis of studies without active stewardship intervention failed to show a statistically significant difference in mortality [39]. Among 9 included studies with the relevant data, time to effective therapy was found to be significantly shorter by a mean difference of −5.03 hours (95% confidence interval, −8.60 to −1.45 hours) with rapid molecular diagnostics compared to conventional microbiology. Lastly, hospital length of stay was shown to be shorter by −2.48 day (95% CI, −3.90 to −1.06 days) [39]. Less understood is the impact that these panels have on antibiotic de-escalation practices, although data suggest that time to first de-escalation is not reduced without active intervention [41].

Given the potential benefit of these tests on critical patient outcomes, antimicrobial stewardship programs should help laboratories advocate for the use of rapid diagnostic testing on blood specimens, as recommended by the Infectious Diseases Society of America (IDSA) antimicrobial stewardship guidelines [42]. Consistent with the Centers for Disease Control and Prevention (CDC)'s Core Elements of Hospital Diagnostic Excellence, we advocate for a team-based approach to selecting and operationalizing these tests, ideally with representation from microbiology, antimicrobial stewardship/pharmacy, infectious diseases, information technology, and infection control [43].

LOWER RESPIRATORY TRACT TEST SYSTEMS

The antimicrobial resistance determinants on mRDT for lower respiratory tract specimens largely follow those available on blood culture systems, with some additions. The Curetis Unyvero Lower Respiratory Tract and bronchoalveolar lavage (BAL) panels include additional OXA targets in *A baumanii* complex, plus *tem* in *Haemophilus influenzae*, and the Cepheid Xpert MTB/RIF assay includes rifampin resistance in *M tuberculosis* (Table 3). Technically, the sensitivity of these panels becomes more important since they cannot rely on the in vitro amplification in a blood culture bottle. The variable dilution of a bronchoalveolar lavage and the potential for polymicrobial specimens, including oropharyngeal contamination, further make these specimens a more challenging analyte. The INHALE study compared a Conformité Européenne - In Vitro Diagnostic-marked Curetis panel (similar, but with additional resistance markers) to the Biofire assay, finding slightly more variable sensitivity of organism target detection in the Unyvero panel relative to Biofire [44]. The performance assessment of the 2 panels for antimicrobial resistance was more complicated, however, given heterogenous resistance mechanisms among gram-negative organisms and presumed higher sensitivity of the PCR assays relative to respiratory culture [44].

Several randomized trials investigating rapid multiplex lower respiratory tract PCR panels compared to standard culture have found improvement in escalation practices and pathogen-directed treatment with the use of PCR [45–48]. Median time-to-escalation has been reported as low as 14 hours from specimen collection [45]. Data on de-escalation are mixed. In spite of active stewardship in conjunction with PCR results, Virk and colleagues [45] detected no improvement in de-escalation with PCR whereas Darie and colleagues [48] found reductions in inappropriate antibiotic therapy with the use of static treatment guidance based on PCR result. The degree of stewardship likely influences the time to de-escalation, which varies between 20 and 48 hours in the literature [45,47,48]. No distinct survival or clinical benefit has been observed with mRDT use compared to conventional culture in the studies reviewed. The available data are heterogenous in terms of study populations, molecular test implemented, and degree of antimicrobial stewardship. Importantly, the detection of resistance markers was infrequent and often not reported in these published studies. Therefore, the effect of mRDTs for resistance determinants on lower respiratory specimens, or "pneumonia panels," on antimicrobial stewardship and patient outcomes remains uncertain.

The Xpert MTB/RIF assay differs from most of the other assays in this review not only in terms of the pathogen but also in the approach to the detection of resistance. Whole genome sequencing has facilitated genotypic-phenotypic correlates of resistance

TABLE 3
Rapid Molecular Lower Respiratory Tract Diagnostics

Panel	Manufacturer	Specimens	Resistance Determinants: Staphylococci	Resistance Determinants: Enterobacterales	Resistance Determinants: *P aeruginosa*	Resistance Determinants: *A baumanii* Complex	Resistance Determinants: *M tuberculosis* Complex	Analytical Turn-Around-Time	FDA Submission
Biofire FilmArray Pneumonia Panel	Biomerieux (formerly Biofire)	Sputum-like specimens (induced or expectorated sputum, endotracheal aspirates), BAL/mini-BAL	mecA/C and MREJ: *S aureus* only	*CTX-M*, KPC, NDM, VIM, IMP, OXA-48-like: Among 7 Enterobacterales species[a]	*CTX-M*, KPC, NDM, VIM, IMP		—	~1 h	K180966, K212727, and K243222
Unyvero Lower Respiratory Tract (LRT)/ Unyvero Lower Respiratory Tract (LRT) BAL	Curetis GmbH[b]	RLT: Tracheal aspirate/RLT BAL: BAL, mini-BAL	mecA: *S aureus* only	*CTX-M* (subgroup 1), KPC, NDM, VIM, IMP, OXA-48-like: Among 9 Enterobacterales species[c]	*CTX-M* (subgroup 1), KPC, NDM, and VIM	*CTX-M* (subgroup 1), KPC, NDM, OXA-23, OXA-24, OXA-48, OXA-58, and VIM	—	~4.5 h	DEN170047 and K191967
Xpert MTB/RIF	Cepheid	"Raw" sputum or processed/ concentrated sputum sediment (induced or expectorated)	—				*Rifampin-resistance region of rpoB*	~2 h	K131706

[a] Includes *E cloacae* complex, *E coli*, *K aerogenes*, *K oxytoca*, *K pneumoniae* group, *Proteus* spp, and *S marcescens*.
[b] Panel also includes tem for *H influenzae*. *Acinetobacter* targets includes additional species other than *A baumannii/calcoaceticus* complex.
[c] Includes *C freundii, E cloacae* complex, *E coli, K oxytoca, K pneumoniae*, *K variicola*, *M morganii*, *Proteus* spp, and *S marcescens*.

TABLE 4
Rapid Molecular Diagnostics: Swabs and Isolates

Panel	Manufacturer	Target	Specimen	Analytical Turn-Around-Time	FDA Submission
BD MAX MRSA XT	BD	mecA/C, SCCmec-MREJ	Nasal swab	~ 3 h (batched)	K120138
BD MAX STAPHSR	BD	mecA/C, SCCmec-MREJ, *S aureus* (nuc)	Nasal swab	~ 3 h (batched)	K071026
Xpert Carba-R	Cepheid	*CTX-M*, KPC, NDM, VIM, IMP, and OXA-48-like	1. Enterobacteriaceae, *A baumannii* complex, or *P aeruginosa* colonies, 2. Rectal and perirectal swabs	~50 min	K152614/S001, K160901, and K173263
Xpert MRSA/SA SSTI	Cepheid	*S aureus (spa), mecA, SCCmec at attB*	Skin and soft tissue infection swab	—	K080837 and K243625
Xpert MRSA NxG	Cepheid	*mecA/C, SCCmec at attB*	Nasal swab	~45 min	K162444
Xpert SA Nasal Complete	Cepheid	*S aureus (spa), mecA, SCCmec at attB*	Nasal swab	~60 min	K100822
Xpert vanA	Cepheid	*vanA*	Rectal swab	~50 min	K092953 and K243405
cobas MRSA/SA (4800 system)	Roche	*S aureus, SCCmec-MREJ*	Nasal swab	~ Hours	K142721
LightCycler MRSA Advanced Test	Roche	SCCmec-orfX	Nasal swab	~ 2 h (batched)	K091409
IMDx VanR for Abbott m2000	Intelligent Medical Devices, Inc.	*vanA, vanB*	Perirectal or rectal swab and stool	~ 3 h (batched)	K123753
BD GeneOhm VanR Assay	BD Diagnostics (GeneOhm Sciences, Inc.)	*vanA, vanB*	Perianal or rectal swabs	~ Hours	K102416
IDI-MRSA Assay	Infectio Diagnostic, Inc.	SCCmec-orfX	Nasal swab	~ Hours	K042357 and K033415
MECA XPRESSFISH	ADVANDX INC.	mecA mRNA	Smears of *S aureus* from blood cultures	~ Hours	K140619

Turn-around times listed as "Hours" indicates less well-documented timing, partially batched, and/or workflow-dependent.

in *M tuberculosis* complex, but this technology is neither yet feasible for a rapid cost-effective diagnostic from a primary specimen nor available as an FDA-approved test on isolates. Targeted assays for multiple resistance targets, including isoniazid, are beginning to be available, but these assays are not FDA-approved. The RNA polymerase gene, *rpoB*, offers both conserved regions for primer binding sites and well-characterized mutations that correlate with rifampin resistance. This facilitates a PCR-based mRDT that then uses 5 different fluorophore-labeled probes to identify mutations within the rifampin-resistance determining region. Rifampin resistance can also be a surrogate for multidrug-resistant (MDR) *M tuberculosis*. Numerous studies and systematic reviews have evaluated the test performance, including a 2019 Cochrane review reporting a pooled sensitivity and specificity for the detection of rifampin resistance of 96% (94–97) and 98% (98–99), respectively [49]. Despite the strong performance characteristics for the detection of rifampin resistance, in regions with low incidence of MDR TB, careful consideration of the positive predictive value is prudent prior to altering therapy from first-line agents.

BONE AND JOINT-RELATED SPECIMENS

A single FDA-approved test system for bone and joint-related specimens is available at the time of this publication, the BioMérieux BIOFIRE Joint Infection (JI) Panel (FDA submission DEN200066). The resistance determinants included are the same as Biofire's other test offerings. Most pertinent to this specimen type is the detection of *mecA*, particularly for MRSA and *S lugdunensis*, although there is little evidence to support the added value of the panel compared to culture specifically for the detection of resistance [50,51]. The detection of the other resistance determinants on the panel (*vanA/B*, *CTX-M*, KPC, OXA-48, NDM, IMP, and VIM) is likely to be rare for most institutions.

SWABS AND DIRECT ISOLATE TESTING

Additional categories of mRDTs for the detection of resistance include screening swabs and culture isolates (Table 4). The colonization of patients with MDR pathogens presents an infection prevention and control risk. To identify these patients for subsequent placement in contact precautions, molecular screening assays have been developed for *S aureus*/MRSA (nares), *Enterococcus* and *vanA* (rectal), and carbapenemases (rectal/perirectal). Cepheid has also adopted their assay for MRSA to skin and soft-tissue infections and carbapenemases to culture isolates. Compared to the other assays discussed, additional key factors to consider include the use of a screening test to guide therapy, acceptable swab/specimen type, and verification/validation considerations. Some older assays for MRSA are included in Table 4 for historical and educational purposes related to the evolution of the target design in the context of staphylococcal genetics, as discussed in the *mecA* section earlier.

Most swab-based screening assays are not FDA-approved as a diagnostic test, yet nares screening for *mecA* has been well-documented to facilitate de-escalation from vancomycin for community-acquired pneumonia [52]. In theory, manufacturers and the FDA could have different thresholds for what is an adequate sensitivity for a test designed as a screening assay versus a diagnostic one. In lieu of appropriately designed studies, uses of these assays outside of the narrow indication for pneumonia de-escalation for managing individual patient therapy may come with risks, ranging from de-escalation of MRSA coverage for non-pneumonia indications to unnecessary escalation for gram-negative infections. It is, therefore, prudent for the laboratory and antimicrobial stewardship/infectious disease to understand the test performance, potential uses, and the potential for overinterpretation of a screening test result to help educate the provider population at large.

The FDA-approved specimen type(s) can also impact specimen collection and laboratory workflows. For example, some test systems may be approved for both spun polyester swabs in Stuart media and flocked Eswabs in Amies media, while others may be approved for only a single swab type. Similar workflow challenges can occur for isolates per package instruction. For example, the Cepheid Xpert Carba-R system is approved for isolated colonies from blood or MacConkey's agar—following subculture with a meropenem disk in the primary streak. This is an obvious contrast for the same assay used as a diagnostic test (isolates) versus a screening test (swab), where this nuance can add an additional day to a result from an isolate.

SUMMARY AND FUTURE DIRECTIONS

The changing antibiotic resistance landscape has spurred advances in rapid resistance detection to expedite the selection of antimicrobial therapy and patient screening. Within this review, we have provided a framework for actionable considerations for incorporating FDA-approved panels for rapid molecular detection of resistance into clinical practice. A multidisciplinary team-based approach is necessary for proper LIS building, EHR reporting, interpreting results, and therapeutic decision-making with timely clinical action. This requires engagement from microbiology, information technology, infection prevention, and antimicrobial stewardship. Thoughtful implementation of mRDTs to detect resistance determinants from positive blood cultures, paired with active antimicrobial stewardship intervention, has been shown to improve patient outcomes; however, data supporting enhanced clinical outcomes with detecting resistance mechanisms from nonblood sources are less robust. Future studies should seek to provide clarity on the utility of such tests on nonblood specimens and further identify optimal patient populations in whom testing may be beneficial. As both resistance and technology continue to evolve, we are optimistic for the availability of additional molecular targets available on FDA-approved panels, including additional beta-lactam, macrolide, sulfonamide, and fluoroquinolones resistance targets.

CLINICS CARE POINTS

- FDA-approved rapid molecular assays for the detection of antimicrobial resistance provide clinically-relevent and actionable results are available for a variety of specimen sources.
- Robust data support the benefit of using mRDT on positive blood cultures for the escalation of therapy, while data for other sources and de-escalation is less robust.
- Careful selection and implementation is critical to optimizing actionability of these FDA-approved diagnostics, with particular attention needed to reporting and active stewardship.

ACKNOWLEDGMENTS

We thank our Mayo Clinic Arizona DASTIC work group from our Clinical Microbiology, Antimicrobial Stewardship, and Infection Prevention and Control teams for many helpful discussions and input on our rapid molecular testing, antimicrobial stewardship workflows, and therapeutic guidelines. In particular, we thank Aubrey Nava, M(ASCP), for many hours of work developing our LIS build for rapid molecular testing on blood cultures and our broader Clinical Microbiology and Pharmacy teams who perform and provide recommendations based on results 24/7.

DISCLOSURE

Nothing to disclose.

SUPPLEMENTARY DATA

Supplementary data to this article can be found online at https://doi.org/10.1016/j.yamp.2025.07.002.

REFERENCES

[1] Bai AD, Lo CKL, Komorowski AS, et al. Staphylococcus aureus bacteraemia mortality: a systematic review and meta-analysis. Clin Microbiol Infect 2022;28(8):1076–84.
[2] Liu PY, Huang YF, Tang CW, et al. Staphylococcus lugdunensis infective endocarditis: a literature review and analysis of risk factors. J Microbiol Immunol Infect Wei Mian Yu Gan Ran Za Zhi 2010;43(6):478–84.
[3] Mergenhagen KA, Starr KE, Wattengel BA, et al. Determining the utility of methicillin-resistant Staphylococcus aureus nares screening in antimicrobial stewardship. Clin Infect Dis 2020;71(5):1142–8.
[4] Wolk DM, Struelens MJ, Pancholi P, et al. Rapid detection of Staphylococcus aureus and methicillin-resistant S. aureus (MRSA) in wound specimens and blood cultures: multicenter preclinical evaluation of the Cepheid Xpert MRSA/SA skin and soft tissue and blood culture assays. J Clin Microbiol 2009;47(3):823–6.
[5] Misiura A, Pigli YZ, Boyle-Vavra S, et al. Roles of two large serine recombinases in mobilizing the methicillin-resistance cassette SCCmec. Mol Microbiol 2013;88(6):1218–29.
[6] CDC. Antibiotic resistance threats in the United States, 2019. 2019. Available at: https://www.cdc.gov/antimicrobial-resistance/media/pdfs/2019-ar-threats-report-508.pdf.
[7] Resistance mechanisms, epidemiology, and approaches to screening for vancomycin-resistant Enterococcus in the health care setting. J Clin Microbiol 2016. https://doi.org/10.1128/jcm.00211-16.
[8] Tamma PD, Heil EL, Justo JA, et al. Infectious diseases society of America 2024 guidance on the treatment of antimicrobial-resistant gram-negative infections. Clin Infect Dis Off Publ Infect Dis Soc Am 2024;ciae403. https://doi.org/10.1093/cid/ciae403.
[9] Castanheira M, Simner PJ, Bradford PA. Extended-spectrum β-lactamases: an update on their characteristics, epidemiology and detection. JAC-Antimicrob Resist 2021;3(3):dlab092.
[10] Bush K, Jacoby GA. Updated functional classification of beta-lactamases. Antimicrob Agents Chemother 2010;54(3):969–76.
[11] Mushtaq A, Chasan R, Nowak MD, et al. Correlation between identification of β-lactamase resistance genes and antimicrobial susceptibility profiles in gram-negative bacteria: a laboratory data analysis. Microbiol Spectr 2022;10(2):e0148521.

[12] Harris PNA, Tambyah PA, Lye DC, et al. Effect of piperacillin-tazobactam vs meropenem on 30-day mortality for patients with E coli or Klebsiella pneumoniae bloodstream infection and ceftriaxone resistance: a randomized clinical trial. JAMA 2018;320(10):984–94.
[13] Lee NY, Lee CC, Li CW, et al. Cefepime therapy for monomicrobial Enterobacter cloacae bacteremia: unfavorable outcomes in patients infected by cefepime-susceptible dose-dependent isolates. Antimicrob Agents Chemother 2015;59(12):7558–63.
[14] Hawkey PM, Warren RE, Livermore DM, et al. Treatment of infections caused by multidrug-resistant gram-negative bacteria: report of the British society for antimicrobial chemotherapy/healthcare infection society/British infection association joint working party. J Antimicrob Chemother 2018;73(suppl_3):iii2–78.
[15] Antimicrobial Resistance Collaborators. Global burden of bacterial antimicrobial resistance in 2019: a systematic analysis. Lancet Lond Engl 2022;399(10325): 629–55. https://doi.org/10.1016/S0140-6736(21)02724-0.
[16] Satlin MJ, Chen L, Gomez-Simmonds A, et al. Impact of a rapid molecular test for Klebsiella pneumoniae carbapenemase and ceftazidime-avibactam use on outcomes after bacteremia caused by carbapenem-resistant Enterobacterales. Clin Infect Dis 2022;75(12):2066–75.
[17] Hammoudi Halat D, Ayoub Moubareck C. The current burden of carbapenemases: review of significant properties and dissemination among gram-negative bacteria. Antibiot Basel Switz 2020;9(4):186.
[18] In vitro activity of ceftolozane-tazobactam, imipenem-relebactam, ceftazidime-avibactam, and comparators against Pseudomonas aeruginosa isolates collected in United States hospitals according to results from the SMART surveillance program, 2018 to 2020. Available at: https://pubmed.ncbi.nlm.nih.gov/35491836/. Accessed March 19, 2025.
[19] Reyes J, Komarow L, Chen L, et al. Global epidemiology and clinical outcomes of carbapenem-resistant Pseudomonas aeruginosa and associated carbapenemases (POP): a prospective cohort study. Lancet Microbe 2023;4(3):e159–70.
[20] Gupta N, Angadi K, Jadhav S. Molecular characterization of carbapenem-resistant acinetobacter baumannii with special reference to carbapenemases: a systematic review. Infect Drug Resist 2022;15:7631–50.
[21] CDC. Carbapenem-resistant Acinetobacter baumannii (CRAB): an urgent public health threat in United States healthcare facilities | A.R. & Patient Safety Portal. Available at: https://arpsp.cdc.gov/story/cra-urgent-public-health-threat. Accessed March 19, 2025.
[22] Zilberberg MD, Kollef MH, Shorr AF. Secular trends in Acinetobacter baumannii resistance in respiratory and blood stream specimens in the United States, 2003 to 2012: a survey study. J Hosp Med 2016;11(1):21–6.
[23] Sabour S, Huang JY, Bhatnagar A, et al. Detection and characterization of targeted carbapenem-resistant health care-associated threats: findings from the antibiotic resistance laboratory network, 2017 to 2019. Antimicrob Agents Chemother 2021;65(12):e0110521.
[24] Sader HS, Mendes RE, Carvalhaes CG, et al. Changing epidemiology of carbapenemases among carbapenem-resistant Enterobacterales from United States hospitals and the activity of aztreonam-avibactam against contemporary Enterobacterales (2019-2021). Open Forum Infect Dis 2023;10(2):ofad046.
[25] CLSI. Performance standards for antimicrobial susceptibility testing. 35th edition CLSI supplement M100. Clinical and Laboratory Standards Institute; 2025.
[26] Tseng AS, Kasule SN, Rice F, et al. Is it actionable? An evaluation of the rapid PCR-based blood culture identification panel on the management of gram-positive and gram-negative blood stream infections. Open Forum Infect Dis 2018;5(12):ofy308.
[27] Cairns KA, Udy AA, Peel TN, et al. Therapeutics for vancomycin-resistant enterococcal bloodstream infections. Clin Microbiol Rev 2023;36(2):e00059–122.
[28] Bryant S, Almahmoud I, Pierre I, et al. Evaluation of microbiological performance and the potential clinical impact of the ePlex® blood culture identification panels for the rapid diagnosis of bacteremia and fungemia. Front Cell Infect Microbiol 2020;10:594951. https://doi.org/10.3389/fcimb.2020.594951.
[29] Smith RD, Johnson JK, Ernst RK. Comparison of 3 diagnostic platforms for identification of bacteria and yeast from positive blood culture bottles. Diagn Microbiol Infect Dis 2023;107(2):116018.
[30] Caméléna F, Péan de Ponfilly G, Pailhoriès H, et al. Multicenter evaluation of the FilmArray blood culture identification 2 panel for pathogen detection in bloodstream infections. Microbiol Spectr 2023;11(1): e0254722.
[31] Berinson B, Both A, Berneking L, et al. Usefulness of BioFire FilmArray BCID2 for blood culture processing in clinical practice. J Clin Microbiol 2021;59(8): e0054321.
[32] Mauri C, Consonni A, Briozzo E, et al. Microbiological assessment of the FilmArray blood culture identification 2 panel: potential impact in critically ill patients. Antibiot Basel Switz 2023;12(8):1247.
[33] Simner PJ, Dien Bard J, Doern C, et al. Reporting of antimicrobial resistance from blood cultures, an antibacterial resistance leadership group survey summary: resistance marker reporting practices from positive blood cultures. Clin Infect Dis 2023;76(9):1550–8.
[34] Fabre V, Carroll KC, Cosgrove SE. Blood culture utilization in the hospital setting: a call for diagnostic stewardship. J Clin Microbiol 2022;60(3):e0100521.
[35] Bunn JD, Cornish NE. Blood culture contamination and diagnostic stewardship: from a clinical laboratory quality monitor to a national patient safety measure. J Appl Lab Med 2025;10(1):162–70.
[36] Pliakos EE, Andreatos N, Shehadeh F, et al. The cost-effectiveness of rapid diagnostic testing for the diagnosis

of bloodstream infections with or without antimicrobial stewardship. Clin Microbiol Rev 2018;31(3):e00095–117.
[37] Box MJ, Sullivan EL, Ortwine KN, et al. Outcomes of rapid identification for gram-positive bacteremia in combination with antibiotic stewardship at a community-based hospital system. Pharmacotherapy 2015;35(3):269–76.
[38] Perez KK, Olsen RJ, Musick WL, et al. Integrating rapid diagnostics and antimicrobial stewardship improves outcomes in patients with antibiotic-resistant Gram-negative bacteremia. J Infect 2014;69(3):216–25.
[39] Timbrook TT, Morton JB, McConeghy KW, et al. The effect of molecular rapid diagnostic testing on clinical outcomes in bloodstream infections: a systematic review and meta-analysis. Clin Infect Dis 2017;64(1):15–23.
[40] Nakagawa R, Jain R, Bryan AB, et al. Optimization of antimicrobial therapy in vancomycin-resistant enterococcal bacteraemia using a rapid detection Gram-positive blood culture assay. J Hosp Infect 2018;99(2):153–7.
[41] Banerjee R, Teng CB, Cunningham SA, et al. Randomized trial of rapid multiplex polymerase chain reaction-based blood culture identification and susceptibility testing. Clin Infect Dis 2015;61(7):1071–80.
[42] Barlam TF, Cosgrove SE, Abbo LM, et al. Implementing an antibiotic stewardship program: guidelines by the infectious diseases society of America and the society for healthcare epidemiology of America. Clin Infect Dis 2016;62(10):e51–77.
[43] CDC. Core elements of hospital diagnostic excellence (DxEx). Patient Safety 2025. Available at: https://www.cdc.gov/patient-safety/hcp/hospital-dx-excellence/index.html. Accessed March 19, 2025.
[44] Enne VI, Aydin A, Baldan R, et al. Multicentre evaluation of two multiplex PCR platforms for the rapid microbiological investigation of nosocomial pneumonia in UK ICUs: the INHALE WP1 study. Thorax 2022;77(12):1220–8.
[45] Virk A, Strasburg AP, Kies KD, et al. Rapid multiplex PCR panel for pneumonia in hospitalised patients with suspected pneumonia in the USA: a single-centre, open-label, pragmatic, randomised controlled trial. Lancet Microbe 2024;5(12):100928.
[46] Enne VI, Stirling S, Barber JA, et al. INHALE WP3, a multicentre, open-label, pragmatic randomised controlled trial assessing the impact of rapid, ICU-based, syndromic PCR, versus standard-of-care on antibiotic stewardship and clinical outcomes in hospital-acquired and ventilator-associated pneumonia. Intensive Care Med 2025;51(2):272–86.
[47] Markussen DL, Serigstad S, Ritz C, et al. Diagnostic stewardship in community-acquired pneumonia with syndromic molecular testing: a randomized clinical trial. JAMA Netw Open 2024;7(3):e240830.
[48] Darie AM, Khanna N, Jahn K, et al. Fast multiplex bacterial PCR of bronchoalveolar lavage for antibiotic stewardship in hospitalised patients with pneumonia at risk of Gram-negative bacterial infection (Flagship II): a multicentre, randomised controlled trial. Lancet Respir Med 2022;10(9):877–87.
[49] Horne DJ, Kohli M, Zifodya JS, et al. Xpert MTB/RIF and Xpert MTB/RIF Ultra for pulmonary tuberculosis and rifampicin resistance in adults. Cochrane Database Syst Rev 2019;6(6):CD009593.
[50] Moran A, Arellano J, Bregman K, et al. Evaluation of a BioFire multiplex PCR panel for detection of joint infections using retrospective and prospectively collected specimens. J Clin Microbiol 2024;62(8):e00182–224.
[51] Pascual S, Noble B, Ahmad-Saeed N, et al. Potential value of a rapid syndromic multiplex PCR for the diagnosis of native and prosthetic joint infections: a real-world evidence study. J Bone Jt Infect 2024;9(1):87–97.
[52] Parente DM, Cunha CB, Mylonakis E, et al. The clinical utility of methicillin-resistant Staphylococcus aureus (MRSA) nasal screening to rule out MRSA pneumonia: a diagnostic meta-analysis with antimicrobial stewardship implications. Clin Infect Dis 2018;67(1):1–7.

SECTION: HOT TOPICS

Advances in Molecular Pathology 8 (2025) 163–173
ADVANCES IN MOLECULAR PATHOLOGY

Health Disparities and Precision Medicine

Sherin Shaaban, MD, PhD[a,b,*], Yuan Ji, MS, PhD, MBA[a,b]
[a]Department of Pathology, University of Utah School of Medicine, Salt Lake City, UT, USA; [b]ARUP Laboratories, Salt Lake City, UT, USA

KEYWORDS
• Disparities • Equity • Precision medicine • Inclusion • Diversity

KEY POINTS

- Health disparities are related to race, ethnicity, gender, and various social determinants of health.
- Precision medicine carries a lot of promise of individualizing patient treatment and care yet could exacerbate existing health disparities.
- Concerted efforts are required in the research and implementation of precision medicine initiatives for the benefits to be reaped by all segments of the society.

INTRODUCTION

Health disparities (HDs) are defined as preventable differences in the burden of disease, injury, or opportunities to achieve optimal health that are experienced by socially disadvantaged populations [1]. Such disparities are measured by the differences in incidence, prevalence, mortality, disease burden, and other adverse health conditions [2]. HDs exist due to unequal allocation of power and resources that result in unequal social, economic, and environmental conditions including the mechanisms that organize the distribution of power and resources differentially along the lines of race and ethnicity, gender, sexual orientation, age, disability status, socioeconomic status (SES), and geographic location [3] (Box 1).

Precision medicine (PM), according to the US Food and Drug Administration (FDA), is an innovative approach to tailoring disease prevention and treatment that considers differences in people's genes, environments, and lifestyles. The goal of PM is to target the right treatments to the right patients at the right time [4]. The promise PM carried of transforming patient care is gradually being realized by advances in identifying genomic causes of cancer and rare diseases through next-generation sequencing (NGS) technologies, or by developing molecularly targeted therapies, or through utilizing massive computational capabilities to decipher large datasets using machine learning (ML) and artificial intelligence (AI). PM also carries the promise of addressing the conundrum of HDs through transformative changes in diagnostics, therapeutics, and preventive medicine practices. Yet such promise could become unattainable without concerted efforts toward inclusion of minorities and disadvantaged populations in the research and development of PM initiatives. On the contrary, without a deliberate approach to inclusivity in PM, the potential for deepening the already existing disparities only increases. The current status of biomedical research, when both testing and the translation of results into therapeutic options are unequally distributed means that marginalized communities disproportionately experience harm and garner fewer benefits due to, for example, barriers in health care access or lack of representation in

*Corresponding author. ARUP laboratories, 500 Chipeta Way, Salt Lake City, UT 84108. *E-mail address:* Sherin.shaaban@aruplab.com

https://doi.org/10.1016/j.yamp.2025.05.008 www.advancesinmolecularpathology.com
2589-4080/25/ © 2025 Elsevier Inc. All rights are reserved, including those for text and data mining, AI training, and similar technologies.

ABBREVIATIONS	
ADR	adverse drug reactions
AI	artificial intelligence
CVD	cardiovascular disease
FDA	Food and Drug Administration
HDs	health disparities
ML	machine learning
NGS	next-generation sequencing
NIH	National Institute of Health
PGx	pharmacogenomics
PM	precision medicine
SES	socioeconomic status

reference databases used in PM [5]. A review of HD as they relate to race and ethnicity, sex and gender, age, SES, and geographic location, will follow, to highlight hurdles that still exist as well as efforts that are being taken toward equitable health for all.

HEALTH DISPARITIES RELATED TO RACE, ETHNICITY, AND GENETIC ANCESTRY

It is imperative to start this section by definitions differentiating between race, ethnicity, and genetic ancestry. Race has historically been defined based on the physical characteristics of a group such as skin color, eye shape, and so forth, and later as a method for demographic categorization of people. Race is a socially constructed term, reflecting the scientific and sociopolitical climate from which it originated to describe biology [6]. Ethnicity is similarly a social construct that is related to cultural factors such as language, religion, and nationality that people within a specific community share [7]. Genetic ancestry, on the other hand, refers to the people that an individual is biologically descended from, including their genetic relationships [8] (Fig. 1). So, while race and ethnicity are social constructs, they offer a crude method of providing information about genetic ancestry and consequently about disease prevalence and risk [9]. Racial disparities in disease should be investigated in light of structural racism alongside careful measures of genetic factors in relevant disease pathways, rather than only relying on genetic ancestry or race as a proxy for disease-causing alleles [10]. To do so, understanding the demographic and socioeconomic composition of racial and ethnic groups is fundamental since such characteristics are associated with health risk factors, disease prevalence, and access to care.

In the United States, the Agency for Healthcare Research and Quality uses measures of different factors

BOX 1
Health disparity and health equity definitions [106,107]

Health disparity:

Definition: A health difference that adversely affects disadvantaged populations, based on one or more of the following health outcomes:

- Higher incidence and/or prevalence and earlier onset of disease
- Higher prevalence of risk factors, unhealthy behaviors, or clinical measures in the causal pathway of a disease outcome
- Higher rates of condition-specific symptoms, reduced global daily functioning, or self-reported health-related quality of life using standardized measures
- Premature and/or excessive mortality from diseases where population rates differ
- Greater global burden of disease using a standardized metric

Populations that experience health disparities include

- Racial and ethnic minority groups
- People with lower SES
- Underserved rural communities
- Sexual and gender minority groups
- People with disabilities

Health equity:

Definition: Equity in health is the absence of systematic disparities in health (or in the major social determinants of health) among groups with different levels of underlying social advantage/disadvantage—that is, wealth, power, or prestige.

Race: Social construction and categorization of people based on perceived shared physical traits that result in the maintenance of a sociopolitical hierarchy. The term is also loosely applied to geographic, cultural, religious, or national groups.

Ethnicity: A characterization of people based on having a shared culture (e.g., language, food, music, dress, values, and beliefs) related to common ancestry and shared history.

Genetic Ancestry: Genetic ancestry refers to information about the people that an individual is biologically descended from, including their genetic relationships. Genetic information can be combined with historical information to infer where an individual's distant ancestors lived

FIG. 1 Definitions of race, ethnicity, and genetic ancestry.

to assess the health status of the population. In the last decade, HDs by race and ethnicity were found for almost all measures analyzed such as infant mortality, childhood obesity, hypertension, insurance coverage, or low-risk births delivered by cesarean section, to name a few measures. For example, infant mortality rates were highest among infants born to black women; Hispanic children had the highest prevalence of obesity; Black men and women were the most likely to have hypertension; lack of health insurance coverage was highest among Hispanic adults, and Black mothers experienced the highest percentage of low-risk cesarean deliveries [11]. Studies of the mortality disparities across races and counties in the United States found that the gap between the life expectancy of Black males in high-risk urban areas and the life expectancy for Asian females was 20.7 years and concluded that the disparities in mortality in the United States are enormous by all international standards [12]. Racial and ethnic minority groups were also overrepresented among the millions of Americans who have inadequate access to a primary care physician [13]. Disparities also occur in quality of care and barriers in seeking preventive care and acute or chronic disease management [11]. Black and Hispanic patients are more likely to lose Medicaid supplemental insurance eligibility, resulting in increased cost-related barriers to care, fewer outpatient visits, and fewer medication fills [14]. More examples could be found in the application of pharmacogenomics (PGx), which is a corner stone of PM. In the United States, the fastest growing minority are the Hispanics, which made up 18.9% of the population based on the latest census [15]. Hispanics and African Americans are at an especially high risk for poor outcomes after anticoagulation therapy with warfarin [16,17], yet they remain largely underrepresented in trials aiming at developing dosing algorithms [18]. Similarly, the development of therapeutics relies on clinical trials conducted mainly in non-Hispanic Whites or less frequently among Asians. Therefore, African, Hispanic, or Native American-specific variants are often missed during drug development and the significance of these variants is only realized upon the release of such drugs to individuals of the underrepresented populations with the development of adverse reactions [19].

While there exists a moral justification and social justice argument to call for minimizing or eliminating racial HD, there is also an economic incentive. The estimated economic burden of racial and ethnic HD in 2018 was estimated to exceed US$421 billion, mostly due to the poor health of the Black population [20]. The economic costs of disparities affect individuals in terms of adverse impacts on employment and greater out-of-pocket health expenditures, and affect the general population through increased direct and indirect cost of health care in addition to the cost of lost productivity [20,21].

To understand the causes of HD related to race and ethnicity, revealing the genetic determinants of these disparities and their interactions with environmental, behavioral, and social factors is needed [22,23]. While the latest US census found that 52.7% of US population aged under 18 years belong to an ethnic or minority group [15], representation of minorities in scientific research including studies investigating genetic determinants of disease remains limited [22,24]. Without such inclusivity, the research outcomes would be poorer disease prediction and treatment of individuals of underrepresented ancestries [25]. To increase such representation, the FDA and the National Institute of Health (NIH) published guidelines and policies encouraging scientists to include minorities, and women, in their research [26]. Moreover, biobanks, and large genomic datasets efforts such as the All-of-Us research program in the United States, attempted at including more minorities [27]. A stated goal of the All-of-Us program is that "*All of Us* should broadly reflect the diversity of the U.S. and ensure inclusion of a broad range of participants, including consideration of biological, social, and other determinants of health that contribute to HD" [28]. Additional efforts such as the Bio-Repository for American Indian Capacity, Education, Law, Economics and Technology project [29] or the *Human Heredity and Health in Africa* project [30] aiming at banking data from populations that have long been ignored, would help build capacity for genomic research in such populations enabling the implementation of PM in such communities.

It is worth noting that recruiting minorities could be hindered by the mistrust of these communities in biomedical research stemming from past experiences of exploitation [25,31], which entails collaboration among the researchers, community leaders, and local authorities to provide a safe environment in which participants feel comfortable taking part in such studies [31,32]. Efforts toward more inclusivity have so far resulted in an increase of inclusion of non-European participants to over 20% in recent studies [33]. More attention to increasing racial and ethnic diversity in the health care workforce, starting with the recruitment of medical students and various health care programs [23,34]. As ML tools are integral to the implementation of PM, efforts toward addressing biases in training datasets for ML should be implemented [35]. This will be discussed later in this review.

HEALTH DISPARITIES RELATED TO SEX AND GENDER

Sex and gender are often conflated assuming that they are one and the same. It is important to have accurate definitions to guide how they relate to the issue of HD. Sex, refers to the biological components, including anatomic and physiologic traits, related to sexual reproduction that classifies individuals to male individuals and female individuals. Gender, on the other hand, is a construct that links language with social and cultural expectations about status and behavior that are associated with sex traits [36,37]. Despite distinct definitions of sex and gender, they remain very closely intertwined.

PM in its pursuit of individualizing patient care and ensuring targeted and equitable health care outcomes, needs to consider the study of sex and gender differences and the development of a gender-specific medicine by studying differences in genes, chromosomes, hormones, and metabolism as well as differences in culture, environment, and society in a multidimensional model [38].

There is a huge gap in knowledge of women health because of decades of exclusion of female subjects from studies outside the study of biology of reproduction [39]. It is estimated that only 2% to 6% of studies are conducted exclusively in female individuals [40]. Consequently, much of our current health care, from drug dosage calculations to diagnostic and treatment protocols, is still based on the study of male individuals [41], translating into inaccurate diagnoses, ineffective treatments, and disparities in health outcomes among female individuals [37]. Efforts to increase inclusion of female subjects have been growing. Funding agencies, such as the NIH or the European commission, have published guidelines to encourage grant recipients to incorporate sex and gender analyses into the design of studies [26,42]. In 2022, Nature Portfolio journals announced that researchers will be prompted to state whether and how sex and gender were considered in their study design [43].

HDs related to sex and gender take many forms. Female patients are reported to have higher rates of adverse drug reactions (ADR) often up to 1.5 to 1.7 fold more than male individuals [44]. In a study that looked at the associations between gender roles and the number of non–life-threatening pain medication ADR reported as severe by people living with chronic pain, stratified analysis by gender roles showed that women reported a greater number of severe ADR than men [45]. Moreover, women often receive diagnosis later than men for most of disorders [46]. Female individuals are also subject to higher rates of misdiagnosis. In a study of autism among adults, compared to male individuals, female individuals showed a significant delay in referral to mental health services and a significantly higher age at diagnosis [47]. Similar patterns were reported for cardiovascular disease (CVD) [48] and cancer diagnosis and care [49]. Women also have an increased risk for unmet health care needs compared to men [50]. A study investigating the gender disparities in health care access found pronounced disparities in younger women, Black women, and women with atherosclerotic CVD [51]. Moreover, women across all age groups experience disproportionately higher out-of-pocket medical expenses compared to men. Out-of-pocket expenses for employed women in the United States are estimated to be US$15 billion higher per year than for employed men [52].

In addition to HD among female individuals compared to male individuals, sexual minorities (eg, gay, lesbian, and bisexual individuals) are more likely to engage in riskier health behaviors, including smoking and heavy drinking and often have poor health outcomes, such as obesity and CVD [53]. These findings were more pronounced among sexual minorities of color in addition to having less access to health care services [14,54].

If PM aims at improving health outcomes through context-sensitive individualization of medical care, it is of paramount importance to integrate the study of sex-related biological variables as they intersect with gender-related social and environmental variables including race, ethnicity, and SES [55].

HEALTH DISPARITIES RELATED TO AGE

The older adult population (>65 years) in the United States and worldwide is growing substantially. Older adults in the United States are about 17% of the population [56,57]. At the same time, according to the 2020 census the population under age 18 showed a decline of 1.4% from the 2010 census data [15]. Such demographic changes come at a cost to the health care systems and individuals, with older adults having higher rates of utilization of medical services while incurring increased medical expenses [58].

Age is considered one of the most important determinants of health, and aging individuals often encounter disadvantages in accessing appropriate, affordable, and quality care [59]. While the decline in health in aging adults is influenced by genetics and natural biological processes, HDs related to age could also reflect the accumulated disadvantages of one's location, gender, and SES, together with one's attitudes and practices and access to or lack of quality health and social services [60].

There are many reasons that lead to inaccessibility of health care services for the elderly, from affordability to lack of specialized centers in rural locations to physical limitations of mobility or lack of transportation access [61]. Health care systems, in addition, are suffering shortages in health care providers, especially those with expertise managing elderly patients [61]. The elderly also face health inequities due to ageism with detrimental effects on health outcomes and quality of life [62]. For example, older patients diagnosed with breast cancer are not treated to the same extent as younger patients and increasing age at diagnosis predicts deviation from guidelines for all treatment modalities. Moreover, older patients are often excluded from clinical trials including those of drug development [63,64]. The prevalence of ADR in the elderly is a major public health concern, although predictable and avoidable, leading to an increase of morbidity, mortality, and health care costs [65]. Polypharmacy (use of $\geq$5 drugs) is another common problem among the elderly leading to higher rates of hospitalizations, especially among elderly patients of lower SES [66]. While PGx could guide treatment regimens, decreasing hospitalizations rates and leading to cost savings, PGx studies in older adults with polypharmacy remain lacking [67].

Differences among the elderly by gender, education and income level, and racial or ethnic background exist. For example, older individuals of lower education level or of lower SES, have less access to health services including cancer screening or vaccinations [59,68]. To reduce HDs in the elderly, there is need for ensuring the availability of affordable and quality social and health services, and an increase in training of geriatrics specialists. Research studies recruitment also needs to be diversified in terms of age as well as gender and SES. Policy and legislative efforts are further needed to ensure various stakeholders play their role in addressing such prevailing disparities.

On the other end of the spectrum, HDs among the pediatric population similarly exist. HDs among children have long-term impact on outcomes, such as adult health, educational attainment, and economic success [69]. HDs in child health outcomes reflect the social and economic conditions in which a child grows [70]. Access to clean air, water, sanitation, shelter, and nutrition is a basic determinant of health. Twenty-six percent of childhood deaths and 25% of the disease burden in children aged under 5 years are attributed to environmental exposures [71]. This means that such burden could be prevented by environmental interventions [72]. Additionally, the lack of access or limited affordability or lack of health insurance is implicated in higher rates of morbidity and mortality among poor children [73]. Moreover, disparities for almost all leading causes of injury and disease are further exaggerated in children of racial minorities [74]. Children's health is a reflection of the family's SES, and children of lower SES show higher rates of body mass index, more behavioral and psychosomatic problems, a lower quality of life, and many other lower indicators of child health [75,76]. To address childhood HDs, changes in economic and social policies are needed [77]. Access to effective health care services is fundamental, and a model of universal health care could address the lack of access to health services [78]. Governments should also ensure the basic determinants of health such as adequate nutrition, education, clean water, and sanitation are available to all children and implement policies to reduce or eliminate poverty [69]. Guidance to clinicians and educators is also needed to identify health inequities in their patients, students, and community, as well as policies to empower them in implementing practices that would address childhood HDs [79,80].

HEALTH DISPARITIES AND ARTIFICIAL INTELLIGENCE

AI has transformative and global implications on medicine and global health, including on addressing HDs [81]. In lower income countries, utilization of AI will enable improvements in health care and decrease the gap between rich and poor countries [82].

While the convergence of AI and PM promises to revolutionize health care through patient-centered, data-driven approach to treatment [83], the potential for amplification of existing HDs remains a major concern. HDs caused by AI systems may stem from data and algorithmic bias propagating deeply rooted societal biases [84]. For a successful implementation of AI systems, the development of algorithms requires large datasets for development and training [81]. Lack of diversity in such training datasets, either in terms of absence of certain groups' representative data or if such data are incorrectly categorized, has detrimental effects once decision support is built relying on such biased data, resulting in underperformance in affected groups such as in inaccurate diagnoses, treatment recommendations, and so forth, and hence have the potential for more harm than benefit [85]. Existing datasets are inherently biased towards European populations, with less representation of women, rural communities, gender and ethnic minorities, and those of lower SES [86]. To give an example, AI models prioritized White patients when treating life-threatening conditions, for example, diabetes, even though Black patients have higher severity indexes [87]. The reason was that the AI algorithms, used health costs as a proxy for health needs and falsely concluded that Black patients are healthier than equally sick White patients, as less money was spent on them [84,87]. Structural inequities can also manifest in datasets through the actions of clinical and data curation teams, while recording, selecting, and labeling data [88]. Human bias in AI can be hard to mitigate, and mainly stem from long-held societal prejudices that are subtle at the level of society yet amplified by AI and large datasets [84].

Relying on datasets inherent with structural biases and deploying AI without systematic ethical considerations may exacerbate HDs [81]. AI implementation guiding principles have been published by the FDA, Health Canada, and the UK Medicines and Healthcare products Regulatory Agency stating that data should be representative of the intended population to "manage any bias, promote appropriate and generalizable performance across the intended patient population, assess usability and identify circumstances where the model may underperform" [89].

HEALTH DISPARITIES RELATED TO SOCIOECONOMIC STATUS

SES, income level, and insurance affordability are known factors impacting patients' access to quality health care, including PM, thus leading to recognizable HDs [90]. Families and individuals with lower incomes are more likely to be uninsured or underinsured without a health care coverage through employer-paid benefits or by public insurance (Medicare or Medicaid), impacting the patient's choice of care based on affordability of the out-of-pocket costs or potential debt they need to bear after care is received [91]. In the 2021 National Healthcare Quality and Disparities Report by the Agency for Healthcare Research and Quality (United States) and based on the data collected by US Department of Health and Human Services Office of Minority Health in 2018, among individuals aged under 64 years, poor, low-income, and middle-income individuals were more likely to be uninsured compared to high-income people of the same ethnic background, with Hispanic individuals having the highest overall uninsurance rate (>15%) compared to Black (5%–10%) and White individuals (<5%) [92]. Low-income patients in an expensive health care system will inevitably suffer undesired health care outcomes due to under or lack of quality health.

While the goal of PM is to reduce the overall cost of health care through maximizing the desired outcomes and minimizing the adverse effects of therapies, it remains significantly more costly than other preventive and conventional therapies [93]. Tran and Zafar analyzed the adverse financial implications of cancer care in the era of molecular and immune therapies and found that most of the biomarker-based targeted cancer therapies can cost patients greater than US $100,000 annually, not to mention the front cost associated with genomic profiling and interpretation, ranging from a few hundred dollars (targeted mutations or single-gene analysis) to a few thousand dollars (NGS testing) or even more if using a whole genome approach [94]. Even among the insured patients, reimbursement rates for targeted therapies can vary based on the specific therapy, insurance plan, and coding practices [95]. These financial considerations compound patients' decisions when choosing the level and the approach of care, or even whether to see a doctor for routine preventive care.

Other factors, such as education, occupation, language or cultural background, living conditions, and immigration status can play a big part in an individual's or a family's decision about their health care management [96]. Although access to health care is a human right, undocumented immigrants are usually neither able to afford a private insurance plan nor eligible for federally funded public health insurance programs. These immigrant families, therefore, may choose to forgo their basic needs for health care and live with the fear of getting sick or injured [97].

PM requires close and effective dialog between the patients (and families) and an interdisciplinary health care team to provide personalized care based on patient's clinical and family history, genomic profiling, life, and other environmental factors. Patients' education, occupation, language, or cultural background may also affect ability to access and benefit from PM efforts, influencing patients' understanding of information or may cause fear of cultural stigma, concerns of invasion of privacy, discrimination, or general distrust of the health care system. One study found out that despite similar attitudes toward the benefits of PM, patients with African American background were significantly more likely than non-Hispanic Caucasian patients to be concerned about discrimination based on genetic results [98].

With major digital transformation of health care, patients' use of the Internet for health care is no longer limited to making appointments or checking test results but have expanded to functionalities like data sharing, remote consultations, patient education, and access to AI-powered diagnostics. Thus, lack or limited Internet access of patients of low SES is another example of how income inequality affects health care access. Policies are needed to bridge an existing digital divide by ensuring access to Internet and digital services for disadvantaged patients, which in turn could improve health outcomes [99].

HEALTH DISPARITIES RELATED TO GEOGRAPHIC LOCATION

Eighty percent of the United States population reside in urban areas, while the remaining 20% reside in rural areas [15]. HDs are exacerbated among patients living in rural locations due to limited transportation, higher rates of chronic diseases, financial challenges, and other unique socioeconomic characteristics. Individuals in rural communities use health care services at lower rates and often reserve their limited resources to seek health care services for critical needs, than for routine care, potentially leading to delays in diagnosis and treatment [100].

As previously discussed, patient's ability to access Internet is important for PM. It is especially valuable for rural communities to receive remote consultations when timely transportation is a daily challenge. However, most patients living in rural areas do not have or cannot afford reliable broadband Internet, which makes conducting telemedicine challenging [101].

The distribution of rural and urban hospitals varies significantly by state, with most rural hospitals being in the South and the Midwest in the United States. Even in the states where there are more rural than urban hospitals, hospitals differ significantly in bed size, services offered, staffing level, and financial stability, with rural hospitals generally facing challenges in attracting and retaining health care professionals [102]. Many health care providers need to travel to provide care periodically and are often shared by several community hospitals dispersed in the region. Lack of on-site diagnostic testing facilities in rural areas affects ability to provide quality and timely care for patients in these regions [103]. With PM efforts almost entirely focused in large medical centers located near urban areas or in academic institutions where medical and scientific expertise, cutting-edge technologies, and other financial resources are ample, it is rational to project that without innovative approaches to providing similar care to patients within rural and remote communities, such advances would only result in worsening of the already existing HDs in communities [104].

SUMMARY

Addressing HDs requires the inclusion of ethnic minorities and socially disadvantaged populations in the research and in the implementation of PM initiatives. There is utmost need to develop an evidence-based understanding of the factors that cause HD including how such factors differ within and in-between countries [105].

To identify, and address HDs, the scientific community must commit to developing a standard approach to assessing and interpreting data about race, ethnicity, and social determinants of health as they relate to HDs when developing and implementing PM initiatives. Such standards require collaboration between health providers of various specialties and researchers in epidemiology, sociology, public policy, and other related fields [105]. This will ensure that scientific advances and innovations in PM are impactful for all segments of the society through strong partnership between community leaders, professional organizations, academia, health care systems, payers, industry, and charitable foundations [104].

FUNDING

This study has been funded by The University of Utah, United States, Department of Pathology, United States, University Development Funds and ARUP Research and Development funds.

DISCLOSURE

The authors report there are no competing interests to declare.

REFERENCES

[1] CDC. Health disparities: CDC. 2020. Available at: https://www.cdc.gov/healthyyouth/disparities/. Accessed October 24, 2022.
[2] Health NIo. Health disparities. 2014. Available at: https://www.nhlbi.nih.gov/health/educational/health-disp/. Accessed February 3, 2025.
[3] Baciu A, Negussie Y, Geller A, et al, editors. Communities in action: pathways to health equity. Washington (DC): National Academies Press (US); 2017.
[4] Precision medicine FDA.gov. 2018. Available at: https://www.fda.gov/medical-devices/in-vitro-diagnostics/precision-medicine. Accessed February 3, 2025.
[5] Popejoy AB, Fullerton SM. Genomics is failing on diversity. Nature 2016;538(7624):161–4.
[6] Ford CL, Airhihenbuwa CO. Critical race theory, race equity, and public health: toward antiracism praxis. Am J Publ Health 2010;100(Suppl 1):S30–5.
[7] Wang VO, Sue S. In the eye of the storm: race and genomics in research and practice. Am Psychol 2005;60(1):37–45.
[8] Institute NHGR. Genetic ancestry. Available at: https://www.genome.gov/genetics-glossary/Genetic-Ancestry. Accessed February 4, 2025.
[9] Burchard EG, Ziv E, Coyle N, et al. The importance of race and ethnic background in biomedical research and clinical practice. N Engl J Med 2003;348(12):1170–5.
[10] Cerdena JP, Grubbs V, Non AL. Genomic supremacy: the harm of conflating genetic ancestry and race. Hum Genom 2022;16(1):18.
[11] National healthcare quality and disparities report. Rockville (MD): National Healthcare Quality & Disparities Report Chartbooks; 2023.
[12] Murray CJ, Kulkarni SC, Michaud C, et al. Eight Americas: investigating mortality disparities across races, counties, and race-counties in the United States. PLoS Med 2006;3(9):e260.
[13] National healthcare quality and disparities report. Rockville (MD): National Healthcare Quality & Disparities Report Chartbooks; 2021.
[14] Roberts ET, Kwon Y, Hames AG, et al. Racial and ethnic disparities in health care use and access associated with loss of medicaid supplemental insurance eligibility above the federal poverty level. JAMA Intern Med 2023;183(6):534–43.
[15] Bureau USC. U.S. Census Bureau, U.S. Department of Commerce. "Age and sex." American community survey, ACS 5-year estimates subject tables, table S0101. 2023. Available at: https://data.census.gov/table/ACSST5Y2023.S0101?q=S0101. Accessed February 26, 2025.
[16] Birman-Deych E, Radford MJ, Nilasena DS, et al. Use and effectiveness of warfarin in Medicare beneficiaries with atrial fibrillation. Stroke (1970) 2006;37(4):1070–4.
[17] Shen AY, Yao JF, Brar SS, et al. Racial/Ethnic differences in ischemic stroke rates and the efficacy of warfarin among patients with atrial fibrillation. Stroke (1970) 2008;39(10):2736–43.
[18] Duconge J, Cadilla CL, Seip RL, et al. Why admixture matters in genetically-guided therapy: missed targets in the COAG and EU-PACT trials. P R Health Sci J 2015;34(3):175–7.
[19] Venkatakrishnan K, Benincosa LJ. Diversity and inclusion in drug development: rethinking intrinsic and extrinsic factors with patient centricity. Clin Pharmacol Ther 2022;112(2):204–7.
[20] LaVeist TA, Perez-Stable EJ, Richard P, et al. The economic burden of racial, ethnic, and educational health inequities in the US. JAMA 2023;329(19):1682–92.
[21] Asif Dhar JB, Neal Batra, Rush Brian, et al. US health care can't afford health inequities: deloitte US. 2022. Available at: https://www2.deloitte.com/us/en/insights/industry/health-care/economic-cost-of-health-disparities.html. Accessed November 7, 2025.
[22] Edwards TL, Breeyear J, Piekos JA, et al. Equity in health: consideration of race and ethnicity in precision medicine. Trends Genet 2020;36(11):807–9.
[23] Genevieve LD, Martani A, Shaw D, et al. Structural racism in precision medicine: leaving no one behind. BMC Med Ethics 2020;21(1):17.
[24] Fisher ER, Pratt R, Esch R, et al. The role of race and ethnicity in views toward and participation in genetic studies and precision medicine research in the United States: a systematic review of qualitative and quantitative studies. Mol Genet Genomic Med 2020;8(2):e1099.

[25] Sirugo G, Williams SM, Tishkoff SA. The missing diversity in human genetic studies. Cell 2019;177(1):26–31.
[26] NIH. NIH policy and guidelines on the inclusion of women and minorities as subjects in clinical research 2017. Available at: https://grants.nih.gov/policy/inclusion/women-and-minorities/guidelines.htm. Accessed October 26, 2022.
[27] All of Us Research Program Genomics I. Genomic data in the all of us research program. Nature 2024;627(8003):340–6.
[28] Mapes BM, Foster CS, Kusnoor SV, et al. Diversity and inclusion for the All of Us research program: a scoping review. PLoS One 2020;15(7):e0234962.
[29] BRAICELET. Bio-repository for American Indian capacity, education, Law, economics and Technology. Available at: https://med.stanford.edu/sphere/research-intiatives/braicelet.html. Accessed February 7, 2025.
[30] Mulder N, Abimiku A, Adebamowo SN, et al. H3Africa: current perspectives. Pharmgenomics Pers Med 2018; 11:59–66.
[31] Ejiogu N, Norbeck JH, Mason MA, et al. Recruitment and retention strategies for minority or poor clinical research participants: lessons from the Healthy Aging in Neighborhoods of Diversity across the Life Span study. Gerontol 2011;51(Suppl 1):S33–45.
[32] Bolen S, Tilburt J, Baffi C, et al. Defining "success" in recruitment of underrepresented populations to cancer clinical trials: moving toward a more consistent approach. Cancer 2006;106(6):1197–204.
[33] Sirugo G, Williams SM, Tishkoff SA. The missing diversity in human genetic studies. Cell 2019;177(4):1080.
[34] Stanford FC. The importance of diversity and inclusion in the healthcare workforce. J Natl Med Assoc 2020; 112(3):247–9.
[35] Huang J, Galal G, Etemadi M, et al. Evaluation and mitigation of racial bias in clinical machine learning models: scoping review. JMIR Med Inform 2022; 10(5):e36388.
[36] Sex and gender identification and implications for disability evaluation. Washington (DC): The National Academies Press. National Academies of Sciences, Eng Med; 2024. p. 293–4.
[37] Subramaniapillai S, Am Galea L, Einstein G, et al. Sex and gender in health research: intersectionality matters. Front Neuroendocrinol 2023;72:101104.
[38] Kautzky-Willer A. [Gender medicine. Sex- and gender-specific aspects of clinical medicine]. Bundesgesundheitsblatt Gesundheitsforschung Gesundheitsschutz 2014;57(9):1022–30.
[39] Beery AK, Zucker I. Sex bias in neuroscience and biomedical research. Neurosci Biobehav Rev 2011; 35(3):565–72.
[40] de Lange AG, Jacobs EG, Galea LAM. The scientific body of knowledge: whose body does it serve? A spotlight on women's brain health. Front Neuroendocrinol 2021;60:100898.
[41] J L. Why women have been excluded from medical studies about their own bodies. MaRS Magazine 2020. Available at: https://www.marsdd.com/magazine/why-women-have-been-excluded-from-medical-studies-about-their-own-bodies/. Accessed February 10, 2025.
[42] Accounting for sex and gender makes for better science. Nature 2020;588(7837):196.
[43] Nature journals raise the bar on sex and gender reporting in research. Nature 2022;605(7910):396.
[44] Rademaker M. Do women have more adverse drug reactions? Am J Clin Dermatol 2001;2(6):349–51.
[45] Nguena Nguefack HL, Gabrielle Page M, Guenette L, et al. Gender differences in medication adverse effects experienced by people living with chronic pain. Front Pain Res (Lausanne) 2022;3:830153.
[46] Sun TY, Hardin J, Nieva HR, et al. Large-scale characterization of gender differences in diagnosis prevalence and time to diagnosis. medRxiv 2023. https://doi.org/10.1101/2023.10.12.23296976.
[47] Gesi C, Migliarese G, Torriero S, et al. Gender differences in misdiagnosis and delayed diagnosis among adults with autism spectrum disorder with no language or intellectual disability. Brain Sci 2021;11(7).
[48] Bosomworth J, Khan Z. Analysis of gender-based inequality in cardiovascular health: an umbrella review. Cureus 2023;15(8):e43482.
[49] Dean D, Smith AW. Addressing sexual and gender minority disparities in cancer research. J Natl Cancer Inst 2023;115(10):1125–7.
[50] Bryant T, Leaver C, Dunn J. Unmet healthcare need, gender, and health inequalities in Canada. Health Policy 2009;91(1):24–32.
[51] Daher M, Al Rifai M, Kherallah RY, et al. Gender disparities in difficulty accessing healthcare and cost-related medication non-adherence: the CDC behavioral risk factor surveillance system (BRFSS) survey. Prev Med 2021;153:106779.
[52] Deloitte. 2023. Available at: https://www2.deloitte.com/us/en/pages/life-sciences-and-health-care/articles/womens-health-equity-disparities.html?utm_source=newsletter&utm_medium=email&utm_campaign=newsletter_axiosvitals&stream=top. Accessed February 20, 2025.
[53] Trinh MH, Agenor M, Austin SB, et al. Health and healthcare disparities among U.S. women and men at the intersection of sexual orientation and race/ethnicity: a nationally representative cross-sectional study. BMC Public Health 2017;17(1):964.
[54] Hsieh N, Ruther M. Sexual minority health and health risk factors: intersection effects of gender, race, and sexual identity. Am J Prev Med 2016; 50(6):746–55.
[55] Nielsen MW, Stefanick ML, Peragine D, et al. Gender-related variables for health research. Biol Sex Differ 2021;12(1):23.

[56] Roman Y. The United States 2020 Census data: implications for precision medicine and the research landscape. Per Med 2022;19(1):5–8.
[57] Teruel Camargo J, Smith JT, Rodriquez EJ, et al. Advancing aging research through a health disparities perspective. J Gerontol A Biol Sci Med Sci 2024; 79(9).
[58] Chen J, Zhao M, Zhou R, et al. How heavy is the medical expense burden among the older adults and what are the contributing factors? A literature review and problem-based analysis. Front Public Health 2023;11: 1165381.
[59] United Nations DoeaSA. Health inequalities in old age 2018. 2025. Available at: https://www.un.org/development/desa/ageing/news/2018/04/health-inequalities-in-old-age/. Accessed February 27, 2025.
[60] Jain S, Bey GS, Forrester SN, et al. Aging, race, and health disparities: recommendations from the research centers collaborative network. J Gerontol B Psychol Sci Soc Sci 2024;79(6).
[61] Jones CH, Dolsten M. Healthcare on the brink: navigating the challenges of an aging society in the United States. NPJ Aging 2024;10(1):22.
[62] Chang ES, Kannoth S, Levy S, et al. Global reach of ageism on older persons' health: a systematic review. PLoS One 2020;15(1):e0220857.
[63] Markopoulos C, van de Water W. Older patients with breast cancer: is there bias in the treatment they receive? Ther Adv Med Oncol 2012;4(6):321–7.
[64] Lau SWJ, Huang Y, Hsieh J, et al. Participation of older adults in clinical trials for new drug applications and biologics license applications from 2010 through 2019. JAMA Netw Open 2022;5(10):e2236149.
[65] Shaaban S, Ji Y. Pharmacogenomics and health disparities, are we helping? Front Genet 2023;14:1099541.
[66] Iqbal A, Richardson C, Iqbal Z, et al. Are there socioeconomic inequalities in polypharmacy among older people? A systematic review and meta-analysis. BMC Geriatr 2023;23(1):149.
[67] Finkelstein J, Friedman C, Hripcsak G, et al. Potential utility of precision medicine for older adults with polypharmacy: a case series study. Pharmgenomics Pers Med 2016;9:31–45.
[68] Terraneo M. Inequities in health care utilization by people aged 50+: evidence from 12 European countries. Soc Sci Med 2015;126:154–63.
[69] Spencer N, Raman S, O'Hare B, et al. Addressing inequities in child health and development: towards social justice. BMJ Paediatr Open 2019;3(1):e000503.
[70] Victorino CC, Gauthier AH. The social determinants of child health: variations across health outcomes - a population-based cross-sectional analysis. BMC Pediatr 2009;9:53.
[71] (WHO) WHO. WHO. Don't pollute my future! The impact of the environment on children's health. Geneva. 2017. Available at: https://www.who.int/publications/i/item/WHO-FWC-IHE-17.01.
[72] Hartinger SM, Lanata CF, Hattendorf J, et al. Improving household air, drinking water and hygiene in rural Peru: a community-randomized-controlled trial of an integrated environmental home-based intervention package to improve child health. Int J Epidemiol 2016;45(6):2089–99.
[73] Barros AJ, Ronsmans C, Axelson H, et al. Equity in maternal, newborn, and child health interventions in Countdown to 2015: a retrospective review of survey data from 54 countries. Lancet 2012;379(9822):1225–33.
[74] Slopen N, Chang AR, Johnson TJ, et al. Racial and ethnic inequities in the quality of paediatric care in the USA: a review of quantitative evidence. Lancet Child Adolesc Health 2024;8(2):147–58.
[75] Poulain T, Vogel M, Sobek C, et al. Associations between socio-economic status and child health: findings of a large German cohort study. Int J Environ Res Publ Health 2019;16(5).
[76] Veldhuis L, Vogel I, van Rossem L, et al. Influence of maternal and child lifestyle-related characteristics on the socioeconomic inequality in overweight and obesity among 5-year-old children; the "Be Active, Eat Right" Study. Int J Environ Res Publ Health 2013; 10(6):2336–47.
[77] Goldhagen JL, Shenoda S, Oberg C, et al. Rights, justice, and equity: a global agenda for child health and wellbeing. Lancet Child Adolesc Health 2020;4(1): 80–90.
[78] Fisher M, Freeman T, Mackean T, et al. Universal Health Coverage for Health Equity: from principle to practice; a response to the recent commentaries. Int J Health Pol Manag 2022;11(8):1601–3.
[79] Cheng TL, Emmanuel MA, Levy DJ, et al. Child health disparities: what can a clinician do? Pediatrics 2015; 136(5):961–8.
[80] Knopf JA, Finnie RK, Peng Y, et al. School-based health centers to advance health equity: a community guide systematic review. Am J Prev Med 2016;51(1):114–26.
[81] Yu L, Zhai X. Use of artificial intelligence to address health disparities in low- and middle-income countries: a thematic analysis of ethical issues. Public Health 2024;234:77–83.
[82] Ciecierski-Holmes T, Singh R, Axt M, et al. Artificial intelligence for strengthening healthcare systems in low- and middle-income countries: a systematic scoping review. npj Digit Med 2022;5(1):162.
[83] Rothlisberger PN. AI-powered patient-centered care: a call to action for innovation. J Healthc Manag 2024; 69(4):255–66.
[84] Norori N, Hu Q, Aellen FM, et al. Addressing bias in big data and AI for health care: a call for open science. Patterns (N Y) 2021;2(10):100347.
[85] Park Y, Hu J. Bias in artificial intelligence: basic primer. Clin J Am Soc Nephrol 2023;18(3):394–6.
[86] Fatumo S, Chikowore T, Choudhury A, et al. A roadmap to increase diversity in genomic studies. Nat Med 2022;28(2):243–50.

[87] Obermeyer Z, Powers B, Vogeli C, et al. Dissecting racial bias in an algorithm used to manage the health of populations. Science 2019;366(6464):447–53.

[88] Ganapathi S, Palmer J, Alderman JE, et al. Tackling bias in AI health datasets through the STANDING Together initiative. Nat Med 2022;28(11):2232–3.

[89] US food and drug administration (FDA) HCatUMaH-pRAM. Good machine learning practice for medical device development: guiding principles 2021 cited March/12/2025. Available at: https://www.fda.gov/medical-devices/software-medical-device-samd/good-machine-learning-practice-medical-device-development-guiding-principles.

[90] Kim Y, Vazquez C, Cubbin C. Socioeconomic disparities in health outcomes in the United States in the late 2010s: results from four national population-based studies. Arch Public Health 2023;81(1):15.

[91] Magge H, Cabral HJ, Kazis LE, et al. Prevalence and predictors of underinsurance among low-income adults. J Gen Intern Med 2013;28(9):1136–42.

[92] Disparities in healthcare. 2021 National Healthcare Quality and Disparities Report 2021. 2025. Available at: https://www.ncbi.nlm.nih.gov/books/NBK578532/. Accessed March 12, 2025.

[93] Cutler DM. Early returns from the era of precision medicine. JAMA 2020;323(2):109–10.

[94] Kumar S, Bennett A, Campbell PA, et al. Costs of next-generation sequencing assays in non-small cell lung cancer: a micro-costing study. Curr Oncol 2022; 29(8):5238–46.

[95] Siddiqui M, Rajkumar SV. The high cost of cancer drugs and what we can do about it. Mayo Clin Proc 2012;87-(10):935–43.

[96] Latif AS. The importance of understanding social and cultural norms in delivering quality health care-a personal experience commentary. Trop Med Infect Dis 2020;5(1).

[97] Alarcon FJ. The migrant crisis and access to health care. Dela J Public Health 2022;8(4):20–5.

[98] Diaz VA, Mainous AG 3rd, Gavin JK, et al. Racial differences in attitudes toward personalized medicine. Public Health Genom 2014;17(1):1–6.

[99] Yu J, Meng S. Impacts of the internet on health inequality and healthcare access: a cross-country study. Front Public Health 2022;10:935608.

[100] Coombs NC, Campbell DG, Caringi J. A qualitative study of rural healthcare providers' views of social, cultural, and programmatic barriers to healthcare access. BMC Health Serv Res 2022;22(1):438.

[101] Butzner M, Cuffee Y. Telehealth interventions and outcomes across rural communities in the United States: narrative review. J Med Internet Res 2021;23(8): e29575.

[102] Hatten JM, Connerton RE. Urban and rural hospitals: how do they differ? Health Care. Financ Rev (Buffalo, N Y) 1986;8(2):77–85.

[103] Maganty A, Byrnes ME, Hamm M, et al. Barriers to rural health care from the provider perspective. Rural Remote Health 2023;23(2):7769.

[104] Khoury MJ, Bowen S, Dotson WD, et al. Health equity in the implementation of genomics and precision medicine: a public health imperative. Genet Med 2022;24(8):1630–9.

[105] Fuentes-Afflick E. Are we serious about addressing health disparities through research? J Pediatr 2022; 247:10–1.

[106] Disparities NIoMHaH. Minority health and health disparities: definitions and parameters. Available at: https://www.nimhd.nih.gov/about/strategic-plan/nih-strategic-plan-definitions-and-parameters.html.

[107] Braveman P, Gruskin S. Defining equity in health. J Epidemiol Community Health 2003;57(4):254–8.

Advances in Molecular Pathology 8 (2025) 175–187
ADVANCES IN MOLECULAR PATHOLOGY

The Near Future of Cancer Cytogenetics

Whole Genome Sequencing, Long-Read Sequencing, or Optical Genome Mapping?

Madina Sukhanova, PhD[a], **Elena A. Repnikova, PhD**[b,*]
[a]Department of Pathology, Division of Molecular Pathology, Feinberg School of Medicine, Northwestern University, 710 N Fairbanks Ct, Suite 2-453, Chicago, IL 60611, USA; [b]Department of Pathology and Laboratory Medicine, Children's Mercy Kansas City, University of Missouri Kansas City Medical School, 2401 Gillham Road, Kansas City, MO 64108, USA

KEYWORDS
• Cytogenetics • DNA • High molecular weight DNA • Whole-genome sequencing • Short-read sequencing • Long-read sequencing • Optical genome mapping (OGM)

KEY POINTS
- Conventional cytogenetics (often referred to as karyotyping) has traditionally served as an essential tool in the diagnostic evaluation of hematological malignancies and solid tumors.
- Contemporary cancer diagnostics necessitates the adoption of advanced high-resolution testing modalities that facilitate simultaneous assessment of genomic variations across the entire genome.
- Modern technologies include nonsequencing optical genome mapping as well as sequencing technologies such as whole genome short-read DNA sequencing and long-read sequencing.
- Each diagnostic method has advantages and limitations. Ultimately, the selection of a diagnostic pipeline should align with clinical therapy guidelines and be tailored to the specific circumstances of each laboratory and health care institution.

INTRODUCTION

Genetic markers are not only increasingly recognized as critical components in cancer diagnosis and risk assessment but also as targets for specific therapies. This allows to increasingly incorporate genetic alterations into tumor classification systems to refine diagnoses and guide treatment strategies [1–3]. Conventional cytogenetics, often referred to as G-banded chromosome analysis, has served for decades as an important diagnostic method in oncology, aiding in the identification of canonical diagnostic chromosomal abnormalities, such as t(8;21)/*RUNX1::RUNX1T1* in acute myeloid leukemia (AML) or t(11;22)/*EWSR1::FLI1* in Ewing sarcoma, reduced number of chromosomes in hypodiploid B-cell acute lymphoblastic leukemia (B-ALL), or an unbalanced der(1;19) resulting in combined loss of 1p/19q in oligodendroglioma. Chromosome analysis has also proven to be a valuable tool in cancer risk assessment, enabling the identification of cases with complex karyotypes in hematologic malignancies and cases exhibiting *MYCN* amplification in neuroblastoma, both of which are recognized as indicators of poor prognosis. The discovery of the Philadelphia chromosome through conventional cytogenetics, followed

*Corresponding author. *E-mail address:* erepnikova@cmh.edu

https://doi.org/10.1016/j.yamp.2025.05.009 www.advancesinmolecularpathology.com
2589-4080/25/ © 2025 Elsevier Inc. All rights are reserved, including those for text and data mining, AI training, and similar technologies.

ABBREVIATIONS	
AML	Acute Myeloid Leukemia
APL	Acute Promyelocytic Leukemia
B-ALL	B-cell Acute Lymphoblastic Leukemia
CNAs	Copy Number Alterations
CN-LOH	Copy-Neutral-Loss of Heterozygosity
ctDNA	circulating tumor DNA
FFPE	Formalin-Fixed Paraffin-Embedded
FISH	Fluorescence *in situ* Hybridization
HRD	Homologous Recombination Deficiency
LRS	Long-Read DNA Sequencing
MRD	Minimal Residual Disease
MSI	Microsatellite Instability
OGM	Optical Genome Mapping
PCR	Polymerase Chain Reaction
SNP	Single Nucleotide Polymorphism
SNVs	Single Nucleotide Variants
SVs	Structural Variants
TAT	Turnaround Time
TMB	Tumor Mutational Burden
WGS	Whole Genome Sequencing

by the development of the first targeted therapies, marked the beginning of a new era in precision medicine, wherein treatments are customized based on the unique genetic profile of each patient's tumor [4].

Chromosome analysis continues to be an important tool **in the diagnosis and management of hematologic malignancies**; however, its limitations—such as low resolution and difficulties associated **with culturing process** or the limited proliferative capacity of tumor cells—have prompted a gradual shift toward the adoption of molecular methods **in solid tumors diagnostics**. Furthermore, improved **understanding of** genomic alterations, **including the clinical significance of promoter region changes and noncanonical fusions with novel partner genes**, tandem duplications, and intragenic deletions has led to a concerted effort to develop high-resolution, genome-wide molecular technologies, such as long-read DNA sequencing (LRS), optical genome mapping (OGM), and short-read whole genome sequencing (WGS). These **techniques** aim to comprehensively assess genetic changes that are frequently cryptic and difficult to identify using traditional cytogenetic **methods**.

As the adoption of these advanced high-resolution technologies increases, a common question is whether any of these innovative methods can replace the wide menu of clinical tests, including traditional chromosome analysis, to serve as a stand-alone clinical test. This review focuses on three genome-wide DNA-based techniques (WGS, LRS, and OGM) and analyzes their respective advantages and limitations in a clinical setting. At the time of this publication, it is evident that there is no definitive superior or inferior technique. Each method may have unique edge cases where genetic abnormalities are identified by one technique but missed by another. However, although utilization of all available techniques could provide the most comprehensive characterization of tumor molecular profile in the setting with unlimited resources, in real clinical practice this approach would be financially burdensome. Thus, it is critical to have a thorough understanding of the advantages and limitations of each technology prior to its implementation to address the clinical question at hand. Ultimately, the selection of a diagnostic pipeline should align with clinical therapy guidelines and be tailored to the specific circumstances of each laboratory and health care institution.

Conventional Cytogenetic Methods

G-banded chromosome analysis and fluorescence *in situ* hybridization (FISH) are well-established complementary clinical tests utilized in oncology. G-banded chromosome analysis has been used in clinical diagnostics for more than 70 years [5]. Despite its low resolution, this method provides a robust overview of the entire human genome packed in a complete set of chromosomes known as karyotype at the single cell level. It enables the detection of polyploidy and aneuploidy (abnormal number of a complete set of chromosomes or any individual chromosome), large size translocations, deletions, insertions, supernumerary marker chromosomes, and so forth [6]. FISH enhances the resolution of chromosome analysis by using fluorescently labeled probes to target specific DNA sequences. Incorporating FISH testing alongside conventional karyotyping allows to identify genetic alterations cryptic to resolution of chromosome analysis, including submicroscopic deletions and atypical gene rearrangements. FISH is particularly valuable for clarification of ambiguous chromosomal alterations, including but not limited to atypical rearrangements or amplification of the *KMT2A* or *MYC* genes in myeloid neoplasms [7–9].

In contrast to karyotype analysis, FISH does not require fresh material and is an effective and rapid diagnostic method in solid tumors, applicable to both touch preparations of fresh tumor tissue and formalin-fixed paraffin-embedded (FFPE) tissue sections. Notable applications include the assessment of *HER2* amplification in breast cancer, *MYCN* amplification in neuroblastoma, and *ALK* or *ROS1* rearrangements in lung cancer, which are critical for informing targeted therapy decisions.

However, both methods have limitations; that is, chromosome analysis has a resolution of approximately 3 to 5 Mb and strongly depends on viability and proliferative rate of tumor cells, whereas a major pitfall of FISH is its targeted nature and restricted number of commercially available probes. Furthermore, the banding resolution of chromosome analysis presents difficulties in accurately identifying abnormalities and is sometimes linked to subjective interpretations [10].

Nevertheless, a combined use of G-banded chromosome analysis and FISH provides a robust assessment of chromosomal integrity and specific well-characterized genetic alterations, often yielding sufficient information for diagnosis, risk stratification, and identifying targets for personalized treatment even nowadays.

Implementation of Whole-Genome Methods in Current Clinical Practice

The substantial decrease in sequencing costs allowed to incorporate WGS into clinical oncology practices across multiple institutions, frequently complemented by comprehensive transcriptome profiling via whole-genome RNA sequencing [11–15]. This success prompted further development of sequencing-based methods, leading to implementation of novel third-generation methodologies interrogating high molecular weight DNA (often referred in literature to as long-read DNA), which confidently detect not only SNVs, CNAs, and SVs but also methylation profiles in its native state without the need of bisulfite conversion and amplification, eliminating artifacts induced by these steps and increasing the accuracy of data. OGM is a nonsequencing technology that is gaining traction in cancer diagnostics; it has the capability to detect not only CNAs but also SVs with presumably higher accuracy compared to the short-read WGS, which still depends on analysis pipelines.

In light of advancements in diagnostic technologies, an obvious question is if any of these molecular methodologies can be utilized as a stand-alone test in cancer diagnostics. What would it take to transition from conventional cancer cytogenetics to a molecular-based diagnostics only, taking into account technical limitations, abnormality detection rates, timeline to a final diagnostic report, and resources needed for clinical validation and implementation? Does traditional cytogenetics, that is, chromosome and FISH analyses, still have a place in cancer diagnostics? This review aims to compare emerging methodologies and evaluate their clinical utility. While we acknowledge the substantial benefits of the emerging new technologies for patient care, we must also address the challenges that need to be resolved before moving away from traditional methodologies.

Landscape of the Modern Whole-Genome Methods

Sequencing-based approaches

Short-read whole genome sequencing. Implementation of WGS in clinical cancer diagnostic setting has become a primary goal since the human genome project completion due to its proven capability to detect a wide range of genomic abnormalities, from SNVs, CNAs, and gene fusions, to pangenomic markers, such as tumor mutational burden (TMB), homologous recombination deficiency (HRD), or mismatch repair deficiency [11,13]. Several reports from various large-scale sequencing programs have highlighted that the combination of genome-wide transcriptome analysis (RNA-seq) and WGS offers a significant capability for detecting clinically actionable variants in patients with hematologic malignancies and solid tumors, including gene expression profile and alternative splicing events [11,16–24]. Some studies have suggested that WGS combined with the whole-genome transcriptome analysis might replace existing cascades of clinical tests in the nearest future [15,25].

One recognized limitation of the existing advanced sequencing technologies in solid tumor diagnostics is the requirement for a significant quantity of DNA extracted from tumor tissue, which is typically acquired through invasive procedures such as needle biopsy or surgical tumor resection. The drastic shift in molecular diagnostics has happened with the understanding that predictive genetic markers in tumor DNA can be detected not only in the biopsies obtained from tumor primary or metastatic sites, but also in body fluids, including but not limited to plasma, urine, saliva, or stool [26], all easily available for collecting through noninvasive methods. Although the discovery that circulating tumor DNA (ctDNA) "shed" into bloodstream due to cell death followed by cell breakdown was made over 75 years ago [27], it took decades before improved library preparation methods with polymerase chain reaction (PCR) enrichment and reduced sequencing cost brought sensitivity of variant detection in ctDNA (sized <150 bp) to 0.01%. This progress enabled the clinical application of short-read sequencing of ctDNA, utilizing various body fluids as sample types for the diagnosis of specific tumor types. Thus, analysis of ctDNA extracted from urine of patients with genitourinary cancers revealed various SNVs or epigenetic markers of clinical significance, such as mutations in **FGFR3** or hypomethylation of *IRAK3, L1-MET,* and *SOX1* [28]. Stool samples can be used for early detection of colorectal cancer [29,30], whereas lavage samples can be tested for the diagnosis of lung cancer [29]. Various clinical trials applying analysis of ctDNA revealed notable concordance between DNA variants detected in circulating tumor cells versus tumor biopsies with a drastic reduction in turnaround time (TAT) [31] revolutionizing the field of solid tumor diagnosis and opening new perspectives for early cancer detection.

With full recognition of many advantages of WGS in cancer diagnostics and clinical research compared to conventional cytogenetics, implementation of WGS should be performed with understanding of potential barriers. First of all, conventional short-read WGS methodologies, despite their robustness, encounter significant challenges in accurate detection of complex structural genomic rearrangements and repetitive sequences, which are frequently associated with cancer. WGS is generally more costly and requires significant bioinformatics support and expertise in variant interpretation to allow careful separation of clinically actionable variants from variants of uncertain clinical significance, making true genome-wide analysis a time-consuming process with the involvement of sophisticated bioinformatics tools to ensure quality and accuracy of variant calling [32]. WGS undoubtedly identifies significantly more genetic markers of known and potential clinical significance compared to accepted standard-of-care tests, such as next-generation sequencing (NGS) panels and conventional cytogenetics; however, when deciding to implement WGS, each institution should take into consideration a substantial upfront investment in instrumentation, laboratory infrastructure, laboratory personnel training, and development and incorporation of bioinformatics analysis pipelines [33].

Long-read sequencing: PacBio and Oxford Nanopore. Long-read sequencing (LRS) technology (often referred to as third-generation sequencing) has recently emerged as a promising tool that is capable of generating significantly longer contiguous DNA sequences (~1 kb–30 kb), overcoming a recognized limitation of short-read WGS known for notable false-positive rate of calling of CNAs and SVs [34,35]. Although characterized by high error rate at the beginning, both major commercially available platforms, PacBio and Oxford Nanopore after recent improvements in chemistry and base-calling bioinformatics tools, reported the sequencing accuracy at up to 99.9% at Q30 providing a promising approach that can capture structural chromosomal abnormalities besides sequence-level variants and CNAs [36,37].

Nowadays, LRS technology facilitates more accurate detection of various structural variations, including translocations, inversions, and large insertions/deletions simultaneously in one test, providing molecular karyotyping data at the superior resolution compared to standard cytogenetics with an improved accuracy and reduced sequencing bias compared to short-read WGS due to no need for amplification in the former. Long-read sequencing provides methylation and hydroxymethylation data without the requirement for bisulfite conversion, which can sometimes introduce errors [38]. The methylation profile has been identified as one of the diagnostic criteria for central nervous system tumors by the World Health Organization [2] and is increasingly valued for its role in the diagnostic differentiation of various solid tumor types, particularly in complex cases involving metastatic processes of unknown primary origin [39–41].

TAT might be variable due to the need of comprehensive analysis pipelines, nevertheless, portable and ultrarapid long-read sequencing (MinION) provides an opportunity for point-of-care detection of clinically targetable genetic markers in less than 10 hours [42,43].

Furthermore, LRS improves the resolution of repetitive regions, enabling better characterization of complex genomic loci and potentially revealing novel cancer-associated variants that are missed by short-read sequencing. It addresses the limitations of short-read WGS by enabling accurate analysis of challenging sequences, including GC-rich regions and tandem repeats. This technology facilitates the precise identification of pseudogenes [44] and often enables phasing the identified variants [45].

Clinical research studies consistently identified LRS as a diagnostic tool with the potential to supersede conventional karyotyping, short-read WGS, and methylation sequencing. However, due to its relative novelty, data on the extent of additional clinical information generated by this methodology, as well as its impact on patient treatment plans compared to standard-of-care tests, remain limited. Further evidence is necessary to fully evaluate its potential.

Nonsequencing-based technology. OGM is a nonsequencing approach that involves analysis of fluorescently labeled DNA molecules, ranging in size from 150 kbp to several megabases in size, linearized for imaging in nanoarrays. Since being pioneered by Schwartz and colleagues [46] in 1993, the technology used in optical mapping has improved substantially. This method now provides the capability to detect CNAs and can detect most SVs with an additional confirmatory sequencing needed to pinpoint precise breakpoints [47]. In contrast to conventional techniques such as karyotyping and FISH, OGM is capable of discerning a broad spectrum of SVs, including large deletions, insertions, translocations, inversions, and complex structural rearrangements, with enhanced resolution and precision. This capability is pivotal given that SVs play a significant role in oncogenesis and tumor progression, affecting gene expression, protein function, and drug responsiveness. OGM is particularly adept at identifying novel gene fusions, potentially influencing further characterization of cancer pathogenesis. Thus, multiple studies have suggested that this technology may serve as a replacement for conventional cytogenetics testing [17,18,20,22].

Based on the current cancer literature review, OGM has the best application in the diagnostics of acute leukemias. While this technology demonstrates distinct advantages in detecting CNAs and SVs across the entire genome over the karyotyping method, it has several recognized limitations that may impede its broader adoption in clinical diagnostics. First, to achieve accurate mapping, OGM requires high molecular weight DNA. Therefore, DNA quantity, degradation, or fragmentation has a significant impact on the quality of the results. Second, the minimum allele fraction threshold for detection is 5% for CNAs and 10% for SVs [48]. Thus, the presence of abnormal cells in less

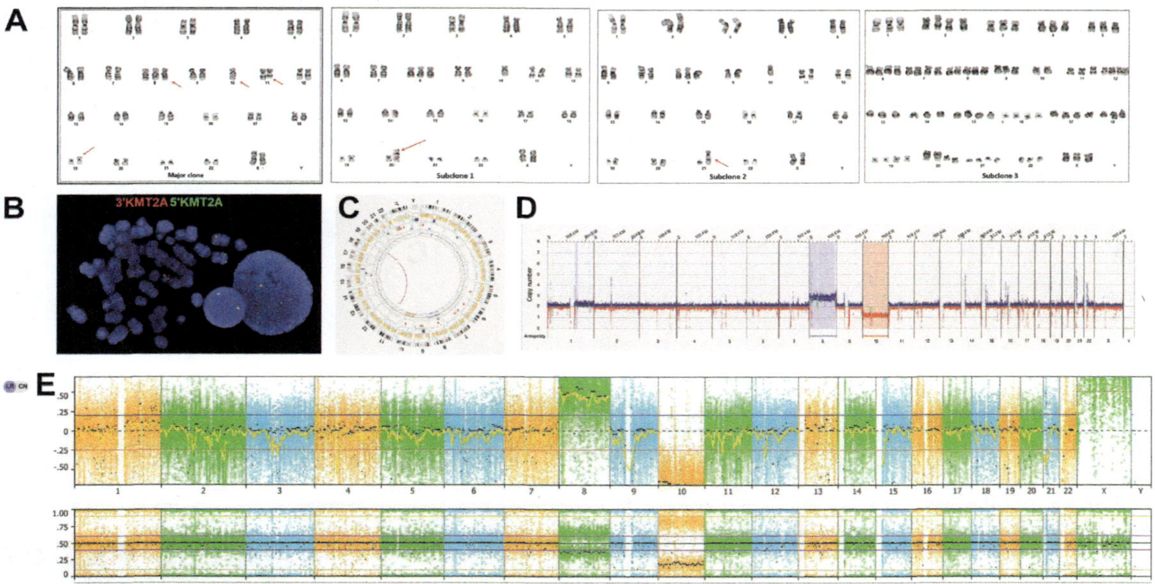

FIG. 1 Genomic analysis of a bone marrow sample from the patient with acute myeloid leukemia. (**A**) G-banding chromosome analysis shows primary clone with the t(11;19) (q23;p13.3), gain of chromosome 8, and loss of chromosome 10 in 12 cells; subclone 1 shows an additional derivative chromosome 20, der(20)t(1;20)(q21;p13) in 5 cells; subclone 2 shows an additional translocation between the long arm of chromosome 1 and the short arm of chromosome 21, and absent derivative chromosome 20 in 2 cells; subclone 3 derived from subclone 2 shows 80 chromosomes with the same structural abnormalities as subclone 2 including gains/losses of several chromosomes in 3 cells. (**B**) FISH analysis shows *KMT2A* rearrangement using break-apart probe. (**C**) OGM Circos plot view showing t(11;19) consistent with the *KMT2A::MLLT1* fusion. (**D**) OGM whole genome view showing gain of the 1q21.1q44 region (~105 Mb) and the chromosome 8, losses of the 1p36.11 region (~1 Mb) and the entire chromosome 10. Other subclonal changes identified by chromosome analysis are not detected by OGM. (**E**) WGS (short-read) whole genome view showing gain of the entire 1q, 8, and loss of 10. Loss of 1p36.11 is detected but not shown in the whole genome view. Sensitivity for chromosomal mosaicism detection is significantly reduced by WGS. The red arrow indicates abnormal chromosomes identified in the major clone. Subsequent subclones 1 and 2 display new abnormalities, marked by red arrows, that were not present in the major clone. The third subclone exhibits additional chromosomal gains observed consistently across the major clone and subclones 1 and 2.

than approximately 10% of the sample may result in normal findings, rendering this technology unsuitable for the detection of minor clones and minimal residual disease (MRD) monitoring and necessitating the use of alternative techniques [49] (Fig. 1A–E).

Many acute and chronic leukemias are often characterized by a high cell count and a significant proportion of abnormal cells, making the implementation of OGM in blood or bone marrow samples relatively straightforward. Nevertheless, the technology may encounter challenges when applied to other sample types (eg, lymph nodes in extramedullary hematologic malignancies) or samples with low and insufficient number of cells, such as pleural fluid (eg, T-cell lymphocytic lymphoma), CD138$^+$ sorted cells (eg, for the diagnosis of a plasma cell disorder) [50]. Additionally, highly repetitive regions, such as centromeric regions, short arms of acrocentric chromosomes, pseudoautosomal regions, and telomeric regions, are often poorly covered by OGM. Consequently, recurrent rearrangements such as the *P2RY8::CRLF2* and *IGH::CRLF2* fusions, which are associated with B-ALL with *BCR::ABL1*-like features, often go undetected [49].

Robertsonian translocations as well as other whole-arm translocations involving centromeric regions cannot be currently detected by OGM [51]. Also, OGM may not accurately detect ploidy—which is important in hypodiploid B-ALL with doubling (Fig. 2A–D). Furthermore, the detection of copy neutral loss of heterozygosity, which is essential information in the diagnosis of certain solid tumors (eg, Wilms tumors and neuroblastoma), is restricted to regions of 20 Mb or greater. The inability to identify critical aberrations affecting treatment decisions requires laboratories to implement additional alternative methods to ensure the comprehensive detection of the full range of abnormalities.

Overall, OGM serves as a highly effective methodology for the identification and characterization of the diagnostic CNAs and SVs. However, its implementation as a frontline diagnostic method necessitates not only expertise in interpretation and an understanding of potential artifactual findings but also a considerable effort in conducting additional testing and confirmations for both hematological malignancies and solid tumors.

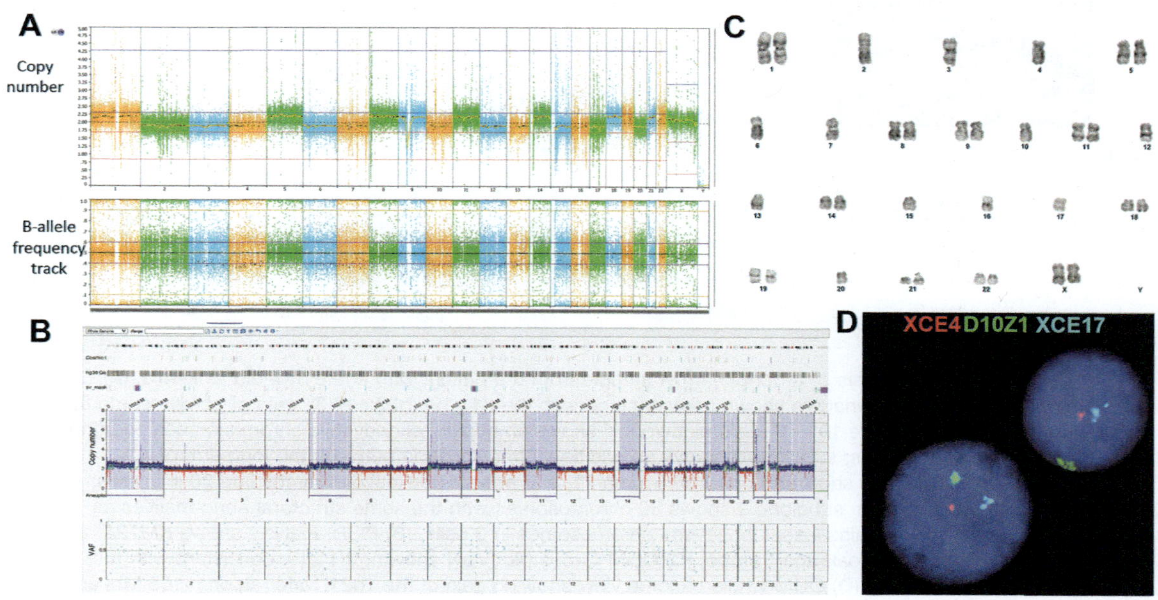

FIG. 2 Comprehensive genomic analysis of a bone marrow specimen obtained from the patient diagnosed with B-cell acute lymphoblastic leukemia. Analysis of the DNA profile utilizing novel molecular techniques necessitates the integration of flow cytometry data, and "**traditional cytogenetic technology to assess ploidy**". (**A**) Short-read WES analysis (**B**) OGM whole genome view. SV Key: Dark blue: CNA gain, Red: CNA loss (**C**) G-banding karyotype analysis showing hypodiploid cell. (**D**) Nuclei FISH analysis using centromeric probe to chromosomes 4, 10, and 17 is consistent with monosomy for chromosomes 4, 10, and 17.

Limitations of advanced molecular technologies employing bulk DNA methods

Ploidy detection. Although advanced technologies such as WGS, LRS, and OGM offer significant benefits in identifying various genomic anomalies associated with cancer, it is crucial to evaluate the limitations of these methods regarding the detection of certain abnormalities prior to implementing them as first-line or standalone diagnostic tools. For example, these technologies may inaccurately assess alterations in ploidy, particularly in cases where modifications impact the entire chromosomal set or several chromosomes, rather than merely the gain or loss of individual chromosomes (Fig. 2A–D). An illustrative case pertains to the precise distinction between hypodiploid B-ALL, classified as a high-risk subtype due to the frequent doubling of the entire leukemia genome (referred to as masked hypodiploidy) and hyperdiploid B-ALL, recognized as a lower-risk disease. In such scenarios, the use of orthogonal testing would be advantageous for an accurate ploidy status assessment. For instance, the Children's Oncology Group recommends incorporating a method with single nucleotide polymorphism (SNP) genotyping capabilities for masked hypodiploid B-ALL. In other cases, FISH, which is applicable to virtually all cancer samples, including tumor touch preparations and FFPE tissue sections, or conventional chromosome analysis, which is limited by the requirement of fresh specimens, can still be employed. Aneuploidy is not exclusive to hematological malignancies (eg, B-ALL or plasma cell neoplasms)—it is also a recurrent finding in many solid tumors (Fig. 3A–D); thus, an

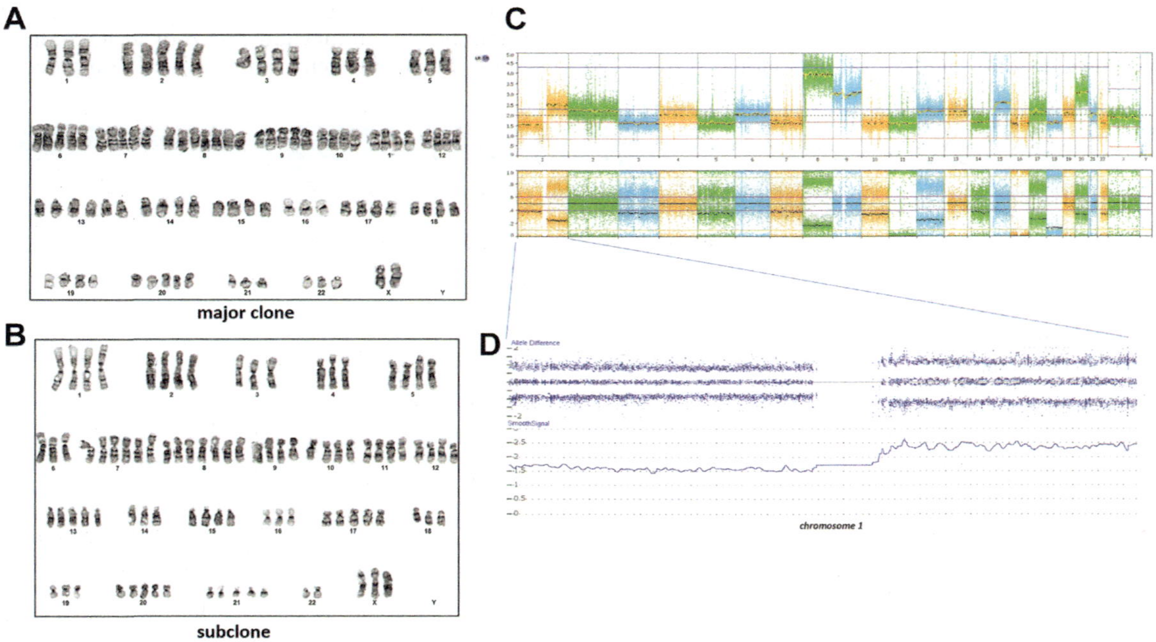

FIG. 3 Genomic characterization of a renal neoplasm with a pathologic diagnosis of metastatic Wilms tumor. G-banding chromosome analysis showed a near-tetraploid karyotype in two clonal populations of cells: (A) the consistent abnormalities in a major clone include a relative loss of chromosomes 1, 4, 5, 16, 21, 22, and X, and a relative gain of chromosomes 2, 6, 7, 8, 9, 13, and 20 in ten cells; (**B**) a subclone contained an additional isochromosome 1q resulting in relative gain of 1q with loss of 1p in eight cells; (**C**) WGS shows average of two clonal populations and identified losses of 1p, 3, 5, 7, 10, 11, 14, 16, 18, and 22 and gains of 1q, 2, 4, 6, 8, 9, 12, 13, 15, 17, 19, and 20 in addition to copy-neutral loss of heterozygosity (cnLOH) involving the entire chromosomes 11 and 16. The findings are consistent with metastatic Wilms tumor. Combined loss of heterozygosity involving 1p and 16q would necessitate augmenting therapy. From genomic analysis only, it appears that there is a loss of the entire 1p. (**D**) The observed loss of 1p is relative to a tetraploid genome and the tumor contains two distinct copies of 1p, with no indications of copy-neutral loss of heterozygosity, as evidenced by SNP microarray analysis of the same tumor.

accurate detection of ploidy is critical not only for precise diagnosis but also for risk assessment and subsequent treatment decisions.

Detection of subclonal abnormalities and complex karyotypes

Another major pitfall for any of the above-mentioned new technologies that utilize bulk DNA lies in their inability to assign detected abnormalities to distinct clones that may be handy in unique cases with multiple neoplasms present in one biopsy or a limited sensitivity in the detection of subclonal abnormalities (Fig. 1) [49]. Examples include either concurrent chronic lymphocytic leukemia in a patient with multiple myeloma [52] or evolving myeloid malignancy in a patient with plasma cells disorder postcytotoxic treatment [53], or a coexistence of chronic myelogenous leukemia and chronic lymphocytic leukemia originated from different clonal cells [54], as well as detection of a complex karyotype (defined based on presence of 3 or more cytogenetic abnormalities in one clone), which is considered an adverse risk factor in myeloid neoplasms (World Health Organization [WHO], International Consensus Classification [ICC], and Revised International Prognostic Scoring System [R-IPSS]). The latest National Comprehensive Cancer Network (NCCN) guidelines currently under review (2025) recommend WGS for the diagnostic evaluation of adult patients with acute myeloid leukemia (AML). However, traditional cytogenetics testing remains included as part of the diagnostic assessment. We believe that wider implementation of WGS following NCCN guidelines recommendations will result in consensus on how to assess genomic complexity from genome-wide sequencing data, an alternative criterion for complex karyotype.

Cost. Despite continuous reduction of cost of sequencing, short-read WGS and long-read sequencing remain expensive technologies to set up in the laboratory with an inevitable need of strong bioinformatics support. Even more, when compared to

TABLE 1
Comparison of Variant Type Detection Between Whole-Genome DNA-Based Methods

	Chromosome Analysis	Short-Read WGS	Long-Read WGS	OGM
Large-scale CNAs (>5 Mb)	Y	Y	Y	Y
Small-to-medium CNAs (<5 Mb)	N	Y	Y	Y
SNVs	N	Y	Y	N
Indels	N	Y	Y	N
Tandem repeats	N	Sequence and size dependent	Y	N
SVs	Y (>5 Mb)	N	Y	>500 bp–5 kb; excluding whole arm and repetitive
TMB	N	Y	Y	N
MSI	N	Y	Y	Y* (requires an additional bioinformatic analysis)
HRD	N	Y	Y	Y* (requires an additional bioinformatic analysis)
CN-LOH	N	Y	Y	>20 Mb
Aneuploidy	Y	Y	Y	Y
Polyploidy	Y	N	N	N
Methylation defects	N	N	Y	N

Abbreviations: CNA, copy number alterations; CN-LOH, copy-neutral loss of heterozygosity; HRD, homologous recombination deficiency; MSI, microsatellite instability; SNV, single nucleotide variant.

TABLE 2
Comparison of Clinical Utility and Other Considerations for Whole-Genome DNA-Based Methods

	Chromosome Analysis	Short-Read WGS	Long-Read WGS	OGM
Mosaicism/tumor purity detection sensitivity	~5%–10%	~10%	~20%–30%	10%
Single cell resolution	Y	N	N	N
Sample/tissue type requirement	Fresh (liquid/solid)	Fresh/Frozen/FFPE (liquid/solid)	Fresh/Frozen (liquid/solid)	Fresh/Frozen (liquid/cell lines)
Minimal sample size	10,000 cells	1 µg DNA	>500 ng DNA	1.5×10^6 cells
Clinical utility	Diagnosis and relapse	Diagnosis, relapse, and MRD (deep sequencing)	Diagnosis and relapse	Diagnosis and relapse
Approximate TAT for laboratory work and reporting of the data (laboratory dependent)	4–21 d	~10–60 d [15,57]	~2–30 d [42,58,59]	~4–28 d [51,60]
Ability to multiplex	Low to medium	High	High	Low to medium
Staffing requirement	Cytogenetic technologist	Molecular genetics technologists and Bioinformatics support	Molecular genetics technologists and Bioinformatics support	Molecular genetics technologists and Bioinformatics support
Minimal number of samples required to be processed together (in one run)	1	16~17 (10B) 24~38 (25B) (depends on the sequencing platform and flow cell capacity)	1~4 (depends on the platform and SMRT cell capacity)	>3
Cost of the test	++	++++	++++	++
Capital investment	+++	+++++	+++++	++

short-read WGS, the third-generation sequencing requires specialized computing algorithms to handle long read length, and is characterized by lower throughput, higher price per base, and more stringent sample requirements in order to obtain high-molecular weight DNA [37].

Throughput. A major current pitfall of OGM and LRS is their lower throughput, which will require an investment in additional instruments for large-scale laboratories processing a significant number of cancer samples every day. On the other hand, laboratories with low sample volumes would face the need to batch several samples for one run, leading to considerably longer TAT.

Turnaround time. Obtaining results in a timely manner is particularly crucial in hematology oncology, as the knowledge of genomic markers facilitates appropriate treatment planning. One such example is acute promyelocytic leukemia (APL) that is driven by hallmark genetic rearrangement, most frequently the t(15;17) resulting in the *PML::RARA* fusion. This leukemia subtype is classified as a medical emergency due to the significant risk of early mortality associated with severe hemorrhagic complications arising from a distinct coagulopathy. Availability of highly effective targeted treatment, which includes all-trans retinoic acid revolutionized the clinical management of patients with APL. As a result, a rapid diagnosis of APL characterized by the t(15;17) is essential. The fastest TAT for this fusion detection can be provided by FISH or reverse transcription polymerase chain reaction (RT-PCR) (<6 hours), followed by rapid karyotyping (~2 days).

Not a minimal residual disease test. Despite the broad range of abnormalities that can be identified through optical genome mapping (OGM) and long-read sequencing, these methods currently do not achieve a sensitivity threshold of 0.01%. Due to these sensitivity limitations, their applications are primarily restricted to diagnostic purposes and relapse assessment, rather than minimal residual disease (MRD) monitoring, which is now considered the standard of care. Consequently, routine molecular MRD assessment using quantitative PCR or digital droplet PCR is recommended by the European Leukemia Network guidelines [55], not only for patients with acute promyelocytic leukemia (APL) but also for those with AML harboring *RUNX1::RUNX1T1* and *MYH11::CBFB* fusions. Although MRD monitoring can be technically performed using short-read WGS, reverse transcription PCR (RT-PCR) remains a highly effective and significantly more cost-efficient method for evaluating treatment response and early disease relapse detection [56].

"Quantity not sufficient" samples. In the diagnosis of solid tumors, the initial biopsy often involves a limited sample size, which can pose challenges in obtaining sufficient quantities of nucleic acids needed for high-throughput molecular tests. When the morphology examination of a limited biopsy is highly indicative of a specific cancer, utilizing FISH or RT-PCR on a touch preparation or FFPE tumor sections can still provide much needed results. In the evaluation of hematologic malignancies, initial bone marrow biopsy assessments for acute leukemias may sometimes be inconclusive. In these cases, analysis of peripheral blood samples serves as a valuable diagnostic tool; however, blood transfusions administered to stabilize the patient can reduce the detectable level of blasts. Considering that the sensitivity of advanced second- and third-generation molecular tests for detecting abnormalities may be limited under these conditions, cytogenetic testing—even with a minimal presence of leukemic blasts—can often play a valuable role in establishing an accurate diagnosis and informing treatment strategies.

SUMMARY

The field of genetic diagnostics has undergone a remarkable transformation since its inception, evolving from conventional chromosome analysis in cultured preparations to the complex and sophisticated whole-genome technologies we have today. This journey has revolutionized the way various cancers are diagnosed and treated, significantly impacting patient care worldwide. The implementation of molecular diagnostic tools marked a new era, improving the diagnostic rate, clarity, and accessibility of data. This innovation has opened new doors for early disease detection and personalized medicine. For many years, conventional chromosome analysis has been serving as an important tool for the diagnosis of many hematological malignancies and solid tumors. Since the introduction of sequencing methods, it has become clear that one of evolving molecular high-throughput technologies supplemented by transcriptome analysis will eventually obsolete conventional chromosome analysis as a frontline diagnostic test. As our comparison tables show (Tables 1 and 2), we are close to the point of transition. However, we hope that our overview demonstrates that there is still scope for conventional chromosome analysis in diagnostic clinical oncology.

It is crucial to carefully evaluate all parameters beginning from the types of malignancies analyzed by the laboratory, clinical guidelines recommendations, expected TAT, staff availability, and financial considerations for each institution to establish the optimal diagnostic pipeline with inevitable periodic reassessment due to rapid advancements in methodologies. The coming years will certainly see major changes. In the interim, the transition period can include proper use of available diagnostic tools for ongoing patient care combined with validation conducted by qualified laboratory personnel. Even if the utility of conventional chromosome analysis as a diagnostic tool is undergoing gradual reduction, some elements of this test, such as visualization of the entire genome at a large scale at a single cell resolution remain valuable. Indeed, while newer high-throughput molecular technologies allow more comprehensive characterization of genomic abnormalities in cancer, it is also important to remember that both hematological malignancies and solid tumors are often composed of a mixture of clones, sometimes with different genetic build. While WGS, LRS, and OGM provide a combined picture of the tumor's genetic makeup, neither technology can currently capture the map of tumor heterogeneity. This can be important for understanding how the tumor evolves and responds to treatment. Therefore, the development of molecular-based technologies that provide genomic information on a single cell level, similar to chromosome analysis and FISH, and coupled with transcriptomics and proteomics analysis would be vital to make major advances in accurate characterization of the cancer genome.

CLINICS CARE POINTS

- Conventional cytogenetics (often referred to as chromosome analysis or karyotyping) is frequently used in the diagnosis of hematologic malignancies and less in the diagnosis of solid tumors.
- Contemporary cancer diagnostics necessitate the adoption of advanced high-resolution testing modalities that facilitate simultaneous assessment of genomic variations across the entire genome. These methodologies include nonsequencing OGM as well as sequencing-based techniques, including whole genome short-read DNA sequencing and long-read sequencing.
- Currently, there is no one-size-fit-all diagnostic method or comprehensive set of methods that can be applied to all clinical scenarios. The selection of a diagnostic pipeline should align with clinical therapy guidelines and be tailored to the specific circumstances of each laboratory and health care institution.

DISCLOSURE

Authors have nothing to disclose.

REFERENCES

[1] Moch H, Cubilla AL, Humphrey PA, et al. The 2016 WHO classification of tumours of the urinary system and male genital organs-part A: renal, penile, and testicular tumours. Eur Urol 2016;70(1):93–105.
[2] Louis DN, Perry A, Wesseling P, et al. The 2021 WHO classification of tumors of the central nervous system: a summary. Neuro Oncol 2021;23(8):1231–51.
[3] Jung Y, Kim J, Shin A, et al. Association of adiposity with periodontitis and metabolic syndrome: from the third national health and nutrition examination survey of United States. Int J Environ Res Public Health 2023; 20(3):2533.
[4] Nowell PC, Hungerford DA. A minute chromosome in human chronic granulocytic leukemia. Science 1960; 142:1497.
[5] Hsu TC. Mammalian chromosomes in vitro: I. the karyotype of man. J Hered 1952;43(4):167–72.
[6] Wan TSK. Cancer cytogenetics: methodology revisited. Ann Lab Med 2014;34(6):413–25.
[7] Safranauskas RMdSO, Cordeiro MG, Velloso EDRP. MYC amplification in leukemia detected by cytogenetics. EJH 2021;2(2):297–8.
[8] Ittel A, Vey N, Mozziconacci M. Multiple cytogenetics forms of KMT2A amplification and jumping translocation in a case of myelodysplastic syndrome. EJH 2021; 2(4):905–6.
[9] L'Abbate A, Tolomeo D, Cifola I, et al. Correction: MYC-containing amplicons in acute myeloid leukemia: genomic structures, evolution, and transcriptional consequences. Leukemia 2018;32(10):2304–y.
[10] Vanderscheldon RK, Sukov WR, Gardner J, et al. Conventional cytogenetic analysis of solid tumor abnormalities: a 25-year review of proficiency test results from the college of american pathologists/american college of medical genetics and genomics cytogenetics committee. Genes 2024;15(12):1612.
[11] Sosinsky A, Ambrose J, Cross W, et al. Insights for precision oncology from the integration of genomic and clinical data of 13,880 tumors from the 100,000 genomes cancer programme. Nat Med 2024;30(1): 279–89.
[12] Din M, Babar KM, Shah D, et al. Dissemination of NDM-1 in pseudomonas aeruginosa and klebsiella pneumoniae isolated from pus samples in tertiary care hospitals of quetta, Pakistan. J Pak Med Assoc 2021;71-(1B):228–32.
[13] Roepman P, de Bruijn E, van Lieshout S, et al. Clinical validation of whole genome sequencing for cancer diagnostics. J Mol Diagn 2021;23(7):816–33.
[14] Wrzeszczynski KO, Felice V, Abhyankar A, et al. Analytical validation of clinical whole-genome and transcriptome sequencing of patient-derived tumors for reporting targetable variants in cancer. J Mol Diagn 2018;20(6):822–35.
[15] Cuppen E, Elemento O, Rosenquist R, et al. Implementation of whole-genome and transcriptome sequencing into clinical cancer care. JCO Precis Oncol 2022;6: e2200245.
[16] Ma X, Liu Y, Liu Y, et al. Pan-cancer genome and transcriptome analyses of 1,699 paediatric leukaemias and solid tumours. Nature 2018;555(7696):371–6.
[17] Valkama A, Vorimo S, Kumpula TA, et al. Optical genome mapping as an alternative to FISH-based cytogenetic assessment in chronic lymphocytic leukemia. Cancers (Basel) 2023;15(4):1294.
[18] Coccaro N, Anelli L, Zagaria A, et al. Feasibility of optical genome mapping in cytogenetic diagnostics of hematological neoplasms: a new way to look at DNA. Diagnostics 2023;13(11):1841.
[19] Kukurba KR, Montgomery SB. RNA sequencing and analysis. Cold Spring Harb Protoc 2015;2015(11):951–69.
[20] Soler G, Ouedraogo ZG, Goumy C, et al. Optical genome mapping in routine cytogenetic diagnosis of acute leukemia. Cancers (Basel) 2023;15(7):2131.

[21] Choo Z, Behr JM, Deshpande A, et al. Most large structural variants in cancer genomes can be detected without long reads. Nat Genet 2023;55(12):2139–48.

[22] Barseghyan H, Eisenreich D, Lindt E, et al. Optical genome mapping as a potential routine clinical diagnostic method. Genes 2024;15(3):342.

[23] Priestley P, Baber J, Lolkema MP, et al. Pan-cancer whole-genome analyses of metastatic solid tumours. Nature 2019;575(7781):210–6.

[24] Pleasance E, Bohm A, Williamson LM, et al. Whole-genome and transcriptome analysis enhances precision cancer treatment options. Ann Oncol 2022;33(9):939–49.

[25] Gagnon M, Tonk SS, Carcamo B, et al. False positive NUP98 fluorescence in situ hybridization rearrangements in B-acute lymphoblastic leukemia. Cancer Genet 2025;292-293:57–64.

[26] Wu X, Zhu L, Ma PC. Next-generation novel noninvasive cancer molecular diagnostics platforms beyond tissues. Am Soc Clin Oncol Educ Book 2018;38(38):964–77.

[27] Mandel P, Metais P. Nuclear acids in human blood plasma. C R Seances Soc Biol Fil 1948;142(3–4):241–3.

[28] Su S, de Castro Abreu AL, Chihara Y, et al. A panel of three markers hyper- and hypomethylated in urine sediments accurately predicts bladder cancer recurrence. Clin Cancer Res 2014;20(7):1978–89.

[29] Minamoto T, Mai M, Ronai Z. K-ras mutation: early detection in molecular diagnosis and risk assessment of colorectal, pancreas, and lung cancers–a review. Cancer Detect Prev 2000;24(1):1–12.

[30] A stool DNA test (cologuard) for colorectal cancer screening. JAMA 2014;312(23):2566.

[31] Parisi C, Tagliamento M, Belcaid L, et al. Circulating tumor DNA in clinical trials for solid tumors: challenges and current applications. J Liq Biopsy 2023;1:100007.

[32] Alfares A, Aloraini T, Subaie LA, et al. Whole-genome sequencing offers additional but limited clinical utility compared with reanalysis of whole-exome sequencing. Genet Med 2018;20(11):1328–33.

[33] Akkari YMN, Baughn LB, Dubuc AM, et al. Guiding the global evolution of cytogenetic testing for hematologic malignancies. Blood 2022;139(15):2273–84.

[34] Nanopore sequencing accuracy. Oxford Nanopore Technologies. Available at: https://nanoporetech.com/platform/accuracy. Accessed February 20, 2025.

[35] Wenger AM, Peluso P, Rowell WJ, et al. Accurate circular consensus long-read sequencing improves variant detection and assembly of a human genome. Nat Biotechnol 2019;37(10):1155–62.

[36] Sakamoto Y, Xu L, Seki M, et al. Long-read sequencing for non-small-cell lung cancer genomes. Genome Res 2020;30(9):1243–57.

[37] Ermini L, Driguez P. The application of long-read sequencing to cancer. Cancers (Basel) 2024;16(7):1275.

[38] Liu Y, Rosikiewicz W, Pan Z, et al. DNA methylation-calling tools for oxford nanopore sequencing: a survey and human epigenome-wide evaluation. Genome Biol 2021;22(1):295–z.

[39] Martisova A, Holcakova J, Izadi N, et al. DNA methylation in solid tumors: functions and methods of detection. Int J Mol Sci 2021;22(8):4247.

[40] Buckley DN, Tew BY, Gooden C, et al. A comprehensive analysis of minimally differentially methylated regions common to pediatric and adult solid tumors. NPJ Precis Oncol 2024;8(1):125.

[41] Duckett D, Vormittag-Nocito ER, Jamshidi P, et al. Accurate identification of primary site in tumors of unknown origin (TUO) using DNA methylation. npj Precis Oncol 2025;9(1):8–z.

[42] Goenka SD, Gorzynski JE, Shafin K, et al. Accelerated identification of disease-causing variants with ultra-rapid nanopore genome sequencing. Nat Biotechnol 2022;40(7):1035–41.

[43] Ultrarapid nanopore genome sequencing speeds up diagnosis in a critical care setting. Am J Med Genet 2022;188(6):1656–7.

[44] Stratton MR, Campbell PJ, Futreal PA. The cancer genome. Nature 2009;458(7239):719–24.

[45] Suzuki A, Suzuki M, Mizushima-Sugano J, et al. Sequencing and phasing cancer mutations in lung cancers using a long-read portable sequencer. DNA Res 2017;24(6):585–96.

[46] Schwartz DC, Li X, Hernandez LI, et al. Ordered restriction maps of saccharomyces cerevisiae chromosomes constructed by optical mapping. Science 1993;262-(5130):110–4.

[47] Yuan Y, Chung CY, Chan T. Advances in optical mapping for genomic research. Comput Struct Biotechnol J 2020;18:2051–62.

[48] Sahajpal NS, Mondal AK, Fee T, et al. Clinical validation and diagnostic utility of optical genome mapping in prenatal diagnostic testing. J Mol Diagn 2023;25(4):234–46.

[49] Shim Y, Koo Y, Shin S, et al. Comparison of optical genome mapping with conventional diagnostic methods for structural variant detection in hematologic malignancies. Ann Lab Med 2024;44(4):324–34.

[50] Giguȓe A, Raymond-Bouchard I, Collin V, et al. Optical genome mapping reveals the complex genetic landscape of myeloma. Cancers (Basel) 2023;15(19):4687.

[51] Dremsek P, Schwarz T, Weil B, et al. Optical genome mapping in routine human genetic diagnostics-its advantages and limitations. Genes 2021;12(12):1958.

[52] Chang H, Wechalekar A, Li L, et al. Molecular cytogenetic abnormalities in patients with concurrent chronic lymphocytic leukemia and multiple myeloma shown by interphase fluorescence in situ hybridization: evidence of distinct clonal origin. Cancer Genet Cytogenet 2004;148(1):44–8.

[53] Boquoi A, Banahan SM, Mohring A, et al. Therapy-related myeloid neoplasms following treatment for multiple myeloma-a single center analysis. Ann Hematol 2022;101(5):1031–8.

[54] Gargallo P, Cacchione R, Chena C, et al. Chronic lymphocytic leukemia developing in a patient with chronic

myeloid leukemia: evidence of distinct lineage-associated genomic events. Cancer Genet Cytogenet 2005;161(1): 74–7.

[55] Heuser M, Freeman SD, Ossenkoppele GJ, et al. 2021 update on MRD in acute myeloid leukemia: a consensus document from the european LeukemiaNet MRD working party. Blood 2021;138(26):2753–67.

[56] Ramos Perez JM, Patel KP, Loghavi S, et al. Value of measurable residual disease monitoring in patients with acute promyelocytic leukemia in the era of frontline 'chemotherapy-free' therapy. Leuk Lymphoma 2022;63(3):672–5.

[57] Samsom KG, Schipper LJ, Roepman P, et al. Feasibility of whole-genome sequencing-based tumor diagnostics in routine pathology practice. J Pathol 2022;258(2):179–88.

[58] Hansen MH, Cdile O, Kjeldsen MLG, et al. Toward cytogenomics: technical assessment of long-read nanopore whole-genome sequencing for detecting large chromosomal alterations in mantle cell lymphoma. J Mol Diagn 2023;25(11):796–805.

[59] Djirackor L, Halldorsson S, Niehusmann P, et al. Intraoperative DNA methylation classification of brain tumors impacts neurosurgical strategy. Neurooncol Adv 2021;3(1):vdab149.

[60] Sahajpal NS, Barseghyan H, Kolhe R, et al. Optical genome mapping as a next-generation cytogenomic tool for detection of structural and copy number variations for prenatal genomic analyses. Genes 2021; 12(3):398.

Advances in Molecular Pathology 8 (2025) 189–196
ADVANCES IN MOLECULAR PATHOLOGY

Economics of Molecular Pathology

Fang Zhao, MD, PhD[a,*], Yuan Ji, MS, PhD, MBA[b]

[a]Department of Pathology and Laboratory Medicine, University of Cincinnati, College of Medicine, 3188 Bellevue Avenue, Cincinnati, OH 45219, USA; [b]Department of Pathology, University of Utah School of Medicine, ARUP Laboratories, 500 Chipeta Way, Mail code 115, Salt Lake City, UT 84108, USA

KEYWORDS

• Economics • Molecular pathology • Cost-effectiveness and cost-benefit analysis • Test implementation

KEY POINTS

- Key players in molecular pathology economics—health care providers, payers, and patients—impact test accessibility and cost.
- Molecular testing advances precision medicine, offering economic value, with tests like next-generation sequencing shown to be cost-effective, though more long-term studies are needed.
- Accurate coding is crucial for reimbursement, but coding challenges can create financial barriers.
- Molecular tests vary in cost, with larger panels offering savings; in-house or outsourced testing depends on patient volume.
- Economic assessments help laboratories evaluate cost-effectiveness and sustainability, with tools like Break-even Analysis aiding decision-making.
- Molecular testing faces reimbursement and access challenges, with return on investment analysis helping laboratories assess financial feasibility and choose between in-house or outsourced testing.

INTRODUCTION

Molecular pathology is a rapidly advancing field within laboratory medicine. The genomic information provided by molecular testing plays a key role in shaping precision medicine. Thanks to the advance of genomic sequencing technology, molecular testing has become more accessible and affordable, enabling its use in clinical settings for targeted therapies and personalized patient care. However, molecular testing is inherently complex, with a variety of testing modalities and a vast range of targets. The diversity of tests offered by commercial, reference, and academic laboratories adds further complexity to the economic landscape of molecular pathology practice. Moreover, evolving regulations are critical to the direction of laboratories offering molecular services. As a result, understanding economic factors of molecular pathology is essential for successfully implementing molecular tests and healthy growth of molecular laboratories. This review examines the economic aspects of molecular pathology, the economic value and health benefits of molecular diagnostics, key considerations in test implementation. We also address challenges related to reimbursement, policy frameworks, and equitable access, while offering strategies for evaluating the health economics of molecular testing, including return on investment (ROI) analysis and decisions regarding in-house versus outsourced testing.

DISCUSSION

Key players within the economic landscape of molecular pathology

Within the economic system of molecular pathology, key players include health care providers, payers, and patients

*Corresponding author. *E-mail address:* zhaofh@ucmail.uc.edu

https://doi.org/10.1016/j.yamp.2025.05.010 www.advancesinmolecularpathology.com
2589-4080/25/ © 2025 Elsevier Inc. All rights are reserved, including those for text and data mining, AI training, and similar technologies.

ABBREVIATIONS

ACLA	American Clinical Laboratory Association
ACMG	American College of Medical Genetics and Genomics
AI	artificial intelligence
AMA	American Medical Association
AMC	academic medical center
AMP	Association for Molecular Pathology
aNSCLC	advanced nonsmall-cell lung cancer
BIA	budget impact analysis
CAP	College of American Pathologists
CBA	cost-benefit analysis
CEA	cost-effectiveness analysis
CGP	comprehensive genomic profiling
CML	chronic myelogenous leukemia
CMS	Centers for Medicare & Medicaid Services
CLFS	Clinical Laboratory Fee Schedule
CPT	Current Procedural Terminology
KPI	key performance indicator
mNSCLC	metastatic nonsmall cell lung cancer
NGS	next-generation sequencing
NSCLC	nonsmall cell lung cancers
PCR	polymerase chain reaction
ROI	return on investment
SGT	single-gene testing
TAT	turnaround times

[1]. Health care providers in the domain of molecular pathology include molecular pathologists (typically board-certified MD pathologists), clinical molecular geneticists (typically board-certified PhD laboratorians), and medical technologists. These professionals are often collectively referred to as molecular professionals. They play a crucial role by providing molecular testing and interpretation to assist in diagnosis, inform prognosis, and guide-targeted therapies. Additionally, many professional organizations actively shape and influence the economic landscape of molecular pathology by participating in coding, coverage, and reimbursement discussions at both local and national levels. These organizations include the Association for Molecular Pathology (AMP), the College of American Pathologists (CAP), the American College of Medical Genetics and Genomics (ACMG), the American Clinical Laboratory Association (ACLA), and the American Medical Association (AMA).

Payers are an integral part of the economics of medicine. In molecular pathology, third-party payers are classified as either governmental (public) or commercial (private). The 2 major public payers in the United States are the nationwide Medicare program and state-specific Medicaid programs. The Centers for Medicare & Medicaid Services (CMS) sets reimbursement rates and coverage policies for molecular tests (Billing and Coding: Molecular Pathology and Genetic Testing; https://www.cms.gov/medicare-coverage-database/view/article.aspx?articleid=58,917).

Most laboratory tests are reimbursed under the Clinical Laboratory Fee Schedule (CLFS). However, tests that require physician interpretation (eg, biopsies and immunohistochemical studies) are paid under the Physician Fee Schedule. Among commercial payers, there are numerous private health insurers offering a variety of plans. These insurers determine which molecular tests are covered and at what cost, directly influencing patient access and affordability [1].

Patients are the ultimate beneficiaries of molecular pathology. The utilization of molecular pathology services varies based on disease type and several other factors, and the proportion of patients benefiting from these services continues to grow. Advances in identifying clinically useful genetic markers, diagnostic methods, and related pharmaceutical interventions are increasing, particularly in the oncology space. Patients are also more aware than ever of the value of molecular genetic testing. Furthermore, patient advocacy organizations are increasingly recognizing the role of molecular pathology and the need to engage with and respond to reimbursement policies that affect patient access to these procedures. Many of these organizations, often disease-centric nonprofits, work diligently to monitor both Medicare and private payer policies that may influence patient access to appropriate molecular testing. The growing patient voice has become crucial in shaping and responding to reimbursement policies, particularly in discussions of coverage and the standards of evidence required to justify the coverage of medical services.

Economic value and health benefits of molecular testing

Molecular testing brings significant economic value and health benefits by advancing the practice of precision medicine. Since its introduction into clinical laboratories, it has transformed patient care by identifying targeted therapy markers for patients, evaluating genetic risk factors to aid in disease risk stratification and monitoring, and guiding personalized treatment plans. Many studies have been conducted to assess the overall economic value and health benefits of molecular testing.

A European group conducted a systematic review of the health economic evidence for the use of molecular biomarker tests in hematological malignancies, aiming to identify and assess the existing economic data on these tests [2]. As we know, molecular biomarker tests play a key role in personalizing treatment strategies for hematological malignancies by tailoring therapies to a patient's specific molecular profile. Their clinical benefits are well-established, with evidence supporting their use in both predictive and prognostic applications. The findings of this study highlight the emerging but still limited economic evidence supporting the use of molecular biomarker tests in the management of hematological malignancies. While half of the reviewed studies demonstrated that companion diagnostics for therapies targeting conditions such as acute myeloid leukemia, chronic myelogenous leukemia (CML), diffuse large B-cell lymphoma, and multiple myeloma are likely cost-effective, the overall body of evidence remains relatively sparse. Notably, the identification of cost-saving potential for treatment monitoring in CML suggests that molecular biomarker tests could offer both clinical and financial benefits. However, the predominance of nonlifetime time horizons and the lack of comprehensive long-term evaluations indicate that current assessments may not fully capture the enduring value of these technologies. The findings underscore the need for more extensive health economic evaluations to support the broader implementation of molecular biomarker testing in routine hematology care.

The economic value of different testing methodologies has also been examined [3–8]. Several studies have evaluated the economic impact of next-generation sequencing (NGS) testing versus single-gene testing (SGT) for detecting targetable biomarkers in nonsmall cell lung cancers (NSCLC).

Pennell and colleagues assessed the economic impact of NGS versus SGT for metastatic nonsmall cell lung cancer (mNSCLC) from the perspective of US payers. NGS provided faster test results (2 weeks) compared with exclusionary and sequential testing (4.7–4.8 weeks) and led to significant cost savings for both Medicare (CMS) and commercial payers. In a hypothetical 1,000,000-member health plan, NGS saved $1.4M to $2.1M for CMS and $3.8K to $250.8K for commercial payers compared with other testing methods. The findings support NGS as a more efficient and cost-effective approach for identifying targetable genomic alterations in mNSCLC patients [4]. Vanderpoel and colleagues compared the costs and time efficiency of NGS versus polymerase chain reaction (PCR) testing for mNSCLC from US payer perspectives. NGS resulted in faster time to targeted therapy (2 weeks) compared with PCR strategies (3–9 weeks) and was the least costly option, with an average per-patient cost of $4932 versus $6605 for PCR. NGS was more cost-effective for both Medicare and commercial payers, despite higher overall costs in commercial plans. The findings support NGS as the preferred strategy due to its lower costs and quicker results [6].

Coding for molecular pathology

Coding, the language of laboratory economics, directly influences the practice of molecular laboratories. Accurate coding for molecular pathology is essential for proper billing, reimbursement, and tracking of these specialized tests [1].

Molecular pathology procedures are primarily billed using Current Procedural Terminology (CPT) codes, which describe specific genetic or molecular tests. The CMS published an article Billing and Coding: Molecular Pathology Procedures (Article ID: A56199) that offers detailed instructions to help providers follow correct billing procedures for molecular pathology services. It was originally effective on January 1, 2019, and revised on January 1, 2025 (https://www.cms.gov/medicare-coverage-database/view/article.aspx?articleid=56,199). Coding guidance was categorized into 4, distinct CPT/HCPCS sections:

Group 1-Tier 1 Covered Codes for which limited coverage may be provided for the genetic tests and for which specific International Classification of Diseases, Tenth Revision, Clinical Modification (ICD-10-CM) diagnosis to CPT procedure groupings may be listed;

Group 2-Tier 1 Codes that require Individual Review for which coverage may be provided for the genetic tests submitted, if documentation supports medical necessity, and for which specific ICD-10-CM diagnosis to CPT procedure groupings may be listed;

Group 3-Tier 1 Noncovered Codes for which genetic testing is unlikely to impact therapeutic decision-making in the clinical management of the patient and will be denied automatically as not medically necessary;

Group 4-Tier 2/NOC Covered Code/Gene Combinations for which limited coverage may be provided for specific genes listed in the Group 4 paragraph; Tier 2/NOC Individual Review Code/Gene Combinations; Tier 2/NOC Noncovered Code/Gene Combinations.

Furthermore, CMS clarifies that when gene panels are ordered, providers should use the appropriate panel CPT codes rather than individual gene codes. For panels with 5 to 50 genes, the correct codes are 81445, 81449, 81450, or 81451, while panels with 51 or more genes should be billed using 81455 or 81456. If a panel includes 1 to 4 genes, the Article recommends using the corresponding panel code or CPT 81479 (unlisted molecular pathology procedure) if no specific code exists. The guidance also notes that claims may be subject to National Correct Coding Initiative or Outpatient Prospective Payment System packaging edits, making it important for providers to review these requirements before submitting claims. Documentation requirements were also outlined, emphasizing the need for thorough records to support coverage eligibility. This includes maintaining physician requisitions, test reports, and quality control records. For laboratory-developed tests, documentation should include assay details, laboratory information, and evidence of clinical and analytical validity. Providers are reminded to include the name and National Provider Identifier (NPI) of the referring or ordering physician on claims and to use Modifier 91 when the same test is performed more than once on the same day, when clinically necessary. Claims missing valid ICD-10-CM diagnosis codes will be returned as incomplete.

Molecular pathology coding presents several challenges due to the complexity and variability of the tests. Molecular assays can differ significantly in their design, methodology, and level of complexity, making it difficult to apply consistent and standardized coding practices. Additionally, the rapidly evolving nature of the field introduces new tests and technologies at a fast pace, necessitating frequent updates to coding standards. This continuous evolution creates a lag between the introduction of new tests and the establishment of appropriate codes. Reimbursement issues further complicate coding, as payers may limit coverage for certain molecular tests due to inconsistent guidelines or a lack of sufficient clinical evidence. These challenges highlight the need for ongoing education, standardized coding protocols, and collaboration between laboratories, payers, and regulatory bodies to ensure accurate billing and appropriate reimbursement for molecular testing.

Adopting best practices for molecular pathology coding is essential to ensure accurate billing, proper reimbursement, and effective data tracking. It is important to use precise CPT and ICD-10 codes that clearly reflect the specific test performed and the patient's diagnosis, helping to justify medical necessity. Keeping up with frequent coding updates is also critical, as the field of molecular diagnostics evolves rapidly, requiring professionals to stay informed through organizations like the AMA and the CMS. Thorough documentation of medical necessity in patient records further supports reimbursement claims. Finally, utilizing reliable coding resources, such as manuals, databases, and guidance from professional organizations, promotes accuracy and consistency. As molecular testing advances, following these best practices is key to effectively capturing the clinical and economic value of these tests.

Economic considerations for molecular test implementation

Molecular tests can be classified into 2 main categories based on the number of genes analyzed: single-gene tests and large-panel tests. Single-gene tests detect mutations in individual genes, such as *KRAS* mutation analysis for colorectal cancer, while large-panel tests, including NGS, whole-exome sequencing, and whole-genome sequencing, simultaneously assess multiple genes and are widely used in oncology and rare disease diagnostics. These tests can also be grouped by methodology, with common techniques including PCR, fluorescence in situ hybridization, NGS, and Sanger sequencing. When implementing molecular testing, both clinical value and economic factors are critical in decision-making. The cost-effectiveness, reimbursement landscape, and downstream financial impact heavily influence whether health care providers opt for single-gene tests, smaller panels, or more comprehensive NGS approaches.

Cost-effectiveness: Single-gene tests and small panels generally have lower upfront costs, making them more attractive in budget-limited settings or when reimbursement is restricted. In contrast, comprehensive panels (eg, NGS), though more expensive initially, offer greater value by detecting multiple genetic alterations in a single test. This streamlined approach reduces the need for sequential testing, which can expedite access to targeted therapies and ultimately lead to downstream cost savings by minimizing the need for repeat biopsies, additional tissue sampling, reflex testing, and ineffective or empiric treatments. While sequential testing may seem more cost-effective at first, it can drive up expenses over time due to repeat testing and delayed access to appropriate therapies. Studies indicate that, despite its higher upfront cost, NGS testing can lower the overall cost of care by accelerating precise therapy selection and avoiding unnecessary interventions [3–8].

Reimbursement and Insurance Coverage: Reimbursement rates heavily influence test selection, as payers are more likely to cover tests with proven clinical utility and regulatory approval (eg, FDA-cleared companion diagnostics). While single-gene tests are often covered by insurers, broader multigene panels may face reimbursement challenges, especially for off-label use or investigational biomarkers. In oncology, coverage for NGS testing is gradually expanding under Medicare and commercial insurance policies. Recent studies show that the cost and coverage of genetic testing are changing, making NGS panel tests for hereditary cancer more common [9]. Providers from safety-net clinics and academic medical centers (AMCs) in California and North Carolina report that they now order NGS panels more frequently than single-gene tests, mainly from a few commercial laboratories. Safety-net clinics face fewer cost barriers thanks to laboratory-sponsored payment assistance programs that reduce or eliminate out-of-pocket expenses. In contrast, AMCs struggle more with insurance issues, especially prior authorization. However, despite improved access through payment assistance, the lack of coverage for genetic counseling remains a major challenge, highlighting the need for better support to ensure fair access to genetic testing.

Testing Efficiency and Turnaround Time: Faster turnaround times (TAT) can lead to cost savings by reducing the duration of ineffective treatments and hospital stays. Single-gene tests typically have a quicker TAT compared with large panel testing. However, a stepwise single-gene approach can prolong the overall TAT, potentially increasing health care costs due to delays in initiating appropriate therapies. In contrast, large NGS gene panel testing generally takes around 2 to 3 weeks but offers the advantage of detecting multiple mutations simultaneously, enabling faster alignment with targeted treatments [10]. In medical emergencies, such as diagnosing acute promyelocytic leukemia (APL), a rapid TAT is essential for life-saving interventions. In such cases, using tests with faster TAT is critical to meeting urgent clinical needs.

Additional factors to consider: Patient population size and complexity, the practice model, and whether to outsource or perform testing in-house should also be considered in the planning phase of test implementation.

The economic feasibility of molecular testing is heavily influenced by the size and characteristics of the patient population. In large health systems or cancer centers with a high patient volume, in-house testing can be more cost-effective, as broader NGS panels become justifiable for diverse patient groups where multigene profiling is clinically relevant. Conversely, smaller practices or niche populations may find outsourcing more economical, as third-party laboratories often offer lower per-sample costs compared with maintaining in-house infrastructure with low utilization. Disease complexity and test frequency also play a key role. In oncology or rare disease settings, comprehensive NGS panels are often more cost-effective due to the need for broader profiling in complex cases. However, for routine genetic screening (eg, *BRCA1/2* or Lynch syndrome genes), smaller panels or single-gene tests may be more viable. Community practices and private clinics are more likely to outsource testing due to lower patient volumes and limited laboratory capabilities. Partnering with reference laboratories or commercial providers reduces capital investment costs, as these laboratories offer bulk pricing and absorb validation and quality control expenses, making outsourcing a financially favorable option.

The decision between in-house and outsourced molecular testing involves several economic trade-offs. In-house testing is typically more cost-effective for large, high-volume practices or academic centers equipped with expertise and infrastructure, as it offers faster TATs, better quality control, and potential revenue opportunities. In contrast, outsourcing is often more practical and economical for smaller practices or those with low testing volumes, as it involves lower upfront costs and reduces operational complexity. A hybrid model can strike a balance between cost-efficiency and scalability, with frequent, routine tests performed in-house, while rare or complex panels are outsourced to reference laboratories.

Essential tools for economic evaluation of molecular testing

Economic assessments, such as cost-effectiveness analysis (CEA) and cost-utility analysis, are used to evaluate the value of in vitro diagnostic (IVD) tests by comparing their costs to outcomes in terms of effectiveness or quality of life. Some frameworks suggest assessing the value of laboratory tests by considering factors like technical accuracy, TAT, utility, and costs. Additionally, multicriteria decision analysis helps compare diagnostic strategies based on benefits, costs, and risks. These evaluations aim to identify tests that offer the greatest health care benefits within available resources. Without clear evidence of cost-effectiveness, laboratories may lean toward cost-cutting measures, potentially limiting patient access to vital services [11].

To evaluate the economic aspects of molecular testing and ensure a sustainable laboratory, various tools and strategies can be used. These methods assess economic feasibility, cost-effectiveness, and long-term viability of integrating molecular diagnostics into laboratory services. Below are key tools and approaches that can assist in these evaluations.

Cost-effectiveness and cost-benefit analysis

CEA: Compares the cost of molecular tests to their health outcomes, using metrics like Incremental Cost-Effectiveness Ratio or cost per diagnosis, to determine whether implementing these tests offers value [12]. CEA calculate the incremental cost per health outcome (eg, deaths prevented and life-years saved), while cost-utility analyses use preference-based health state measures, such as quality-adjusted life-years. These analyses assume that decision makers aim to maximize health within resource constraints.

Cost-Benefit Analysis (CBA): Converts all benefits (improved diagnosis, reduced health care costs, etc) into monetary terms to assess if the molecular tests generate enough benefits to justify the costs. CBA incorporates monetary values for genetic testing, including the perceived value of information beyond health outcomes. However, traditional measures may not fully capture the broader outcomes of genetic testing that are important to decision makers and consumers. Grosse and colleagues recommended that health policy makers take into account the value of information and other nonhealth aspects of genetic testing when making decisions [12].

CEA/CBA analyses are essential for determining whether molecular testing implementation provides value to both the laboratory and the health care system. By evaluating the costs of molecular tests against the benefits they offer, such as improved diagnostics and patient outcomes, laboratories can assess whether these tests are financially viable.

Budget impact analysis

The budget impact analysis (BIA) tool helps laboratories assess the financial implications of introducing molecular testing by accounting for both direct and indirect costs. It considers initial investments, such as equipment, reagents, training, and infrastructure, as well as ongoing operational expenses like maintenance, staffing, and consumables. The tool also evaluates potential long-term savings, including reduced re-testing, improved treatment outcomes, and fewer diagnostic errors. By providing a comprehensive financial overview, the BIA helps laboratories make informed decisions about adopting molecular testing and understand its potential impact on their overall budget and patient care efficiency. For example, a recent study used BIA tool to assess the effects of increasing comprehensive genomic profiling (CGP) for advanced nonsmall-cell lung cancer (aNSCLC) in a US health plan. They found that raising CGP use from 20% to 30% led to 3.11 additional life-years gained and a $0.01 in US dollars per member per month budget impact, most of which was attributable to prolonged survival associated with increased use of more effective treatments [13].

Break-even analysis

A break-even analysis helps laboratories determine when they will start making a profit from molecular tests by calculating the minimum number of tests or volume of services needed to cover implementation costs. It is particularly useful when evaluating new tests or technologies to assess how soon they will become financially sustainable. Key inputs for this analysis include fixed and variable costs, the price per test or service provided, and the projected testing volume. A recent study used break-even analysis to compare NGS-based and SGT-based testing for aNSCLC and mCRC patients [14]. NGS was cost-saving in 15 of 16 cases, with savings up to €1249 per patient. It became more cost-effective after a certain patient threshold, depending on molecular alterations tested. In one case, NGS was more expensive by €25. Overall, NGS was generally less costly, with savings increasing as patient numbers grew.

Key performance indicators and dashboards

Regular monitoring of key performance indicators (KPIs) enables laboratories to assess their financial health and performance in real time, allowing laboratory managers to make informed decisions about molecular test implementation. KPIs such as cost per test, test turnaround time [15], test utilization rate, patient satisfaction, and clinical outcomes, and profit margins can be tracked through dashboards to provide insights into financial, operational, and quality metrics. This helps ensure that laboratories optimize their operations while maintaining high standards of care and profitability.

Challenges and strategies in the health economics of molecular testing

The implementation of molecular testing in health care systems faces several economic challenges, particularly concerning reimbursement, policy frameworks, and equitable access. Reimbursement policies for molecular diagnostics vary widely across regions and payers, often lacking consistency or sufficient coverage. This can create financial barriers for both laboratories and patients, limiting the widespread adoption of innovative tests. Additionally, existing policy frameworks may struggle to keep pace with the rapid advancements in molecular technology, leading to outdated regulations and ambiguous billing codes. This can result in delayed payments, under-reimbursement, or denied claims. Equitable access also remains a challenge, as rural and underserved populations often have limited access to molecular testing due to logistical constraints or lack of insurance coverage, creating disparities in early diagnosis and precision treatment.

To overcome these challenges, laboratories need to implement comprehensive strategies for assessing the economic impact of molecular testing. A critical approach is conducting ROI analysis [16,17]. This includes evaluating the savings from improved clinical outcomes, such as fewer hospitalizations and reduced treatment failures, and balancing them with the initial and ongoing costs of testing. ROI analysis enables decision-makers to determine whether molecular testing provides long-term financial value, making its adoption more justifiable. Additionally, laboratories must carefully consider the financial and operational implications of conducting tests in-house versus outsourcing. In-house testing offers faster results and more control over quality but demands significant investment in equipment, staffing, and infrastructure. In contrast, outsourcing may lower capital costs but can result in longer processing times and less oversight. A detailed cost-benefit analysis can help laboratories choose the most economically feasible option based on their testing needs, available resources, and future financial objectives.

FUTURE DIRECTIONS

The economics of molecular pathology is set for significant transformation as technological advancements, personalized medicine, and value-based health care models continue to redefine the landscape. One key future direction is the increased integration of artificial intelligence (AI) and machine learning into molecular diagnostics [18,19]. These technologies can enhance test accuracy, automate data interpretation, and streamline workflows, ultimately reducing labor costs and improving efficiency. As AI-powered tools become more accessible, laboratories may experience reduced TAT and greater cost-efficiency, making molecular testing more scalable and financially sustainable.

Another emerging trend is the shift toward value-based reimbursement models, where payments are increasingly tied to patient outcomes rather than test volume. This model incentivizes laboratories to prioritize clinically impactful tests that offer clear health benefits. To thrive in this framework, molecular pathology laboratories will need to demonstrate the cost-effectiveness and clinical utility of their tests using real-world evidence and health economic data. Additionally, companion diagnostics—molecular tests used to guide targeted therapies—are likely to become more common, particularly in oncology and rare diseases. As precision medicine expands, these tests will play a larger role in treatment decisions, driving demand, and influencing reimbursement policies.

SUMMARY

The economics of molecular pathology is becoming increasingly complex as testing technologies advance and health care systems embrace precision medicine. Laboratories and health care providers will need to continually adapt by conducting thorough economic evaluations, including ROI analyses, cost-effectiveness studies, and break-even assessments. Strategic decisions regarding in-house versus outsourced testing, operational efficiencies, and reimbursement navigation will be critical to ensuring financial sustainability. Looking ahead, molecular testing will continue to shape the future of diagnostics and personalized care, making it essential for laboratories to balance clinical innovation with economic viability to thrive in an evolving health care landscape.

CLINICS CARE POINTS

- Molecular pathology plays a crucial role in health care decisions and patient outcomes, with key stakeholders including health care providers, payers, and patients.
- The economic value and health benefits of molecular testing are significant, particularly in precision medicine, though challenges such as coding complexities, test implementation costs, and securing reimbursement remain.
- Essential economic evaluation tools, such as cost-effectiveness analysis, cost-benefit analysis, and key performance indicators, are necessary for assessing the financial viability of molecular testing.
- Artificial intelligence-powered tools and value-based reimbursement models are pivotal in improving efficiency and sustaining the economics of molecular pathology.

DECLARATION OF AI AND AI-ASSISTED TECHNOLOGIES IN THE WRITING PROCESS

During the preparation of this work the authors used Generative AI. After using this tool/service, the authors reviewed and edited the content as needed and take full responsibility for the content of the publication.

DISCLOSURE

The authors have nothing to disclose.

REFERENCES

[1] Sireci AN, Patel JL, Joseph L, et al. Molecular pathology economics 101: an overview of molecular diagnostics coding, coverage, and reimbursement: a report of the association for molecular pathology. J Mol Diagn 2020; 22(8):975–93 [published Online First: 20200603].

[2] Vu M, Degeling K, Thompson ER, et al. Health economic evidence for the use of molecular biomarker tests in hematological malignancies: a systematic review. Eur J Haematol 2022;108(6):469–85 [published Online First: 20220302].

[3] Bestvina CM, Waters D, Morrison L, et al. Cost of genetic testing, delayed care, and suboptimal treatment associated with polymerase chain reaction versus next-generation sequencing biomarker testing for genomic alterations in metastatic non-small cell lung cancer. J Med Econ 2024;27(1):292–303 [published Online First: 20240224].

[4] Pennell NA, Mutebi A, Zhou ZY, et al. Economic impact of next-generation sequencing versus single-gene testing to detect genomic alterations in metastatic non-small-cell lung cancer using a decision analytic model. JCO Precis Oncol 2019;3:1–9.

[5] Sheffield BS, Eaton K, Emond B, et al. Cost savings of expedited care with upfront next-generation sequencing testing versus single-gene testing among patients with metastatic non-small cell lung cancer based on current Canadian practices. Curr Oncol 2023;30(2):2348–65 [published Online First: 20230215].

[6] Vanderpoel J, Stevens AL, Emond B, et al. Total cost of testing for genomic alterations associated with next-generation sequencing versus polymerase chain reaction testing strategies among patients with metastatic non-small cell lung cancer. J Med Econ 2022;25(1):457–68.

[7] Yang SC, Lin CC, Chen YL, et al. Economic analysis of tissue-first, plasma-first, and complementary NGS approaches for treatment-naive metastatic lung adenocarcinoma. Front Oncol 2022;12:873111. https://doi.org/10.3389/fonc.2022.873111 [published Online First: 20220520].

[8] Zheng Y, Vioix H, Liu FX, et al. Diagnostic and economic value of biomarker testing for targetable mutations in non-small-cell lung cancer: a literature review. Future Oncol 2022;18(4):505–18 [published Online First: 20211206].

[9] Lin GA, Trosman JR, Douglas MP, et al. Influence of payer coverage and out-of-pocket costs on ordering of NGS panel tests for hereditary cancer in diverse settings. J Genet Counsel 2022;31(1):130–9 [published Online First: 20210707].

[10] Ewalt MD, West H, Aisner DL. Next generation sequencing-testing multiple genetic markers at once. JAMA Oncol 2019;5(7):1076.

[11] Bogavac-Stanojevic N, Jelic-Ivanovic Z. The cost-effective laboratory: implementation of economic evaluation of laboratory testing. J Med Biochem 2017;36(3):238–42 [published Online First: 20170714].

[12] Grosse SD, Wordsworth S, Payne K. Economic methods for valuing the outcomes of genetic testing: beyond cost-effectiveness analysis. Genet Med 2008;10(9):648–54.

[13] Harvey MJ, Cunningham R, Sawchyn B, et al. Budget impact analysis of comprehensive genomic profiling in patients with advanced non-small-cell lung cancer. JCO Precis Oncol 2021;5:1611–24.

[14] Pruneri G, De Braud F, Sapino A, et al. Next-generation sequencing in clinical practice: is it a cost-saving alternative to a single-gene testing approach? Pharmacoecon Open 2021;5(2):285–98 [published Online First: 20210304].

[15] Hawkins RC. Laboratory turnaround time. Clin Biochem Rev 2007;28(4):179–94.

[16] Thusini S, Milenova M, Nahabedian N, et al. The development of the concept of return-on-investment from large-scale quality improvement programmes in healthcare: an integrative systematic literature review. BMC Health Serv Res 2022;22(1):1492 [published Online First: 20221207].

[17] Ardon O, Asa SL, Lloyd MC, et al. Understanding the financial aspects of digital pathology: a dynamic customizable return on investment calculator for informed decision-making. J Pathol Inf 2024;15:100376. https://doi.org/10.1016/j.jpi.2024.100376 [published Online First: 20240410].

[18] Dias R, Torkamani A. Artificial intelligence in clinical and genomic diagnostics. Genome Med 2019;11(1):70 [published Online First: 20191119].

[19] Nicora G, Zucca S, Limongelli I, et al. A machine learning approach based on ACMG/AMP guidelines for genomic variant classification and prioritization. Sci Rep 2022;12(1):2517 [published Online First: 20220215].

Moving?

Make sure your subscription moves with you!

To notify us of your new address, find your **Clinics Account Number** (located on your mailing label above your name), and contact customer service at:

Email: journalscustomerservice-usa@elsevier.com

800-654-2452 **(subscribers in the U.S. & Canada)**
314-447-8871 **(subscribers outside of the U.S. & Canada)**

Fax number: 314-447-8029

Elsevier Health Sciences Division
Subscription Customer Service
3251 Riverport Lane
Maryland Heights, MO 63043

*To ensure uninterrupted delivery of your subscription, please notify us at least 4 weeks in advance of move.

ELSEVIER

9780443429293